D1605943

Levine's Conservation Model

A Framework for Nursing Practice

Levine's Conservation Model

A Framework for Nursing Practice

Edited by

Karen Moore Schaefer RN, DNSc
Associate Professor
Allentown College of Saint Francis de Sales
Center Valley, Pennsylvania

Nurse Researcher
The Allentown Hospital—Lehigh Valley Hospital Center
Allentown, Pennsylvania

Adjunct Assistant Professor
University of Pennsylvania
School of Nursing
Science and Role Development Division
Philadelphia, Pennsylvania
and

Jane Benson Pond RNC, MSN, CRNP
Adult Nurse Practitioner
General Internal Medicine
Silverstein Practice
Hospital of the University of Pennsylvania
Philadelphia, Pennsylvania

Lecturer
University of Pennsylvania
School of Nursing
Graduate Program in Primary Care
Philadelphia, Pennsylvania

With special contributions by
Myra E. Levine RN, MSN, FAAN
and
Jacqueline Fawcett PhD, FAAN

 F. A. DAVIS COMPANY • Philadelphia

Printed in the United States of America

Last digit indicates print number: 10 9 8 7 6 5 4 3 2 1

NOTE: As new scientific information becomes available through basic and clinical research, recommended treatments and drug therapies undergo changes. The author(s) and publisher have done everything possible to make this book accurate, up-to-date, and in accord with accepted standards at the time of publication. The authors, editors, and publisher are not responsible for errors or omissions or for consequences from application of the book, and make no warranty, express or implied, in regard to the contents of the book. Any practice described in this book should be applied by the reader in accordance with professional standards of care used in regard to the unique circumstances that may apply in each situation. The reader is advised always to check product information (package inserts) for changes and new information regarding dose and contraindications before administering any drug. Caution is especially urged when using new or infrequently ordered drugs.

Library of Congress Cataloging-in-Publication Data

Levine's conservation model: a Framework for nursing practice /
    edited by Karen Moore Schaefer and Jane Benson Pond; with special
    contributions by Myra E. Levine and Jacqueline Fawcett.
        p. cm.
    Includes bibliographical references.
    Includes index.
    ISBN 0-8036-7747-2 (hardbound: alk. paper)
    1. Nursing. 2. Nursing—Philosophy.   I. Schaefer, Karen Moore,
1994-   . II. Pond, Jane Benson, 1944-   .   III. Levine, Myra E.
IV. Fawcett, Jacqueline.
    [DNLM; 1. Models, Nursing.   WY 100 L665]
RT84.5.L49   1991
610.73—dc20
DLC
for Library of Congress   91-9488
                                                                        CIP

P r e f a c e

Levine's Conservation Model was initially developed to provide an organizing framework for teaching the fundamental principles of nursing. As students of Levine moved into their professional roles, they used these principles (conservation of energy, structural integrity, personal integrity and social integrity) as a basis for the care they provided to patients. Many of them became nursing administrators, teachers, clinical specialists and researchers. Subsequently, those principles, intended to be the basis for a sophomore level course, have gained recognition as a model for nursing.

We are challenged to present you with the first book dedicated to the discussion of Levine's model in practice. The title of the book, *Levine's Conservation Model: A Framework for Nursing Practice*, reflects our belief that the conservation model has universality. The word *practice* is used in its broadest sense and is intended to include clinical practice, administration, education, and research.

To provide the reader with a link to the past, we have included what we believe are the most critical and useful excerpts from the second edition of Levine's book, *Introduction to Clinical Nursing* (Appendix B), and the instructor's guide to that edition (Appendix A)*. We have included a glossary of terms used by Levine in her conceptual model, defined and paraphrased from her work. An annotated bibliography includes the work of Levine and others using her model in practice.

The content of this book is appropriate for the undergraduate student learning about the use of the conservation principles in practice, for the master's student using the conceptual model in practice, and for the doctoral student testing and developing theory in nursing. Finally, this book offers clinicians many practical examples of how the model can be used in their practice. For these reasons the book can function as a supplemental text for courses about theory development and nursing practice.

Levine's chapter, "The Conservation Principles: A Model for Health," provides the reader with her latest thoughts on adaptation and holism. Her discussion of the conservation principles supports the notion that conservation is fundamental to caring and that the principles are appropriate for use in a variety of settings. In Chapter 2 Jacqueline Fawcett incorporates Levine's latest considerations of her model in a comprehensive

---

*Appendixes A and B have been reprinted in their original form. The use of masculine and feminine pronouns in *Introduction to Clinical Nursing* does not reflect F.A. Davis's current policy of avoiding sexism in language.

analysis and evaluation of the conservation model. Readers can use this chapter as a basis for drawing their own conclusions about the model and generating new discoveries from their experiences using the model.

In Chapter 3 Schaefer provides an analysis of the research related to the conservation model. Chapter 13 by Sister Ruth Alyce Cox on "a tradition of caring" at the Alverno Health-Care Facility offers an example of how the model can be used by administrators to organize care delivery systems. Chapter 14 by Grindley and Paradowski and Chapter 15 by Schaefer describe the use of the model in education. The chapters by Foreman and by Roberts, Fleming, and Giese (Chaps. 4 and 10) show how the model can be tested in practice.

We believe that this book will be a valuable addition to the texts on theory development and the use of nursing models in practice. As Levine states, "A textbook . . . establishes a baseline for further study, and should be used as a background against which lecture, discussion, and clinical conferences can be structured. It should never be used as the single source of information available to a student because no text, no matter how excellent, can ever achieve such eminence. It is a stimulant, a guideline, an invitation to further reading. . . ."*

We hope the reader will share our enthusiasm about the book and will be encouraged to explore the use of this model in practice. "But you are the only one who's placing the judgement on it and as long as you're substantiating your argument, they can't—they're not going to disagree with—They can't—It's not a matter of disagreeing, as long as you substantiate what you're saying. They're teaching you a method, and you're applying it for yourself."†

KAREN MOORE SCHAEFER
JANE BENSON POND

*Levine, M.E. (1973). *Instructor's guide to introduction to clinical nursing* (2nd ed., p. 4). Philadelphia: F.A. Davis.

†Belenky, M.F., Clinchy, B.M., Goldberger, M.R., & Tarrule, J.M. (1986). *Women's ways of knowing: The development of self, voice, and mind* (pp. 91–92). New York: Basic Books.

Acknowledgments

We are indebted to Jacqueline Fawcett for believing in our ideas and helping us through the initial processes of putting a book together. Without Myra Estrin Levine there would be no book; we are grateful that she published her ideas in the first place, and for all the support and encouragement she has given us while we put this project together. For sharing their predicaments, we gratefully acknowledge the patients who give us purpose and direction (all names of the patients and families have been changed to protect their personal integrity). To Robert G. Martone, Senior Editor, and to the staff of F.A. Davis, thank you for helping us to develop our creative ideas.

For reviewing impromptu the chapter on congestive heart failure, we thank Constance Molchaney, R.N., M.S.N. To Doris Lewis, who patiently typed multiple drafts of the book, we are grateful. We are deeply indebted to our partners for never complaining about the long hours and quiet time needed to develop the book, and for helping us celebrate our accomplishments.

Contributors

Elizabeth W. Bayley, RN, PhD
Associate Professor
Burn, Emergency and Trauma Nursing
Widener University
School of Nursing
Chester, Pennsylvania

Sister Ruth Alyce Cox, RN, PhD
Nursing Home Administrator/Geriatric Nurse Practitioner
Sisters of Saint Francis
The Alverno Health Care Facility
Clinton, Iowa

Maureen Dever, RN, MSN, CPNP
Nurse Practitioner
Kutztown University
Kutztown, Pennsylvania

Jacqueline Fawcett, PhD, FAAN
Professor
Science and Role Development Division
University of Pennsylvania
School of Nursing
Philadelphia, Pennsylvania

Nancy Fleming, RN, CNM, PhD
Adjunct Nurse Midwife Faculty
Department of Maternal Child Nursing
University of Illinois
Health Science Center
Chicago, Illinois

Marquis D. Foreman, RN, PhD
Assistant Professor
Department of Medical-Surgical Nursing
College of Nursing
University of Illinois at Chicago
Chicago, Illinois

Deborah (Yeates) Giese, RN, CNM, MS
Nurse Midwife
Gunderson Clinic, Ltd.
La Goss, Wisconsin

Joan Grindley, RN, EdD
Associate Professor
Chairperson—Department of Nursing and Health
Allentown College of Saint Francis de Sales
Center Valley, Pennsylvania

Debra Halupa, RN, MSN
Instructor
Geisinger Medical Center
Danville, Pennsylvania

Myra E. Levine, RN, MSN, FAAN
Professor Emerita
Medical-Surgical Nursing
College of Nursing
University of Illinois at Chicago
Chicago, Illinois

Barbara McCall, RN, BSN
Former Staff Nurse
Graduate Hospital
Philadelphia, Pennsylvania

Mary Beth Paradowski, RN, MSN
Assistant Professor
Allentown College of Saint Francis de Sales
Center Valley, Pennsylvania

Angela Pasco, RN, MSN
Instructor
School of Nursing
Pottsville Hospital
Pottsville, Pennsylvania

Joyce E. Roberts, CNM, PhD, FAAN
Head—Maternal-Child Nursing
M-C 802
College of Nursing
University of Illinois at Chicago
Chicago, Illinois

Susan Taney, RN, MSN, CRNP
   Adult Nurse Practitioner
   Emergency Services Department
   Hospital of the University of Pennsylvania
   Philadelphia, Pennsylvania

Table of Contents

Appendixes

Chapter
O N E

The Conservation Principles
A Model for Health

Myra Estrin Levine, R.N., M.S.N., F.A.A.N.

Critics of nursing theory have rarely understood the conceptual base from which the theorists have created their work. They have adopted strategies that ignore the content and concepts, substituting semantics for substance. They have asked, "How do these ideas fit the categories I have chosen as essential?" rather than "What concepts has the theorist employed, what is their provenance, and have they been correctly utilized?"

Some theory analysts in nursing have deplored the use of "borrowed theory" from other disciplines in the formulation of nursing theory (Kim, 1983). The affliction Gould (1981) once called "physics-envy"—a naive belief that it is possible to create theory involving human subjects with the same purity and isolation as the mathematical formulas that describe physical theories and laws. Nursing cannot turn its back on any discipline that deals with human beings and their perturbations. Each and every science that adds information and insight to the human condition is a fit subject for the nurse theorist. Rather than "borrowed," such use of theory is *adjunctive*. It is useful, rational, justifiable, and sensible to share with other disciplines' guidelines for nursing theory. It must be emphasized that nursing theory with antecedents in adjunctive disciplines sustains a responsibility to identify the contributed knowledge.

It is unethical to assume that using a theory from an adjunctive discipline magically transforms it into nursing theory and no further attribution to the source is necessary. It is also imperative that the adjunctive theory be used *correctly*. Too frequently the work from an adjunctive discipline is identified as a source, but no hint of it can be found in the theorist's work. The analysis of nursing theory that focuses on and finally identifies the ad-

1

junctive content upon which it is based—and the accuracy of its usage—will signal the coming of age in nursing scholarship. There is no nursing theory that does not have its roots in other disciplines (Levine, 1988a).

FOLLOWING THE "PROCEDURE"

In the most traditional nursing fashion, the analysts of nursing theory have created evaluation procedures—step-by-step formats—that attempt to put all nursing theories into the same box, whether they fit or not. Person, environment, health, and nursing are described as "metaparadigms" or "concepts" but in fact are neither. They are, in the best Aristotelian sense, *commonplaces*. It would be impossible to create, describe, discuss, or critique nursing activities without these basic constituents. The concepts employed by the theorist need the commonplaces as the building blocks of their discourse, but the soul of the theory rests in the concepts that the theorist has chosen to order those basic parts (Levine, 1988b).

CULTURING BIBLIOGRAPHIC VIRUSES

In the same way a computer "virus" alters, distorts, and may even destroy the knowledge stored in a network, there are "viruses" contaminating the bibliographies of theory "analysts." They perpetuate wrong conclusions, naive assumptions, and misinformed biases. These misconceptions and misunderstandings become the bibliographic basis upon which countless nursing students depend. Errors of fact and judgment are perpetuated by later "analysts" who use published work without questioning its validity. As a result, the original work of the theorist is hidden in secondary sources that have never themselves been subjected to the same rigorous criticism. Ideas are associated with the theorist's work that are utterly foreign transplants of the critic's own viewpoint.

Errors of fact or interpretation range from hilarious to serious misreading. One critic, for example, in describing my use of Gibson's perceptual systems, changed the word *haptic*, which means "touch," to *hepatic* in every instance in which the term *haptic* was appropriate (cited in Meleis, 1985). How many readers are wondering still what the liver has to do with perception? What, in fact, did the author understand about perception? Why should her ignorant error become associated with my work?

That error has not, to my knowledge, been replicated, but a far more serious misinterpretation has been thoroughly established in the literature again and again and rarely questioned. Esposito and Leonard (1980) contributed a chapter on the conservation principles that used as its principal source *Introduction to Clinical Nursing* (Levine, 1969a). The use of an introductory text for critiquing theory led to their conclusion that the conservation principles are useful only with sick patients. They identified the "major limitations" as the "focus on the individual, on illness, and on the dependency of the patient" (Esposito & Leonard, 1980, p. 162). The authors, drawing from their own beliefs, attributed Maslow as a source for my work. My graduate students for the past 20 years will testify to my criticism of Maslow and my rejection of his influence on nursing education. Although Goldstein (1963), Gibson (1966), Dubos (1965), Bates (1967), Hall (1959), Erikson (1968), and Beland (1971) are specifically cited in my text as the authors who most influenced my work, they are not mentioned by Esposito and Leonard.

Peiper (1983) used the beginning text as the major resource for her critique and evaluation of the conservation principles as "limited in scope to the ill, hospitalized person" (p. 115). Peiper extended the use of the text to include within the framework of a "theory" the nine models that were intended to direct the nursing fundamentals essential to a beginning student of nursing. They were part of the textbook but were completely unrelated to the theory, and only by stretching far beyond the text could they be construed as germane to the conservation principles.[1]

CONSERVATION: A HEALTH MODEL

Feynman (1965) describes conservation as one of the "great general principles (which) all detailed laws . . . seem to follow" (p. 59). No sophisticated theorizing can displace the fundamental importance of natural law. Identification by scientists of the universal importance of the concept of conservation makes it an essential component in understanding human life. Implicit in the knowledge of conservation is the fact of wholeness, integrity, unity—all of the structures that are *being conserved*. It is no linguistic accident that the word *health* is a derivative of the same root that also produces *whole* and *hale*. What would be the purpose of conservation except to defend, sustain, maintain, and define the integrity of the system for which it functions? The pursuit of health and the well-being it promises are achieved by each individual in countless ways but with a constant factor always present: conservation of the integrity of the person is essential to ensuring health and providing the strength to confront disability. Indeed, the importance of conservation in the treatment of illness is precisely focused on the reclamation of wholeness, of health.

Conservation is of crucial importance because it focuses its attention on the integrity, the unique oneness of the whole person. Stevens (1979, p. 45) writes:

> Levine's elements are located in the nursing act. Levine's four principles compartmentalize the nursing problems, but they do not compartmentalize man. Therefore Levine is able to assert a holistic view of man. Indeed, the whole man is the subject matter on which each of her discrete nursing problems focuses.

Every nursing act is dedicated to the conservation, or "keeping together," of the wholeness of the individual. The experience of wholeness is the foundation of all human enterprise. It seems strange that the integrity of the individual must be constantly reasserted. The need to compartmentalize in order to understand complex systems has created habits of thinking that are poor preparation for focusing on the unity of the individual. Just as a thermostat turns on the system only when the setting must be restored, conservation allows the living body to thrive on the frugality required for effective functioning. The facts of energy exchange and utilization in living systems demonstrate repeatedly that the paths chosen are the most economic, frugal, and energy-sparing ones available. Countless physiologic systems are regulated by negative feedback in which energy is used only when the system needs to be corrected (Levine, 1989).

While illness challenges the integrity of the person, defending the person's health—his or her unique wholeness—is a continuing endeavor. The popularity of alternative life-styles, pseudoscience, and paranormal psychology is a consequence of the concern every self has for itself. The mysticism and quackery of the marketplace is not required to arouse awareness of selfhood. Inherent in the life experience is a state of being described as "health." Definitions of health are often so diffuse as to be meaningless, and still every individual defines health for himself or herself. Personal definitions come from within the beliefs, values, language, mores, customs, and laws of the groups into which each person is socialized. Every cultural group has defined health on its own terms, and even with the heavy influence of technology, there remain powerful remnants of localized biases that define what is healthy and what is not.

Widely promoted "fitness" behaviors are directed by the individual's conservation efforts. Emphasis on nutrition, exercise, a "stress-free" daily life, and even "safe sex" choices require the active participation of the individual in his or her own best interests. The importance of fitness, however, is clearly dependent upon apprehension of the threat of disease. Fitness choices are health promoting because they promise to maintain health—by preventing noxious disease. It is a paradox that while personal health concerns direct individuals to consumption of soluble fiber, oat bran, and fish oils, the shared environment is increasingly threatened through misuse and indifference. Perhaps no stronger statement of the singular importance of the self can be made. Wholeness is the universal target of selfhood, and conservation is the guardian activity that defends and protects it.

The word *healing* also shares the same root as *whole* and *health*. Healing is the avenue of return to the daily activities compromised by ill health. It is not only the insult or injury that is repaired—*but the person himself or herself*. Indeed, the expectation that healing will restore the conditions that existed before the intrusion persists even in situations where the therapeutic outcome leaves a loss of function or effectiveness. It is not merely the healing of an afflicted part. It is, rather, a return to selfhood, where the encroachment of the disability can be set aside entirely, and the individual is free to pursue once more his or her own interests without constraint.

HIDDEN ADAPTIVE PATTERNS

Every self-sustaining system monitors its own behavior by conserving the use of the resources required to define its unique identity. The ability of every individual not only to survive but to flourish is a consequence of the competence of the person's interactions with the environments in which he or she functions. Every successful living organism has the ability to select from the environment those elements that are essential to its welfare and to exclude those that are repetitive, harmful, or inconsequential. As Bernard (1957) and earlier Cannon (1939) emphasized, the organism must possess the ability to stabilize its internal environment in the face of the uncontrolled factors it may confront in its external environment. Such activity, resulting in the safety and well-being of the individual, was described as a stable state, or *homeostasis*. Waddington (1968) suggested, instead, the term *homeorhesis* to emphasize the constant fluid and changing character of the *milieu interne*. The concept of stability within confined limits of experience fits readily the observation of warm-blooded organisms, but there are countless cold-blooded species that are susceptible to every change in their environment—and still flourish. Homeorhesis and enticstasis are both a consequence of conservation: the frugal, economic, contained, and controlled use of environmental resources by the individual organism in his or her best interest. This is the achievement of adaptation.

Every environment is fraught with dangers and pitfalls. Every species, whether warm-blooded or cold-blooded, survives the challenge of the environment by its ability to overcome threats to its well-being. The environmental "fit" that underscores successful adaptation suggests that every species has fixed patterns of response uniquely designed to ensure success in essential life activities, demonstrating that adaptation is both historical and specific. However, tremendous opportunities for individual accommodations are locked into the gene structure of each species; every individual is one of a kind.

The vast genetic potential and the unmeasurable environmental impact offer a range of independence and free choice that supports the success of countless forms of living creatures. The range of adaptation available to a species is impossible to determine unless, in confronting the threat, its adaptive potential is revealed. This has been remarkably demonstrated by the impact of technology on human survival. Several children have been successfully resuscitated after rescue from prolonged submersion because of the sophistication of the available technology. Their ability to recover seems clearly associated with an adaptation long unused but still present in the human genetic code. Recognition of "immersion hypoxia" and the "dive reflex" as an adaptive pattern allows planning intervention and care of the victims (Shovein, Land, Richter, & Leedom, 1989).

An equally remarkable ability to survive was seen in the rescue of newborn infants buried in the rubble of a hospital after the devastating earthquake in Mexico City in 1988. Several were recovered alive, all reportedly born within the same narrow time period and discovered within 8 days of their birth. An adaptive pattern, long dormant until this unique circumstance brought it to light, seems responsible for the miraculous survival of the infants.

The likelihood that there are other potential adaptive configurations that sustain survival under great duress and are hidden in the genetic code is reinforced by Anderson's work with preterm newborns. She describes the introduction of "skin-to-skin" or "kangaroo" care in poverty-stricken

Colombia as a successful strategy to save preterm infants who would otherwise have failed. The absence of technologic preterm infant care created the urgency of an alternative solution and what Anderson calls "a deep respect for natural processes" (Anderson, Marks, & Wahlberg, 1986, p. 807). In a subsequent paper, Anderson (1989) describes the use of kangaroo care in Western European countries, adding further data for the description of a dormant adaptive pattern in which the preterm newborn actually thrives when the infant, only hours after birth, is placed, skin to skin, in an upright position between the mother's breasts. This facilitates and encourages breastfeeding, but even more remarkable are observations of the quiet calm of the infant and subsequent data suggesting that the infants gain weight, cry less, and show improved physiologic functioning with this technique.

These adaptation patterns were obscured by an altered environment, one in which the technology substituted for "natural processes." Each demonstrates the three characteristics of adaptation: history, specificity, and redundancy (Levine, 1989; Wallace, 1987). Environmental change rendered them no longer necessary, but the fact that they persist testifies to the durability of adaptations available to individuals, rooted in history and awaiting the specific circumstances to which they respond.

The redundancy of adaptations does not always depend on long unused and obscured behavior patterns. The ubiquitous presence of "failsafe" options in the anatomy, physiology, and psychology of individuals represents a redundancy easily identified and often employed in planning health care. The choice of one strategy instead of another rests with the knowledge of the health care planner. Often there is tacit recognition that more than one solution is possible. Achieving health, as the individual experiences it, is predicated on a deliberate selection of redundant options. When the individual loses redundant choices as a consequence of disease, trauma, aging, or environmental circumstances, survival becomes difficult and ultimately fails for lack of fail-safe options—either those that the person possesses or those that can be employed in his or her behalf. The possibility exists that aging itself is a consequence of failed redundancy of physiologic and psychologic processes.

Adaptation has been a concept widely admired by nurses and often invoked by theorists. It poses practical problems of unsolved proportions, but there is little justification for discarding it altogether. However, to speak of "adaptation levels" is glib and useless in the face of the impossibility of measuring or quantifying adaptive behaviors. For example, it is easily demonstrated that the pH of the circulatory system is rigidly limited and that deviations beyond those narrow parameters are destructive to the individual. However, choosing a therapeutic intervention to correct the pH is based on complex factors in the individual and the environment in which he or she is being treated. Success or failure must be monitored cautiously to be certain the best choices have been made. Recognition of the adaptation rests on the ability to define its precise nature—a task that is often impossible. Although certain generalized adaptations can be described—the required oxygen tension, temperature tolerance of living cells, effect of atmospheric pressure on physiologic function, for example—precise identification of the adaptive condition is not possible. Perhaps the time will come when genetic mapping will make such information available, but until then the focus of nursing intervention must be on the consequences of care rather than on algorithms designed to display the adaptive patterns. All discussions of adaptation rest finally on generalizations arising from shared experience and observations. The research necessary to describe adaptation patterns and the therapeutic interventions that will support them has yet to be done.

THE "INTEGRITY" PRINCIPLES

The universality of energy conservation makes it a factor that cannot be ignored in any consideration of the human condition and most specifically in understanding nursing as a humane enterprise. Energy, the life source, cannot be directly observed but the consequences of its exchange are predictable, manageable, and quantifiable. Instruments can monitor, measure, produce, or capture energy. To describe energy in mystical terms and ascribe to its transfer magical powers is poetic and wistful but hardly the stuff of scientific research. Faith in healers who trade in the myths of therapeutic touch has recurred in every generation, a companion to suffering and fear. Faith is often a source of strength for frailty, but it is not nursing science.

The sources of energy available to the individual are finite. Through conservation, energy is spent carefully, with essential priorities served first. The ways in which energy resources are gathered and spent are well documented in fact. Although exact measurement is rarely possible, the effects of energy utilization on the individual are often quite apparent. For example, the extreme fatigue reported by patients undergoing radiation therapy demonstrates how a limited resource and energy conservation can produce clinical symptoms. The cell destruction caused by radiation demands an unusual response from the body's inflammatory system, a costly energy expense. The fatigue that is experienced emphasizes that the available energy sources are limited and the individual is forced to reduce activity to that which is absolutely necessary. Even then, it is difficult to accomplish even ordinary tasks. There are many situations in which the restrictions imposed by extreme fatigue dictate the nursing interventions required. Although the precise energy measure may not be possible, the clinical manifestations are easily recognizable.

An energy resource sufficient to permit free participation in an active life is essential to the wholeness of the individual. Mobility and the freedom to choose activities depend on the structural integrity of the individual. The fact that the skeletal-muscle system must be used in order to ensure its functional capacity has been an empirical given in nursing. It has dictated the necessity for appropriate positioning, range of motion, and mobilization in times of limited activity, but defending structural integrity is not a passive enterprise.

Repair and healing to sustain the wholeness of structure and function are achieved by conservation. The acute inflammatory reaction with its manifestation of intense activity requires a large investment by the body, designed to localize and quickly exclude the source of insult. The damage is limited in place and time so that by a vigorous assault a minimum of functional tissue is sacrificed. However, if the acute attack is not quickly successful, the area is walled off and the investment of the body's resources withdrawn. A chronic lesion may persist, but as long as it is quiescent its cost is minimized. The quickness of the body's response to insult and injury is directed at the limitation of scar tissue, and a minimum of interference with subsequent structure and function. Conservation of structural integrity emphasizes that the individual's defense against the hazards of the environment are achieved with the most economical expense of effort. Nursing cannot do less.

The importance of appropriate exercise and the sense of well-being that accompanies it are a testimony to the role of structural integrity in the achievement of wholeness, of health. Obviously the ability to move freely through each day and to make the active choices that guarantee that freedom depends on an adequate energy resource as well as the structural integrity of the individual. The decisions themselves record the impact of the individual's abilities, desires, goals, and expectations summarized in the self.

Goldstein (1963) described brain-injured soldiers, even those with severe disability, clinging to some semblance of self-awareness. It is not necessary to describe extreme conditions to recognize that every individual defends his or her unique personhood, the individual within known as the self. Wholeness is summarized in that knowledge. It is private, but it has public faces; it is beyond communication with another, and yet it is capable of liaisons of love and friendship and companionship.

Life is a shared experience, and yet the barriers isolate each individual so that participation rests with the interpretation each makes of his or her predicament. In every society, there is an established fashion through which the developing child is turned into a self-sufficient adult. It is expected that independence will permit judgments that protect the security and well-being of each person. To whatever degree such independence is achieved, it is defended and cherished by the person. The expectation that the individual will make acceptable choices is the goal of the entire process, but there are never guarantees that the decisions will always be appropriate. Yet there is a naive belief that the right decisions can be encouraged by a relentless educational effort. If it were so simple, it would be possible to eliminate crime and drug abuse and all the angry behaviors that distort and destroy life. The person is created from birth through childhood and is critically formed during adolescence. Each person arrives on the threshold of adult life with self-definitions that will forever after influence every choice that is made. To whatever degree independence and competence are achieved, the awareness of the self is the strong core of identity that is summarized in personal integrity.

Health belief evangelists often overlook the crucial importance of the uniqueness of the individual's private self. The trust displayed by health belief promoters in diet, exercise, and control of stress, for all its good sense, becomes strident when individuals are accused of failure because they do not follow the rules. The notion that people are inept if they do not choose an approved life-style invites the abuse of blaming the victim. It is naive, and perhaps even immoral, to focus on stress as the underlying cause of all kinds of sickness.

There are therapeutic strategies to assist those who are incompetent in the face of threat, but no general announcement that people should "avoid stress" in order to remain healthy makes sense. Given the option, few people would choose a stressful environment if they had the means— and the strength—to avoid it. It is particularly cruel to blame individuals with serious diagnoses, such as cancer, as victims of their own errors. Too little is known of the etiology of life-threatening illness to allow such self-serving certainty. In good times and bad, the individual confronts life challenges in his or her own way, captured by circumstances that cannot be controlled, a prisoner of his or her physical condition and the lifelong repertoire of choices the individual is able to make.

It is impossible to acknowledge the wholeness of the individual without considering his or her social context. The ethnic and cultural heritage, the economic niche, the opportunities ignored or seized—all of these define the variety of social roles every individual occupies in a lifetime. It is the promise of assistance that creates a community. The health and welfare of the individual are protected by the social organizations into which the person is born, or is chosen, or is elected to participate. Exclusion from membership is equally influential, not only for the individual but also for the establishment of the character of the larger community. The essence of social organization rests with the responsibility of the aggregate for the well-being of its individual members. The community describes the guidelines for individual behavior by establishing the accepted definitions of health—and of illness. The community prescribes the therapeutic interventions that are acceptable, as well as those who are eligible to receive it. It is the social system that, in every place and in every generation, establishes the values that direct it and sets the rules by which its members are judged. The social integrity of the individual mirrors the community to which he or she belongs.

Kolata (1989) asked residents of nursing homes and their nursing providers to rank their concerns according to importance. The expectation that there would be a focus on issues of dying and extraordinary life support technology was not supported. There was, however, a major difference in the focus of the residents as opposed to that of their caregivers. The residents ranked first the ability to go out—to leave the home to shop or go for a walk—and to be free to make that choice. The nursing assistants, on the other hand, ranked as first the activities provided in the residence: recreation, entertainment, and crafts. The second choice in importance for the residents was contacts with family and friends, access to the phone, and receiving mail. The nursing assistants ranked this 10th; in their view it was the least important choice. The nursing home residents ranked visitors in 10th place, but the nurse aides ranked visitors in second place. The residents ranked bathing and other care procedures fourth, whereas the assistants ranked care seventh. Even in the restricted social milieu of a nursing home (there were 45 nursing homes in the study), the residents voted for freedom and those activities that most closely resembled the way in which they had always lived their lives. The importance they placed on their freedom to choose social activities, rather than those activities chosen for them, underlines their demand for respect of their personhood.

The conservation principles address the integrity of the individual. They are not simply turned on and off in the event of illness. The striving for wholeness in every human being is a process that does not end from birth to death. Every activity requires an energy supply because nothing works without it. Every activity must respect the structural wholeness of the individual because well-being depends upon it. Every activity is chosen out of the abilities, life experience, and desires of the self who makes the choices. Every activity is a product of the dynamic social systems to which the individual belongs. The conservation principles may be addressed singly. Indeed, research and scholarly study must focus on discrete issues. But the integrity of the whole person cannot be violated. However narrowed the study problem may be, the influence of all four conservation principles must be acknowledged, and the wholeness of the person sustained.

Gould (1981) says:

> Theories . . . are not inexorable inductions from facts. The most creative theories are often imaginative visions imposed upon facts . . .

He adds:

> . . . a factual reality exists and . . . science . . . though often in an obtuse and erratic manner, can learn about it. (p. 22)

As nursing learns about itself, the importance of theory building cannot be sacrificed to careless scholarship. Both the theorist and the critic are bound to the facts—and to the vision.

REFERENCES

Anderson, G. (1989). Skin-to-skin kangaroo care in western Europe. American Journal of Nursing, 89, 662–666.

Anderson, G., Marks, E., & Wahlberg, V. (1986). Kangaroo care for premature infants. American Journal of Nursing, 86, 807–809.

Bates, M. (1967). Naturalist at large. Natural History, 86, 10.

Beland, I. (1971). Clinical nursing: Pathophysiological and psychosocial implications (2nd ed.). New York: Macmillan.

Bernard, C. (1957). An introduction to the study of experimental medicine. New York: Dover.

Cannon, W.B. (1939). The wisdom of the body. New York: W.W. Norton & Co.

Dubos, R. (1965). Man adapting. New Haven: Yale University Press.

Erikson, E. (1968). Identity: Youth and crisis. New York: W.W. Norton & Co.

Esposito, C., & Leonard, M. (1980). In J. George (Chair), Nursing theories: The base for professional nursing practice (pp. 150–163). Nursing Theories Conference Group, Englewood Cliffs, N.J.: Prentice Hall.

Fawcett, J. (1989). Analysis and evaluation of conceptual models of nursing (2nd ed.). Philadelphia: F.A. Davis.

Feynman, R. (1965). The character of physical law. Cambridge, MA: M.I.T. Press

Gibson, J. (1966). The senses considered as perceptual systems. Boston: Houghton-Mifflin.
Goldstein, K. (1963). Human nature. New York: Schocken Books.
Gould, S. (1981). The mismeasure of man. New York: W.W. Norton & Co.
Hall, E. (1959). Silent language. Greenwich, CT: Fawcett.
Kim, H. (1983). The nature of theoretical thinking in nursing. Norwalk, CT: Appleton-Century-Crofts.
Kolata, G. (1989, January 19). Life's basic problems are still top concern in the nursing homes. New York Times, Section 2, p. 14.
Levine, M.E. (1969a). Introduction to clinical nursing. Philadelphia: F.A. Davis.
Levine, M.E. (1969b). Instructors' guide to introduction to clinical nursing. Philadelphia: F.A. Davis.
Levine, M.E. (1973a). Introduction to clinical nursing (2nd ed.). Philadelphia: F.A. Davis.
Levine, M.E. (1973b). Instructors' guide to introduction to clinical nursing (2nd ed.). Philadelphia: F.A. Davis.
Levine, M.E. (1988a). Antecedents from adjunctive disciplines: Creation of nursing theory. Nursing Science Quarterly, 1, 16–21.
Levine, M.E. (1988b). Review of Parse's nursing science: Major paradigms, theories and critiques. Nursing Science Quarterly, 4, 184–185.
Levine, M.E. (1989). The conservation principles: Twenty years later. In J. Riehl-Sisca (Ed.), Conceptual models for nursing (3rd ed.) (pp. 325–338). Norwalk, CT: Appleton & Lange.
Meleis, A. (1985). Theoretical nursing development and progress. Philadelphia: J.B. Lippincott.
Peiper, B. (1983). Levine's nursing model. In J. Fitzpatrick & A. Whall (Eds.). Conceptual models of nursing analysis and application. Bowie, MD: Robert Brady.
Shovein, J., Land, L., Richter, G., & Leedom, C. (1989). Near drowning. American Journal of Nursing, 89, 680–686.
Stevens, B. (1979). Nursing theory. Boston: Little, Brown & Co.
Waddington, C.H. (Ed.). (1968). Towards a theoretical biology: I. Prolegomena. Chicago: Aldine.
Wallace, D. (Producer). (1987). The nurse theorists, portraits of excellence: Myra Levine (video). The Helene Fuld Health Trust. Oakland, CA: Studio Three Production.

NOTES

1. The publication of *Introduction to Clinical Nursing* in 1969 was a bold venture by F.A. Davis Company. The text was designed as a first course in nursing and represented a radical departure from traditional approaches. It sought to combine in a single beginning text the basics of the course in Fundamentals of Nursing (Nursing Arts, Foundations) with the content of a first course in medical-surgical nursing. The premise was that students would learn more quickly and thoroughly through a first nursing experience with real patients rather than with a giggling classmate in a Nursing Arts laboratory. Since it was a first course, the usual dependence on medical diagnosis as a basis for teaching medical-surgical nursing was abandoned. It was not intended to be an encyclopedia of nursing. Instead, each chapter, using the conservation principles as guidelines, discussed a *prototype nursing problem*, based on the clinical behaviors and signs and symptoms appropriate to the physiologic content. The plan of the book was described in the Instructors' Guide for both the first and second editions. (Levine, 1969b, 1973b) (see Appendix A for Second Edition).

Chapter
T W O

Analysis and Evaluation of Levine's Conservation Model*

Jacqueline Fawcett, Ph.D., F.A.A.N.

Myra E. Levine's conservation model represents a distinctive perspective of the phenomena of interest to the discipline of nursing. The concepts and propositions of the conservation model are at the level of abstraction of a paradigm or conceptual model of nursing. In fact, Levine (1985, 1987) noted that her work is "a generalization" of nursing and agreed that it is indeed a conceptual model.

This chapter presents an analysis and evaluation of Levine's Conservation Model, which were carried out using the framework of questions presented in Table 2-1.

ANALYSIS OF LEVINE'S CONSERVATION MODEL

Levine (1966a) presented the rudiments of her conceptual model in an article titled "Adaptation and Assessment: A Rationale for Nursing Intervention." Additional elements of the model were presented in two other articles: "The Four Conservation Principles of Nursing" (Levine, 1967) and "The Pursuit of Wholeness" (Levine, 1969b). A comprehensive discussion of the model was presented in the book titled *Introduction to Clinical Nursing* (Levine, 1969a). The second edition of this book was published in 1973. Other features of the model were given in Levine's 1971 publication, *Holis-*

---

*Adapted from Fawcett, J. (1989). Analysis and evaluation of conceptual models of nursing (2nd ed.). Philadelphia: F.A. Davis.

TABLE 2-1. A FRAMEWORK FOR ANALYSIS AND EVALUATION OF
CONCEPTUAL MODELS OF NURSING

Questions for analysis
- What is the historic evolution of the conceptual model?
- What approach to development of nursing knowledge does the model exemplify?
- Upon what assumptions was the conceptual model based?
- How are nursing's four metaparadigm concepts explicated in the model?

> How is *person* defined and described?
> How is *environment* defined and described?
> How is *health* defined? How are *wellness* and *illness* differentiated?
> How is *nursing* defined? What is the goal of nursing? How is the nursing process
> described?

- What statements are made about the relationships among the four metaparadigm concepts?
- What areas of concern are identified by the conceptual model?
- What is the source of these concerns?

Questions for evaluation
- Are the assumptions upon which the conceptual model was based made explicit?
- Does the conceptual model provide complete descriptions of all four concepts of nursing's
  metaparadigm?
- Do the relational propositions of the conceptual model completely link the four metapara-
  digm concepts?
- Is the internal structure of the conceptual model logically congruent?

> Does the model reflect more than one contrasting world view?
> Does the model reflect characteristics of more than one category of models?
> Do the components of the model reflect logical translation of diverse per-
> spectives?

- Does the conceptual model generate empirically testable theories?
- Do tests of derived theories yield evidence in support of the model?
- Is the conceptual model socially congruent?

> Does the conceptual model, when linked with relevant theories, lead to nursing
> activities that meet society's expectations or do the expectations created
> by the conceptual model require societal changes?

- Is the conceptual model socially significant?

> Does the conceptual model, when linked with relevant theories, lead to nursing
> actions that make important differences in the person's health status?

- Is the conceptual model socially useful?

> Does the conceptual model include explicit rules for research, practice, educa-
> tion, and administration?
> Is the conceptual model comprehensive enough to provide direction for re-
> search, practice, education, and administration when linked with relevant
> theories?
> Are investigators given sufficient direction about what questions to ask?

TABLE 2–1. *Continued*

Are practitioners able to make pertinent observations, decide that a nursing problem exists, and prescribe and execute a course of action that achieves the goal specified?

Do educators have sufficient guidelines to construct a curriculum, and do they have reasonable understanding of what knowledge and skills are needed?

Do administrators have sufficient guidelines to organize and deliver nursing services?

• What is the overall contribution of the conceptual model to nursing knowledge?

SOURCE: Fawcett, J. (1989). Analysis and evaluation of conceptual models of nursing (2nd ed. pp. 43–44). Philadelphia: F.A. Davis, with permission.

tic Nursing, and her presentations at conferences (Levine, 1978, 1984a, 1986), as well as her responses to a videotaped interview (Levine, 1987). The most recent explications of Levine's conceptual model may be found in the book chapter "The Conservation Principles of Nursing: Twenty Years Later" (Levine, 1989a) and Chapter One of this book, "The Conservation Principles—A Model for Health" (Levine, 1991). Levine (personal communication, July 15, 1987) regarded the 1989a chapter as "a significant restatement of the model . . . a natural evolutionary statement of how the basic concepts are related to each other." Further refinements are evident in Chapter 1 of this book.

Levine (1969a) commented that she developed her model as a starting point for the theory development needed to provide the "whys" of nursing activities. She stated, "The serious study of any discipline requires a theoretical baseline which gives it substance and meaning" (p. ix). Although Levine did not underestimate the importance of technical skills, she pointed out (p. vii):

Nursing . . . remain(s) characterized by a rigid dependence on procedures. The "why" is not entirely neglected, but it is often applied after the fact, as if such justification invested the procedure with a special scientific holiness. Nurses cherish "applied science principles" in an era when nursing is deeply involved in scientific research, but even the lessons learned from nurse researchers are too often ignored.

Levine's attention to the theoretical basis for nurse's actions came at a time when nursing was beginning to recognize the need for substantive knowledge (Newman, 1972). A major feature of her work is the explication of the scientific concepts underlying nursing processes. In fact, she deliberately set out to provide "an intellectual framework for analysis and understanding of the scientific nature of nursing activity" (Levine, 1969a, p. viii).

Levine (1973) developed her model from the basic assumption that nursing intervention is a conservation activity. Drawing from Tillich (1961), she assumed that the "multidimensional unity of life" must be conserved. She also assumed that "the human being responds to the forces in his environment in a singular yet integrated fashion" (p. 6). Elaborating, Levine explained (p. 13):

> The holistic nature of the human response to the environment provides the rationale for substantive principles of nursing. A principle is a fundamental concept that forms the basis for a chain of reasoning. Formulated on a broad base, it establishes the relationships between apparently otherwise unrelated facts. Nursing principles are fundamental assumptions which provide a unifying structure for understanding a wide variety of nursing activities. Nursing principles are all "conservation" principles.

Levine (personal communication, February 2, 1982) stated that she "did not invent the notion of Conservation—I simply live in a natural world where it is a characteristic of experience." Indeed, citing Feynman (1965), Levine (1988b, 1991) pointed out that conservation is a natural law of science. She maintained that the universal importance of conservation made it essential knowledge about human life that must be included in the nursing curriculum. She went on to explain (p. 227):

> The development of the four conservation principles grew naturally out of my desire to organize nursing knowledge so that the student would have a strong organizing basis for interpreting all kinds of nursing situations. It was easy to work with, and in its simplicity it seemed to open many channels of thinking that had not been obvious before. . . . I adopted it as the basis for a textbook in beginning nursing, *Introduction to Clinical Nursing*. I never dreamed that others would see in it a new (conceptual model of) nursing. I was certain it would educate good nurses. That is all I ever wanted to do.

Levine is known for her careful citations of the many scientists from various disciplines whose work has influenced her thinking. She has acknowledged the contributions to her thinking made by the work of Bates (1967), Beland (1971), Dubos (1961, 1965), Erikson (1964), Gibson (1966), Goldstein (1963), Hall (1959), and Sherrington (1906), among others. However, she disclaimed, "even with some vigor," any dependence on Maslow and other more recent authors whose work focuses on holism (Levine, personal communication, February 2, 1982). Moreover, she has rejected Maslow's influence on nursing education (Levine, 1991).

Levine's use of knowledge from a variety of disciplines indicates that she used a deductive approach to develop her conceptual model. This approach is further illustrated in the following comment (Levine, 1969a, p. viii):

> The essential science concepts develop the rationale (for nursing actions), using ideas from all areas of knowledge that contribute to the development of the nursing process in the specific area of the model.

Content of the Model: Concepts

PERSON

Levine's model focuses on the individual person, described as a holistic being. Citing Erikson's (1964) definition of wholeness, Levine (1969b) stated, "From the moment of birth until the instant of death, every individual cherishes and defends his 'wholeness' " (p. 93). Levine (1973, 1989a) pointed out that Erikson's definition emphasizes the mutuality between diversified functions and parts within an entirety. This definition also maintains that the boundaries between parts are open and fluid, such that the parts "have a yearning for each other" (Levine, 1978). Wholeness, according to Levine (1989a, pp. 325–326):

> . . . can be used as a starting point of analysis only if it can be converted into manageable parts . . . but none of the isolated aspects of wholeness can have meaning outside of the context within which the individual experiences his or her life. . . . Only then are the "open and fluid" boundaries established.

Levine (1973) further described the person as an organism that is a system of systems. She stated (pp. 8–9):

> The total life process of the entire organism is dependent upon the interrelatedness of its component systems. In fact, the organism is a system of systems, and in its wholeness expresses the organization of all the contributing parts.

Levine (1973) characterized the life process as unceasing change that has direction, purpose, and meaning. She explained (pp. 9–10):

> The organism represents a pattern of orderly, sequential change. Because it is both ordered and sequential, the pattern is a message. So long as the pattern is consistent, it is also understandable. . . . The change which supports the well-being of the organism can be predicted, measured, and observed, and therefore is a cogent message.

According to Levine (1973), change occurs through adaptation. She explained, "The organism retains its integrity in both the internal and external environment through its adaptive capability" (p. 10). She went on to say (pp. 10–11):

> Adaptation is the process of change whereby the individual retains his integrity within the realities of his environments. Adaptation is basic to survival, and it is an expression of the integration of the entire organism.

In fact, Levine (1989a) maintained that "the life process *is* the process of adaptation" (p. 326).

Further discussion of the person and adaptation within the context of Levine's conceptual model requires consideration of the relationship between the person and the environment. The next section focuses on Levine's view of environment. It is followed by consideration of the person-environment relationship and additional discussion of adaptation.

ENVIRONMENT

Levine referred to an internal environment and an external environment. She maintained that "the integrated response of the individual aris(es) from the internal environment" (Levine, 1973, p. 12). Drawing upon the concept of the *milieu interne* that Claude Bernard discussed in the late 19th century, Levine (1973, p. 7) explained:

Bernard identified the primordial seas, captured within the integument of the human body and providing the organism with a tightly regulated solution of substances essential to its continuing well-being. . . . Man carried the essentials with him, safely packaged inside his skin. But it was apparent to Bernard, and to the army of investigators who followed him, that the internal environment was susceptible to constant change.

Levine (1973) traced the further development of the concept of internal environment to Cannon's (1939) formulation of homeostasis and finally to Waddington's (1968) idea of homeorhesis. Homeostasis, maintained Levine (1989a), should not be viewed as a system of balance and quiescence but rather as "a state of energy-sparing that also provides the necessary baselines for a multitude of synchronized physiological and psychological factors" (p. 329). Levine stated that homeostasis reflects congruence of the person with the environment.

Homeorhesis, as described by Levine (1973, p. 7),

. . . is a stabilized flow rather than a static state. Such a concept emphasizes the fluidity of change within a space-time continuum and more nearly describes the remarkable patterns of adaptation which permit the individual's body to sustain its well-being within the vast changes which encroach upon it from the environment.

The internal environment is subject to continuous change from the challenges of the external environment, which are always a form of energy. The maintenance of the integration of bodily functions in the face of these changes depends on multiple negative-feedback loops, which are control mechanisms that result in autoregulation of the internal environment (Levine, 1973). Collective synchronization of multiple negative-feedback loops is accomplished through homeostasis and "creates the 'stable state' of the internal environment" (Levine, 1989a, p. 329).

Levine (1973) rejected the "simplistic view of the external environment" as "a kind of stage setting against which the individual plays out his life" (p. 12). Rather, she adopted Bates's (1967) formulation of external environment as perceptual, operational, and conceptual.

The perceptual environment encompasses "that portion of the environment to which the individual responds with his sense organs" (Levine, 1973, p. 12). It includes "those factors which can be recorded on the sensory system—the energies of light, sound, touch, temperature, and chemical change that is smelled or tasted, as well as position sense and balance" (Levine, 1989a, p. 326). Levine (1971) pointed out that the person "is not a passive recipient of sensory input. [Rather], he seeks, selects, and tests information from the environment in the context of his definition of himself, and so constantly defends his safety, his identity, and in a larger sense, his purpose" (p. 262).

The operational environment is "that which interacts with living tissues even though the individual does not possess sensory organs that can record the presence of these external factors" (Levine, 1989a, p. 326). Thus, the operational environment is not directly perceived by the individual. It encompasses "every unseen and unheard aspect of the individual's life-space (including) all forms of radiation, microorganisms, (and) pollutants that are odorless and colorless" (Levine, 1989a, p. 326). Although this aspect of the environment cannot be apprehended by the senses or antici- pated symbolically, it is of vital concern because of its potential danger to the well-being of the individual (Levine, 1971).

The conceptual environment is "the environment of language, ideas, symbols, concepts, and invention" (Levine, 1989a, p. 326). It encompasses "the exchange of language, the ability to think and to experience emotion . . . value systems, religious beliefs, ethnic and cultural traditions, and the individual psychological patterns that come from life experiences" (Lev- ine, 1973, p. 12). This aspect of the environment takes into account the fact that "human beings are sentient, thinking, future-oriented and past-aware individuals" (Levine, 1989a, p. 326).

Levine (1973) mentioned the importance of both internal and external environments and noted that the interface between the two is involved in the person's adaptation. She explained (p. 12):

> Separate consideration of either the internal or external environments can provide only a partial view of the complex interaction that is taking place be- tween them. It is, in fact, at the interface where the exchange between internal and external environments occurs that the determinants for nursing interven- tion are found. In this broader sense, all adaptations represent the accommo- dation that is possible between the internal and external environments.

PERSON AND ENVIRONMENT

Levine (1989a) maintained that the person is not separate from the en- vironment. She stated, "The person cannot be described apart from the specific environment in which he or she is found. The precise environment necessarily completes the wholeness of the individual" (p. 325). Levine further stated (p. 326):

> The interaction at the interface between individual and environment is an orderly, sometimes predictable, but always a limited process. The conse- quence of the interaction is invariably the product of the characteristics of the living individual *and* the external factors. . . . The *process* of the interaction is *adaptation*.

Levine (1989a) explained that adaptation can be thought of as a way in which the person and the environment become congruent over time or as the fit of the person with his or her "predicament of time and space" (p. 326). Adaptation is characterized by history, specificity, and redun- dancy. The fundamental nature of adaptation, then, is "a consequence of a historical progression: the evolution of the species through time, reflect- ing the sequence of change in the genetic patterns that have recorded the change in the historical environments" (p. 327).

The specificity of adaptation is exemplified by the synchronized tasks of body systems. In particular, each body system has specific tasks involv- ing biochemical changes in response to environmental challenges. Al- though the tasks are specific, they are synchronized with each other and serve the individual as a whole. Specificity in biochemistry is dependent upon sequential change that occurs in cascades. The cascade "is characterized by the intermingling of the steps with each other—the precursor is not entirely exhausted when the intermediate forms develop and the final stage is congruent with the steps that precede it" (Levine, 1989a, p. 328).

Levine (1989a) explained that the cascade of adaptations is characterized by redundancy, which refers to the series of wavelike adaptive responses that are available to the individual when environmental challenges arise. Examples of redundancy in adaptation include the "ubiquitous . . . 'fail-safe' options in the anatomy, physiology, and psychology of individuals" (Chap. 1, p. 6). Some redundant systems respond instantly to threatened shifts of physiologic parameters. Others are corrective and use the time interval provided by the instantaneous response to correct imbalances. Still other redundant systems function by re-establishing a previously failed response.

Redundancy also is seen in four levels of organismic responses to environmental challenges. These responses are considered to be

> . . . coexistent in a single individual, and in fact, often influence each other. They represent, however, an assembly of parts which have indeed entered into fruitful association and organization. Together they permit the person to protect and maintain his integrity as an individual. (Levine, 1969b, p. 98)

Levine (1989a, p. 330) pointed out that because the responses are redundant,

> . . . they do not follow one another in a prescribed sequence, but are integrated in individuals by their cognitive abilities, the wealth of their previous experience, their ability to define their relationships to the events and the strengths of their adaptive capabilities.

She further noted that although some responses can be considered psychologic and some behavioral,

> . . . the integration of living processes argues that they are one and the same—not merely parallel and not merely simultaneous—but essential portions of the same activity.

The most primitive level of organismic response is the "fight-or-flight" mechanism. This adrenocortical-sympathetic reaction is an instantaneous response to a real or imagined threat. The fight-or-flight mechanism swiftly provides a condition of physiologic and behavioral readiness for sudden and unexplained environmental challenges.

The second level is the inflammatory-immune response. This response to injury is important for maintenance of structural continuity and promotion of healing. It "assures restoration of physical wholeness and the expectation of complete healing" (Levine, 1989a, p. 330).

The third level is the stress response. Drawing from Selye's (1956) description of stress, Levine (1989a) stated that this response is "recorded over time and is influenced by the accumulated experience of the individual" (p. 330).

The fourth level of organismic response is perceptual awareness, as mediated through the sense organs. This sensory response is concerned with gathering information from the environment and converting it to meaningful experience (Levine, 1969b, 1989a). Perceptual awareness is described in some detail by Levine (1973). She stated, "The human being is a sentient being, and the ability to interact with the environment seems ineluctably tied to his sensory organs" (p. 446). Drawing upon Gibson's (1966) formulation of perceptual systems to explain the mediation of behavior by sensory organs, Levine (1969b) commented, "Individual identity arises out of information received through these intact and functional perceptual systems" (p. 97).

Gibson (1966) proposed five perceptual systems. The basic orienting system provides a general orientation to the environment and is essential to the function of the other perceptual systems. The anatomic organ of this system is the balancing portion of the inner ear, which responds to changes in gravity, acceleration, and movement. The visual system permits the person to look, and the auditory system permits listening to sounds as well as identifying the direction from which they are coming. The haptic system responds to touch through reception of sensations of the skin, joints, and muscles. The taste-smell system provides information about chemical stimuli and facilitates safe nourishment (Levine, 1969b, 1973). Levine (1989a) pointed out that for Gibson, "individuals do not merely 'see'—they *look;* they do not merely 'hear'—they *listen.* Thus equipped with the ability to select information from the environment, the individual is an active, seeking participant in it—not merely reacting but influencing, changing, and creating the parameters of his or her life" (p. 330).

The product of adaptation, according to Levine (1989a), is conservation. She explained (p. 329):

> Survival depends on the adaptive ability to use responses that *cost the lease* to the individual in expense of effort and demand on his or her well-being. That is, of course, the essence of *conservation....* Conservation is clearly the consequence of the multiple, interacting, and synchronized negative feedback systems that provide for the stability of the living organism.... [Indeed], homeostasis might be called the state of conservation.

The ultimate purpose of conservation, then, is "to defend, sustain, maintain, and define the integrity of the system for which it functions" (Levine, in press). Indeed, conservation is the "guardian activity that defends and protects [wholeness, which is] the universal target of selfhood" (Chap. 1, p. 4).

HEALTH

Conservation is clearly linked to the health state of the person. Levine explained, "Conservation of the integrity of the person is essential to ensuring health and providing the strength to confront disability. Indeed, the importance of conservation in the treatment of illness is precisely focused on the reclamation of wholeness, of health" (Chap. 1, p. 3).

Levine (1973, 1984a) characterized health and disease as patterns of adaptive change. She commented that adaptation is not an all-or-none process; rather, it is a matter of degree—some adaptations are successful and some are not; some work and some do not. There are, however, no maladaptations. Thus, adaptation has no value attached to it; it just is. Levine (1973) went on to explain (p. 11):

> The measure of effective adaptation is compatibility with life. A poor adaptation may threaten life itself, but at the same time the degree of adaptive potential available to the individual may be sufficient to maintain life at a different level of effectiveness. . . . All the processes of living are processes of adaptation. Survival itself depends upon the quality of the adaptation possible for the individual.

Levine (1989a) further explained, "The most successful adaptations are those that best fit the organism in its environment. A 'best fit' is accomplished with the least expenditure of effort, and with sufficient protective devices built in so that the goal is achieved in as economic and expeditious ɪ manner as possible" (p. 330).

Levine (1984b) indicated that she does not like the term *wellness* and prefers the word *health*. It may be inferred from her description of health as "wholeness" (Levine, 1973, p. 11) and as "successful adaptation" (Levine, 1966a, p. 2452) that she used *health* to mean *wellness*.

It also may be inferred that wellness means social well-being. This inference is supported by the following statement: "One criterion of successful adaptation is the attainment of social well-being, but there is tremendous variation in the degree to which this is achieved" (Levine, 1966a, p. 2452). Indeed, Levine (1984b) has stated that health is socially defined in the sense of "Do I continue to function in a reasonably normal fashion?"

Levine used Wolf's (1961) concept of disease as adaptation to noxious environmental forces for her description of illness. She explained that, "disease represents efforts of the individual to protect his integrity" (Levine, 1971, p. 257). In the same vein, Levine noted that inasmuch as "illness challenges the integrity of the person, defending the person's health—his or her unique wholeness—is a continuing endeavor" (Chap. 1, p. 4).

Disease, for Levine, is undisciplined and unregulated change, a disruption in the orderly sequential pattern of change that is characteristic of life. This anarchy of pattern may not be successful in supporting life. Levine (1973) maintained that "such anarchy, in fact, occurs in disease processes, and unless the pattern can be restored, the organism will die" (p. 9).

The anarchy of disease processes is a positive-feedback mechanism. Levine (1973) noted that positive feedback "results in an increasing rate of function without the regulatory control that restores balance. Thus a 'vicious cycle' is instituted which produces more and more disruption of function" (p. 10).

Levine (1973) pointed out that individuals acknowledge illness through their perceptual systems. She stated (p. 456):

> Physical well-being is dependent upon an experienced body which is communicating the "right" signals. The constancy of awareness of the internal feeling of the body is the baseline against which well-being is measured. . . . Individuals can acknowledge "illness" only in recognizing an alteration in their perception of internal feelings.

Levine has linked healing with wholeness and health. She noted (Chap. 1, p. 4):

Healing is the avenue of return to the daily activities compromised by ill health. It is not only the insult or injury that is repaired—*but the person himself or herself*. . . . It is not merely the healing of an afflicted part. It is, rather, a return to selfhood, where the encroachment of the disability can be set aside entirely, and the individual is free to pursue once more his or her own interests without constraint.

The foregoing description of health indicates that Levine conceptualized this concept as a continuum. This interpretation is supported by the following comment (Levine, 1973, p. 11):

Adaptation . . . is susceptible to an infinite range within the limits of life compatibility. Within that range, there are numerous possible degrees of adaptation. Thus, the dynamic processes establishing balance along the continuum are adaptations.

NURSING

Levine (1973) described nursing as a human interaction: "It is a discipline rooted in the organic dependency of the individual human being on his relationships with other human beings" (p. 1). She further described nursing as "a subculture, possessing ideas and values which are unique to nurses, even though they mirror the social template which created them" (p. 3).

The goal of nursing, according to Levine (1984a), is the promotion of wholeness for all people, well or sick. She maintained (Levine, 1971, p. 258):

The goal of all nursing care should be to promote wholeness, realizing that for every individual that requires a unique and separate cluster of activities. The individual's integrity—his one-ness, his identity as an individual, his wholeness—is his abiding concern, and it is the nurse's responsibility to assist him to defend and to seek its realization.

Levine repeatedly emphasized the importance of deriving nursing processes from scientific knowledge as well as from the messages given by the patient. This is illustrated in the following quotations:

Ultimately, decisions for nursing intervention must be based on the unique behavior of the individual patient. It is the nurse's task to bring a body of scientific principles on which decisions depend into the precise situation which she shares with the patient. (Levine, 1966a, p. 2452)

The integrated response of the individual to any stimulus results in a re-alignment of his very substance, and in a sense this creates a message which others may learn to understand. Each message, in turn, is the result of observation, selection of relevant data, and assessment of the priorities demanded by such knowledge. . . . Understanding the message and responding to it accurately constitute the substance of nursing science. (Levine, 1967, pp. 46–47)

The nursing process of Levine's conceptual model is conservation. Levine (1989a) defined conservation as "keeping together" and stated that conservation—the "keeping together" function—should be the major guideline for all nursing intervention (p. 331). Indeed, "every nursing act is dedicated to the conservation, or 'keeping together,' of the wholeness of the individual" (Chap. 1, p. 3).

Levine emphasized the roles of both nurse and patient in conservation, as illustrated in the following statement (Levine, 1973, p. 13):

"To keep together" means to maintain a proper balance between active nursing intervention coupled with patient participation on the one hand and the safe limits of the patient's ability to participate on the other.

In fact, Levine (1984b) stated that she regards patients as partners or participants in nursing care. She views the person who is a patient as being temporarily dependent on the nurse. The nurse's goal is to end the dependence—that is, the patient status of the person—as quickly as possible. Levine (1989b, pp. 4–5) explained:

Individuals enter into a state of patienthood when they require the expert services that physicians and nurses can provide. The fundamental moral responsibility of patient care is the limitation and relief of suffering. Once individuals are restored, the dependent but willing partnership is dissolved. Their privacy restored to them, individuals cease to be patients.

Levine (1989a) noted that as part of the patient's environment, the nurse brings to nursing care situations his or her "own cascading repertoire of skill, knowledge, and compassion. It is a shared enterprise and each participant is rewarded" (p. 336).

Although Levine did not identify an explicit nursing process, it is possible to extract a format from several of her publications. Levine (1966a) referred to assessment of the patient's nursing requirements, stating: "Sensitive observation and the selection of relevant data form the basis for [the nurse's] assessment of [the patient's] nursing requirements" (p. 2452). The elements of assessment are delineated in Levine's discussion of identification of nursing care needs. She called this "trophicognosis," which is defined as "a nursing care judgment arrived at by the scientific method" (Levine, 1966b, p. 57).

Levine (1966b) presented trophicognosis as an alternative to nursing diagnosis. Tracing the development of nursing diagnosis and its legal interpretation, she pointed out that the term always referred to "diagnosis of disease made by a nurse" (p. 55). Then, citing the only dictionary definition of diagnosis, she maintained that it is "incorrect to use the term diagnosis as a synonym for observations, judgments, problems, needs or assessments" (pp. 56–57). In concluding her argument, Levine stated (p. 57):

Because the term, nursing diagnosis, is now susceptible of legal interpretation, and other usages of the term are semantically incorrect, it is proposed that a new nursing term be used to described the scientific approach in the determination of nursing care. Such a method of ascribing nursing care needs may be called trophicognosis.

The elements of trophicognosis are presented in Table 2–2. Levine (personal communication, August 13, 1987) stated that she and her colleagues are developing a taxonomy of trophicognoses.

According to Levine (1973), "nursing intervention must be designed so that it fosters successful adaptation whenever possible" (p. 13). Indeed, nursing must view individuals so that the 'best fit' available to each person

TABLE 2-2. ELEMENTS OF TROPHICOGNOSIS

I Establishing an objective and scientific rationale for nursing care
  A Basis for implementation of prescribed medical regimen
    1 Knowledge and understanding of the medical diagnosis
    2 Evaluation of the medical history, with specific reference to areas influencing the nursing care plan
    3 Knowledge of laboratory and x-ray reports emphasizing factors that influence nursing care
    4 Consultation with physician to share information and clarify nursing care decisions
    5 Knowledge of aspects of prescribed medical regimen (expected and untoward effects) as contribution to the evaluation of the effectiveness of the therapy
  B Basis for implementation of prescribed paramedical regimen
    1 Knowledge of paramedical diagnoses and prescriptions for care
    2 Clear definition of nurse's role in paramedical prescriptions
  C Determination of nursing processes demanded by medical treatment
    1 Observation of effects of prescribed medical aspects of patient's care on individual progress
    2 Adaptation of nursing techniques to the unique cluster of needs demonstrated in the individual patient
  D Basis for implementation of the unique nursing needs of the individual patient
    1 Knowledge and understanding of the principles of nursing science
    2 Provision for gathering a nursing history, with specific reference to aspects that will influence the nursing care plan
    3 Accurate recording and transmittal of observations and evaluation of patient's response to nursing processes
    4 Utilization of knowledge gained in consultation with family members or other individuals concerned with the patient, including the religious counselor
II Implementation of nursing care within the structure of administrative policy, availability of equipment, and established standards of nursing care

SOURCE: Levine, M.E. (1966b). Trophicognosis: An alternative to nursing diagnosis. In *American Nurses' Association Regional Clinical Conference* (Vol. 2, pp. 59–60). New York: American Nurses' Association, with permission.

can be sustained" (Levine, 1989a). Interestingly, however, adaptation is impossible to measure or quantify. Levine explained, "Although certain generalized adaptations can be described—the required oxygen tension, temperature tolerance of living cells, effect of atmospheric pressure on physiologic function, for example—precise identification of the adaptive condition is not possible" (Chap. 1, pp. 6–7). Inasmuch as adaptation cannot be directly observed, the consequences of care are taken into account (Chap. 1, p. 7).

The consequences of nursing care may be therapeutic or supportive. Levine (1973, p. 13) explained:

> When nursing intervention influences adaptation favorably, or toward renewed social well-being, then the nurse is acting in a therapeutic sense. When nursing intervention cannot alter the course of the adaptation—when her best efforts can only maintain the status quo or fail to halt a downward course—then the nurse is acting in a supportive sense.

Nursing intervention is structured according to four conservation principles: conservation of energy, conservation of structural integrity, conservation of personal integrity, and conservation of social integrity. Conservation of energy, according to Levine (1988b), "refers to balancing energy output and energy input to avoid excessive fatigue, that is, adequate rest, nutrition, and exercise" (p. 227). Levine (1989a) explained that the conservation of energy is a natural law "found to hold everywhere in the universe for all animate and inanimate entities" (p. 331). Energy, according to Levine, is not directly observable, although "the consequences of its exchange are predictable, manageable, and quantifiable. Instruments can monitor, measure, produce, or capture energy" (Chap. 1, p. 7). Energy parameters of concern to nurses include body temperature; pulse, respiratory, and metabolic rates; blood gases; and blood pressure; among others. There are, Levine maintained, finite sources of energy available to the person. Conservation of energy ensures that "energy is spent carefully, with essential priorities served first" (Chap. 1, p. 7). Although individuals conserve their energy, even at perfect rest, energy from life-sustaining activities such as biochemical changes is expended. Levine (1989a, p. 332) commented:

> The conservation of energy is clearly evident in the very sick, whose lethargy, withdrawal, and self-concern are manifested while, in its wisdom, the body is spending its energy resource on the processes of healing.

Conservation of structural integrity focuses on healing. More specifically, this principle of conservation "refers to maintaining or restoring the structure of the body, that is, preventing physical breakdown and promoting healing" (Levine, 1988b, p. 227). Levine pointed out that we expect and have confidence in the ability of our bodies to heal. Healing, according to Levine (1989a), "is the defense of wholeness . . . [and] a consequence of an effective immune system" (p. 333). Conservation of structural integrity "emphasizes that the individual's defense against the hazards of the environment are achieved with the most economical expense of effort" and results in "repair and healing to sustain the wholeness of structure and function" (Chap. 1, p. 8).

Conservation of personal integrity underscores the fact that "every individual defends his or her unique personhood, the individual within known as the self. Wholeness is summarized in that knowledge [of self]" (Chap. 1, p. 8). This conservation principle, then, focuses on the maintenance or restoration of the patient's sense of identity, self-worth, and acknowledgment of uniqueness" (Levine, 1988b, p. 227). The self, according to Levine (1989a), is "much more than a physical experience of the whole body, although it is unquestionably a part of that awareness" (p. 334). Personal integrity emphasizes individuals' perseverance in retaining their identities. "Everyone seeks to defend his or her identity as a self, in both that hidden, intensely private person that dwells within and in the public faces assumed as individuals move through their relationships with others" (Levine, 1989a, p. 334).

Conservation of social integrity, Levine (1988b) noted, "refers to the acknowledgment of the patient as a social being. It involves the recognition and presentation of human interaction, particularly with the patient's significant others" (p. 227). This conservation principle emphasizes the fact that "selfhood needs definition beyond the individual . . . [and that] the individual is created by the environment and in turn creates within it" (Levine, 1989a, p. 335). The principle states that each individual's identity places him or her "in a family, a community, a cultural heritage, a religious belief, a socioeconomic slot, an educational background, a vocational choice" (Levine, 1989a, p. 335). Social context is a necessity of wholeness. Indeed, Levine maintained that "it is impossible to acknowledge the wholeness of the individual without considering his or her social context" (Chap. 1, p. 9). Levine (1988b) noted that the four conservation principles "apply equally to living things, and the derivative meaning of 'conservation' as a 'keeping together' function seemed entirely appropriate as the essential goal of nursing care" (p. 227). She also pointed out that the conservation principles do not operate singly but rather are "joined within the individual as a cascade of life events, churning and changing as the environmental challenge is confronted and resolved in each individual's unique way" (Levine, 1989a, p. 336). The integration of conservation principles is exemplified in the following quotation (Chap. 1, p. 10):

> The conservation principles address the integrity of the individual . . . from birth to death. Every activity requires an energy supply because nothing works without it. Every activity must respect the structural wholeness of the individual because well-being depends upon it. Every activity is chosen out of the abilities, life experience, and desires of the self who makes the choices. Every activity is a product of the dynamic social systems to which the individual belongs.

Use of the four conservation principles in the nursing process is outlined in Table 2–3.

TABLE 2-3. LEVINE'S CONSERVATION PRINCIPLES

I Principle of Conservation of Energy:
Nursing intervention is based on the conservation of the individual patient's energy—balancing energy output and energy input by preventing excessive fatigue and promoting adequate rest, nutrition, and exercise

A Relevant scientific considerations

  1 The ability of the human body to perform work is dependent upon its energy balance—the supply of energy-producing nutrients measured against the rate of energy-using activities

  2 The energy required by alterations in physiologic function during illness represents an additional demand made on the energy production systems

  3 Fatigue, often experienced with illness, is an empiric measure of the additional energy demand

B Nursing intervention

  1 General considerations

    a Nursing intervention is based on the balancing of energy input with energy output

TABLE 2-3. *Continued*

    b Assessment of patient's ability to perform necessary activities without producing excessive fatigue
      1 Vital signs
      2 Patient's general condition
      3 Patient's behavior
      4 Patient's tolerance of nursing activities required by his or her condition
    c Allowable activity for patient based on his or her energy resources
    d Interventions designed to provide an adequate deposit of energy resource and regulate expenditure of energy
  2 Examples of specific nursing interventions
    a Provision for rest
    b Maintenance of adequate nutrition

II Principle of Conservation of Structural Integrity:
Nursing intervention is based on the conservation of the individual patient's structural integrity—maintaining or restoring the structure of the body by preventing physical breakdown and promoting healing
  A Relevant scientific considerations
    1 Structural change results in a change of function
    2 Pathophysiologic processes present a threat to structural integrity
    3 Healing processes restore structural integrity
    4 Surgical procedures are designed to restore structural integrity
    5 Structural integrity is restored when the scar is organized and integrated in the continuity of the part affected
  B Nursing intervention
    1 General considerations
      a Limit amount of tissue involvement in infection and disease
      b Prevent trophicogenic (nurse-induced) disease
    2 Examples of specific nursing interventions
      a Anatomic positioning of patient
      b Physiologic positioning of patient
      c Maintenance of patient's personal hygiene
      d Assist patient with range-of-motion exercises and passive exercises

III Principle of Conservation of Personal Integrity:
Nursing intervention is based on the conservation of the patient's personal integrity—maintaining or restoring the patient's sense of identity, self-worth, and acknowledgment of uniqueness
  A Relevant scientific considerations
    1 There is always a privacy to individual life
    2 Assumption of responsibility for one's own decisions develops with maturation
    3 Self-identify and self-respect are the foundations of a sense of personal integrity
    4 Illness threatens self-identity and self-respect
    5 Hospitalization may compound and exaggerate the threat to personal integrity
    6 Individuals possess a lifetime commitment to the value systems and social patterns of their subcultural affiliations
    7 The patient's family may be deeply affected by the changes resulting from illness
    8 Hospitalization is characterized by isolation from family and friends
  B Nursing intervention
    1 General considerations
      a Respect from the nurse is essential to the patient's self-respect
      b Accept the patient the way he or she is
      c Foster patient participation in decision making within safe limits
      d Determine and take into the account patient's moral and ethical values

TABLE 2-3. *Continued*

  2 Examples of specific nursing interventions
    a Recognize and protect patient's space needs
    b Ensure privacy during performance of body functions and therapeutic procedures
    c Respect importance patient places on personal possessions
    d Use appropriate mode of address when dealing with patient
    e Support patient's defense mechanisms as appropriate
IV Principle of Conservation of Social Integrity:
  Nursing intervention is based on the conservation of the individual patient's social integrity—acknowledging the patient as a social being
  A Relevant scientific considerations
    1 The social integrity of individuals is tied to the viability of the entire social system
    2 Individual life has meaning only in the context of social life
    3 The way in which individuals relate to various social groups influences their behavior
    4 Individual recognition of wholeness is measured against relationships with others
    5 Interactions with others become more important in times of stress
  B Nursing intervention
    1 General considerations
      a A failure to consider the patient's family and friends is a failure to provide excellent nursing care
      b The social system of the hospital is artificial
      c Concern for holistic well-being of individuals demands attention to community attitudes, resources, and provision of health care in the community
      d The nurse-patient interaction is a social relationship that is disciplined and controlled by the professional role of the nurse
    2 Examples of specific nursing interventions
      a Consider patients' social needs when placing them in the nursing unit
      b Position patient in bed to foster social interaction with other patients
      c Avoid sensory deprivation for the patient
      d Promote the patient's use of newspapers, magazines, radio, and television as appropriate
      e Provide family with knowledgeable support and assistance
      f Teach family members to perform functions for the patient as necessary

SOURCE: Adapted from Levine, M.E. (1967). The four conservation principles of nursing. Nursing Forum, 6, 47–59; Levine, M.E. (1973). Introduction to clinical nursing (2nd ed., pp. 13–18). Philadelphia: F.A. Davis; and Levine, M.E. (1988). Myra Levine. In T.M. Schoor & A. Zimmerman, Making choices. Taking chances. Nurse leaders tell their stories (p. 227). St. Louis: C.V. Mosby.

Content of the Model: Propositions

The propositions of Levine's Conservation Model link the metaparadigm concepts of person, environment, health, and nursing. The person is repeatedly placed in the context of the environment, as is illustrated in the following quotations (Levine, 1973):

> The individual is always within an environmental milieu, and the consequences of his awareness of his environment persistently influence his behavior at any given moment. (p. 444)

[The person's] presence in the environment also influences it and thereby the kind of information available from it. (p. 446)

The individual protects and defends himself within his environment by gaining all the information he can about it. (p. 451)

The links among all metaparadigm concepts are stated in the following quotations:

The nurse participates actively in every patient's environment, and much of what she does supports his adaptations as he struggles in the predicament of illness. (Levine, 1973, p. 13)

But even in the presence of disease, the organism responds wholly to the environmental interaction in which it is involved, and a considerable amount of nursing care is devoted to restoring the symmetry of response—symmetry that is essential to the well-being of the organism. (Levine, 1969b, p. 98)

Areas of Concern

The major area of concern addressed by Levine's Conservation Model is the maintenance of the person's wholeness. Levine (1973) focuses on adaptation as the process by which individuals maintain their wholeness or integrity. Thus, the model emphasizes the effectiveness of the person's adaptations. Furthermore, this conceptual model focuses the nurse's attention on the person and the complexity of his or her relationships with the internal and external environments. The model also emphasizes the nurse's responsibility for conservation of the patient's energy, as well as his or her structural, personal, and social integrity.

The source of threats to the person's wholeness or integrity is environmental challenge. Apparently, challenges may come from the internal or external environment. This interpretation of Levine's ideas is supported by the following comment (Levine, 1973, p. 8):

The exquisite internal balance responds constantly to the external forces. . . . There is an intimate relationship between the internal and the external environments, much of it vividly understood in recent years by research in physiological periodicity and the circadian cycles.

This interpretation is supported further by Levine's (1973) reference to positive feedback in the internal environment, which is manifested when pathologic processes occur and can be responsible for pathology.

EVALUATION OF LEVINE'S CONSERVATION MODEL

The evaluation presented in this section is based on the results of the analysis of the model as well as publications and presentations by others who have used or commented on this conceptual model.

Explication of Assumptions

Levine explicitly identified the assumptions underlying her conceptual model. Her presentation of the model indicates that she values a holistic approach to the nursing care of all people, well or sick. She also values the unique individuality of each person, as noted in comments such as those that follow (Levine, 1973):

> Ultimately, decisions for nursing intervention must be based on the unique behavior of the individual patient. . . . A theory of nursing must recognize the importance of unique detail of care for a single patient within a empiric framework which successfully describes the requirements of all patients. (p. 6)
>
> Patient centered nursing care means individualized nursing care. It is predicated on the reality of common experience: every man is a unique individual, and as such he requires a unique constellation of skills, techniques, and ideas designed specifically for him. (p. 23)

Furthermore, although Levine (1973) commented that human beings are dependent on their relationships with other human beings, she values the patient's participation in nursing care. This is attested to by the following comment (p. 13):

> "To keep together" means to maintain a proper balance between active nursing intervention coupled with patient participation on the one hand and the safe limits of the patient's ability to participate on the other.

Comprehensiveness of Concepts and Propositions

Levine's descriptions of the person, the environment, health, and nursing are comprehensive and essentially complete. Consequently, there is little need for inference in this conceptual model.

The nursing process extracted from Levine's writings meets Walker and Nicholson's (1980) criteria. Levine repeatedly emphasized the need for a scientific knowledge base for nursing judgments. Moreover, Levine's frequent citations of relevant research support the consistency of this model with scientific findings on human behavior. These features of the model are evident in statements such as the following (Levine, 1966a):

> It is the nurse's task to bring a body of scientific principles on which decisions depend into the precise situation which she shares with the patient. (p. 2452)
>
> The modern nurse has available rich knowledge of human anatomy, physiology, and adaptability. (p. 2453)

Furthermore, Levine emphasized a concern for the individual person, reflecting the ethical standards of nursing. She expressed her ethical standards in the *American Journal of Nursing* article "Nursing Ethics and the Ethical Nurse." She concluded that publication by stating (Levine, 1977, p. 849):

> The wholeness which is part of our awareness of ourselves is shared best with others when no act diminishes another person, and no moment of indifference leaves him with less of himself. Every moment of moral injustice extracts a price from both patient and nurse, just as every moment of moral responsibility gives each strength to grow in his wholeness.

Levine's attention to ethical standards is reflected in the following statements (Levine, 1967)

Nursing intervention must deal with the rights and privileges of the individual in tangible ways. . . . The emphasis on patient teaching recognizes the individual's right to be assisted in understanding the implications of his disease, his treatment, and his care. He must also be assured that his medical and social problems will remain privileged and confidential. (p. 54)

True conservation demands that the nurse accept the patient the way he is. (p. 55)

The generality of the nursing process is partially documented in Levine's (1973) book. This text includes nursing processes appropriate for patients who have a failure of nursing system integration, hormonal disturbances, fluid and electrolyte imbalances, aberrant cellular growth, and several other pathologic states. In addition, the applicability of the nursing process in various settings is documented later in the chapter in the section on social utility.

The dynamic nature of the nursing process is evident in Levine's (1973) statement that nursing care plans "must allow for progress and change and project into the future the patient's response to treatment" (p. 46), as well as in Levine's (1989a) presentation of nursing care as use of a "cascading repertoire of skill, knowledge, and compassion" (p. 326). Given Levine's explanation of cascades as nonlinear, interacting and evolving processes, the nursing process clearly is dynamic.

The criterion for comprehensiveness of propositions stipulates that all four metaparadigm concepts be linked. The statements presented in the analysis section of this chapter attest to the satisfaction of this criterion.

Logical Congruence

WORLD VIEWS

Levine's conceptual model clearly reflects the organismic view of the world. She regards the person as a holistic being who constantly strives to preserve wholeness and integrity. Furthermore, although Levine (1989a) discusses physiologic and behavioral responses, she regarded these as "one and the same—not merely parallel and not merely simultaneous—but essential portions of the same activity" (p. 330). Moreover, although she identified four principles of conservation, she viewed them as joined, not isolated or separate.

The elements of organicism are exemplified explicitly in the following quotations:

Nursing intervention, traditionally directed by procedures or manifestations of disease symptoms, needs new directions if the holistic approach is to be utilized. The individual must be recognized in his wholeness, and the powerful influence of adaptation recognized as a dynamic and ever-present factor in evaluating his care. Instead of listing "needs" or "symptoms," it should be possible to identify for each individual the patterns of his adaptive response, and to tailor intervention to enhance their effectiveness. (Levine, 1971, pp. 257–258)

All nursing care is focused on man and the complexity of his relationships

with his environment, both internal and external, and common experience
emphasizes that every response to every environmental stimulus results from
the integrated and unified nature of the human organism. In other words, every response is an organismic one—no other kind is possible—and every
adaptive change is accomplished by the entire individual. (Levine, 1967,
p. 46)

Organicism also is reflected in Levine's characterization of the person
as an active participant in interactions with the environment. This is seen
especially in her statement that "the individual can . . . never be passive.
He is an active participant in his environment, not only altering it by his
presence but also actively and constantly seeking information from it"
(Levine, 1969b, p. 96). The active organism viewpoint also is reflected in
Levine's discussion of the perceptual systems. For example, Levine (1973)
commented, "The human being is a sentient being, and the ability to interact with the environment seems ineluctably tied to his sensory organs"
(p. 446). She also noted, "The perceptual systems provide information to
the individual; usually this is knowledge sought by the individual" (Levine,
1973, p. 450).

There is little evidence of a mechanistic world view in the model. In
fact, Levine (1971) explicitly rejected mechanism, stating, "The mechanistic view of the body and mind does little to restore to the individual the
wholeness he recognizes in himself" (p. 254). However, at one point Levine did present a somewhat reactive, mechanistic view of the person. She
stated, "The human being responds to the forces in his environment in a
singular yet integrated fashion" (Levine, 1966a, p. 2452). Here, Levine appears to be attempting to translate the mechanistic idea of reaction to the
environment by bringing in the idea of a more holistic, integrated response.
Furthermore, this comment is offset by Levine's explicit statements about
the active nature of the person, as noted earlier.

Levine's model seems to reflect the world view of change. This viewpoint is evident in statements such as the following, both from Levine
(1973, p. 10):

> Change is the essence of life, and it is unceasing as long as life goes on.
> Change is characteristic of life.

In contrast, the emphasis on homeostasis and conservation suggests
that Levine's model reflects the persistence view of the world. Levine
(1989a) regarded homeostasis as "a state of energy-sparing" (p. 329); it
even "might be called the state of conservation" (p. 320). The essence of
conservation, in turn, is the use of responses "that *cost the least* to the individual in expense of effort and demand on his or her well-being" (p. 329).

Given Levine's primary focus on conservation, it seems more appropriate to classify this conceptual model as within the persistence view of
the world. Apparently, Levine regards the many changes that must occur
as the person faces environmental challenges as necessary for survival.
Conservation facilitates and maintains the patterns and routines of human
behavior, and adaptive changes represent invention of new routines to
avoid extinction.

Classification of the Model

Close examination of the content of Levine's Conservation Model indicates that the systems category is an appropriate classification. The characteristic of integration of parts is reflected in the following quotations:

> The total life process of the entire organism is dependent upon the interrelatedness of its component systems. In fact, the organism is a system of systems. (Levine, 1973, pp. 8–9)

> Human life must be described in the language of "wholes." . . . perceiving the "wholes" depends upon recognizing the organization and interdependence of observable phenomena. (Levine, 1971, p. 255)

Other than her comment regarding the organism as a system of systems, Levine does not explicitly address the characteristic of system. Environment, however, is addressed repeatedly and is viewed as both internal and external. The relationship of the person to environment is expressed clearly in the following statement: "The person cannot be described apart from the specific environment in which he or she is found" (Levine, 1989a, p. 325). Levine (1973) related the idea of "wholeness" to that of the open system. Citing Erikson (1968), she stated that a whole is an open system and explained, "The unceasing interaction of the individual organism with its environments does represent an 'open and fluid' system" (p. 11).

The characteristic of boundary is explicitly addressed in this conceptual model in the discussion of individual territoriality. Levine (1973) commented, "Every individual requires space, and both the establishment of his personal boundaries and their defense are essential components of his behavior" (p. 459). Levine (1973) went on to cite Hall's (1966) work on human territorial behavior, with its identification of the intimate, personal distance, social distance, and public distance zones maintained among people.

The systems model characteristic of tension, stress, strain, and conflict is alluded to by Levine in her discussion of adaptation. She stated (Levine, 1973, pp. 10–11):

> Change is characteristic of life, and adaptation is the method of change. The organism retains its integrity in both the internal and external environment through its adaptive capability. Adaptation is the process of change whereby the individual retains his integrity within the realities of his environments.

Levine's (1989a) use of the term *environmental challenge* suggests that this is what represents the factors or forces that are responsible for initiating change and adaptation.

Levine (1973) referred to the characteristic of steady state when she discussed homeorhesis. This term denotes "a stabilized flow, rather than a static state" (p. 7). Levine (1973) commented, "The concept of stabilized flow more accurately reflects the reality of daily change as well as the alterations in physiological activity that characterize the processes of growth and development" (pp. 7–8). In one of her most recent works, however, Levine (1989a) seemed to favor homeostasis as the best descriptor of internal environment, regarding it as a state that "provides the necessary baselines for a multitude of synchronized physiological and psychological factors," (p. 329) rather than a system of balance and queasiness. In fact, Levine (personal communication, August 13, 1987) indicated that homeostasis is the appropriate view of the internal environment because it captures the notion of the congruence of the person with the environment.

The characteristic of feedback is addressed in this conceptual model in terms of physiologic and pathologic processes. In keeping with systems models, Levine (1973, 1989a) associated negative feedback with autoregulation of physiologic systems and positive feedback with disruption of function seen in pathologic processes.

Meleis (1985) classified Levine's conceptual model within the outcome category. She noted that Levine's work focuses on nursing activities and actions designed to care for people. Marriner (1986) placed Levine's work within her energy fields category. Stevens (1984) classified Levine's model in the conservation category. Interestingly, Levine (cited in Riehl-Sisca, 1989) apparently regarded her conceptual model as an interaction model and Riehl-Sisca (1989) classified it as such. The content of Levine's model does not, however, address any of the characteristics of that category as described by Fawcett (1989). Certainly Levine's work deals with the interaction between person and environment, but that is not the same as the symbolic interactionism, emphasized in the interaction category. When asked about the interaction classification, Levine (personal communication, August 13, 1987) agreed that her conceptual model does not reflect symbolic interactionism and went on to say that hers is "an adaptation model."

Generation and Testing of Theory

Levine (1978a) stated that she was trying to develop two theories, which she called therapeutic intention and redundancy. Work on the theory of therapeutic intention began in the early 1970s. Levine (personal communication to L. Criddle, July 22, 1987) indicated that she "was seeking a way of organizing nursing intervention growing out of the reality of the *biological* realities which nurses had to confront." Her thinking about therapeutic intention is summarized in the following statements (Levine, personal communication to L. Criddle, July 22, 1987) that describe broad areas of therapeutic intervention and create parameters of nursing care:

1. Therapeutic regimens that support the integrated healing processes of the body and permit optimal restoration of structure and function through natural response to disease.
2. Therapeutic regimens that substitute an external servomechanism for a failure of autoregulation of an essential integrating system.
3. Therapeutic regimens that focus on specific causes, and by surgical restructuring or drug therapy, restore individual integrity and well-being.
4. Therapeutic regimens that cannot alter or substitute for the pathology so that only supportive measures are possible to promote comfort and humane concern.
5. Therapeutic regimens that balance a significant toxic risk against the threat of the disease process.

6. Therapeutic regimens that simulate physiologic processes and reinforce or antagonize usual responses in order to create a therapeutic change in function.
7. Therapeutic regimens that manipulate diet and activity to correct metabolic imbalances related to nutrition and/or exercise.

Levine (personal communication, August 13, 1987) regarded the seven areas of therapeutic intention as an "imperfect list that is not yet complete."

Although the theory of therapeutic intention seems to extend the nursing process component of the conservation model, Levine (personal communication to L. Criddle, July 22, 1987) stated that she never associated the idea of therapeutic intention with the principles of conservation. She explained, "I suppose it would be a claim to some greater wisdom to suggest that every idea I ever had was in some way associated with the conservation principles—but that is simply not true. My thought habits are fairly consistent but I have devoted them to many areas which are not organically related."

Levine (1978a) noted that she and a colleague had been working on the theory of redundancy for some time. This "completely untested, completely speculative" theory has "redefined aging and almost everything else that has to do with human life." She proposed that "aging is the diminished availability of redundant systems necessary for effective maintenance of physical and social well-being" (Levine, 1978b). This theory seems to extend the discussion of redundancy related to specificity of adaptation and organismic responses. Indeed, Levine noted that "the possibility exists that aging itself is a consequence of failed redundancy of physiologic and psychologic processes" (Chap. 1, p. 6).

Social Considerations

SOCIAL CONGRUENCE

Although Levine's conceptual model was initially formulated many years ago, it is congruent with the present emphasis on holistic approaches to health care and consideration of the person as a unique individual. Levine developed her model at a time when nursing activities in acute care settings were becoming more mechanical, owing to the rapid increase in medical technology. She spoke out against the growing functionalism of nursing and reoriented nurses to the patient as a whole being, as is evident in the following comment (Levine, 1966a, p. 2453):

> Discovering ways to perceive and cherish the essential wholeness of man becomes imperative with the rapid growth of automation in modern disciplines which possess a technology. Nursing is one of them, and nurses will not escape the sweeping changes that automation promises. But nurses do know that the integrated human being is not merely "programmed" to respond to life in automatic ways. . . . It is the task of nursing to recognize and value the wondrous variety of all mankind while offering ministrations that conserve the unique and special integrity of every man.

Levine (1973) noted that "the whole man is the focus of nursing intervention—in health and sickness, in tragedy and joy, in hospitals and clinics and in the community" (p. vii). Although little discussion of the use of this conceptual model in health promotion and illness prevention situations is available, its broad focus is congruent with society's increasing interest in promotion of health and prevention of illness.

Social Significance

Hirschfeld (1976) provided some evidence of the social significance of Levine's Conservation Model. She noted, "Myra Levine's four principles of conservation are useful in deciding what will help the cognitively impaired aged person and determining what the priorities should be in his or her care" (p. 1981). She went on to describe application of the principles of conservation to the care of several patients who had cognitive impairments. In concluding her article, Hirschfeld (p. 1984) stated,

> Surely, nursing care that incorporates Levine's four conservation principles can make a difference to the individual and family equilibrium that are disturbed by events as devastating as mental impairment.

Additional evidence of social significance was provided by V. G. Lathrop (personal communication, May 5, 1982), who used Levine's model to guide the nursing care of patients in the Intensive Treatment Unit for Mentally Ill Offenders at Saint Elizabeth's Hospital in Washington, D.C. According to Lathrop, nursing audits based on the American Nurses' Association Psychiatric/Mental Health Standards of Nursing Practice revealed that "treatment provided was more holistic in nature."

SOCIAL UTILITY

The utility of Levine's Conservation Model is documented by the publication of this book, as well as by other publications. The specific utility of the conservation model for nursing research is documented by several studies. The rules for research regarding phenomena to be studied have been proposed by Levine (personal communication to L. Criddle, July 22, 1987), who stated, "I do not believe that the Conservation Principles can be used as a research model *one at a time*. They intersect with each other and must be viewed in context." Levine (personal communication, August 13, 1987) did, however, indicate that it would be appropriate to develop instruments that deal with just a conservation principle. Elaborating, Levine (Chap. 1, p. 10) stated:

> The conservation principles may be addressed singly. Indeed, research and scholarly study must focus on discrete issues. But the integrity of the whole person cannot be violated. However narrowed the study problem may be, the influence of all four conservation principles must be acknowledged, and the wholeness of the person sustained.

Levine (1978a) provided further specification of phenomena to be studied when she noted that a needed area of nursing research is the investigation of the interface between the internal and external environments of the person. Other rules must be developed.

Four doctoral dissertations based on Levine's conservation principles were recently completed at the University of Illinois at Chicago. Cox (1988) studied pregnancy, anxiety, and time perception. Fleming (1988) compared women with different perineal conditions after childbirth. Foreman (1988, 1989) described the development of confusion in elderly patients. MacLean (1988) described cues used by nurses for identification of activity intolerance. In addition, Blasage's (1987) dissertation research, at Loyola University of Chicago, examined and identified trends in Levine's writings. Moreover, Cooper's (1989) dissertation research, conducted at the University of Pennsylvania, focused on development of an instrument to assess the status of open, soft tissue wounds healing by secondary intention. Cooper clearly linked her work to the principle of conservation of structural integrity.

Other research based on Levine's conceptual model includes studies by Newport (1984), Yeates and Roberts (1984), and Winslow and her associates (1984, 1985). Newport compared the body temperatures of infants who had been placed on their mothers' chests immediately after birth with infants who were placed in a warmer. Yeates and Roberts compared the effects on labor progress of two bearing-down techniques during the second stage of labor.

Winslow (personal communication to M. E. Levine, October 6, 1982) indicated that her research on energy utilization during toileting and bathing is based on Levine's principle of conservation of energy. However, the published reports of this research do not cite Levine (Winslow, 1983; Winslow, Lane, & Gaffney, 1984, 1985).

Geden's (1982) report of her study of energy expenditure during lifting cited notions of energy mentioned in some nursing models, including Levine's. There is no evidence, however, that this research was an explicit test of Levine's principle of conservation of energy. In fact, Geden (1985) interpreted her work within the context of Orem's general theory of nursing.

Tompkins (1980) cited a few conceptual models of nursing, including Levine's, in the discussion of findings from her study of the effect of restricted mobility and leg dominance on perceived duration of time. This research was not, however, derived from Levine's model.

Schaefer's Chapter 3 of this book extends the discussion of research based on Levine's Conservation Model. Her chapter also presents implications for further development of the research rules.

The utility of Levine's conceptual model for nursing practice has been documented, and rules for practice are becoming evident. First, it is clear that the focus of all nursing care is conservation of the patient's wholeness. Second, it is clear that legitimate recipients of nursing care encompass individuals who are sick and those who are well. Third, it is clear that the nursing process is guided by the principles of conservation.

Levine's conceptual model has been used in various clinical settings and situations. Hirschfeld (1976) linked the principles of conservation with theories of pathophysiology, aging, and cognitive impairment to develop nursing interventions for several patients who were cognitively impaired as a result of illness. Herbst (1981) linked the principles of conservation with knowledge of the pathophysiology of cancer and presented a comprehensive description of nursing that takes into account the wholeness of the patient, the nurse, and the disease process. Brunner (1985) used the conservation principles and knowledge of cardiac pathology to formulate a nursing care plan for cardiac patients. Crawford-Gamble (1986) described the use of the four conservation principles, linked with knowledge of the effects of surgery, in care of a woman undergoing reimplantation of digits of her hand. Fawcett and her associates (1987) used knowledge of end-stage heart disease and critical care unit environments to formulate trophicognoses for a 57-year-old man. Savage and Culbert (1989) described the role and distinctive contributions of the nurse in the care of infants and toddlers at risk for developmental delay. Levine (1989c) discussed ethical issues surrounding the care of the elderly critical care patient.

Furthermore, Cox (1985) described the use of Levine's Conservation Model to guide nursing care of elderly residents of the Alverno Health Care Facility in Clinton, Iowa. Her discussion underscored the utility of Levine's model for health promotion and illness prevention. In addition, Pond (1985) reported her use of the conceptual model in the emergency department of the Hospital of the University of Pennsylvania in Philadelphia. And M. Mercer (personal communication, December 10, 1983) outlined an assessment format she used in the critical care unit at Chester County Hospital in West Chester, Pennsylvania.

Use of the conceptual model as a guide for nursing practice also was reported by V. G. Lathrop and M. J. Stafford. As noted in the section on social significance, Lathrop (personal communication, May 5, 1982) used Levine's Conservation Model in a psychiatric-mental health setting. Furthermore, Stafford (personal communication, June 2, 1982), a clinical specialist in cardiac nursing, used Levine's Conservation Model for nursing care of patients at the Hines Veterans Administration Hospital in Hines, Illinois.

Several chapters in this book focus on use of Levine's conceptual model as a guide for nursing practice. In Chapter 12, Pond, for example, discusses Levine-based nursing care of homeless persons. Furthermore, Pasco and Halupa, in Chapter 8, discuss management of patients in pain based on the conservation principles. Foreman (Chapter 10) describes the care of confused elderly patients, using all the conservation principles. Other examples include Levine-based nursing practice in the areas of pediatric nursing, neuroscience nursing, and burn nursing (see Chapters 5, 6, and 7, respectively).

The utility of Levine's conceptual model for nursing education also is documented. The role for education regarding curriculum content is partially specified in Levine's (1969a, 1973) book. Although her book was written and revised many years ago, the content areas identified as appropriate for an introductory nursing course are just as relevant today. The areas are vital signs, body movement and positioning, personal hygiene, fluids, nutrition, pressure gradient systems, application of heat and cold, medications, and asepsis. Other rules for education have not yet been formulated.

Some publications describing the use of Levine's Conservation Model in nursing education were located. Stevens (1984) offered a hypothetical curriculum design based on Levine's model. Findings from surveys of baccalaureate nursing programs conducted by Hall (1979) and Riehl (1980) revealed that Levine's conceptual model is used as a guideline for curriculum development. In particular, Riehl found that Levine's model is "popular with faculty, especially in the Chicago area" (p. 396). The names of the schools of nursing using Levine's model were not given in the survey reports. In Chapter 14 of this book, Grindley and Paradowski present a description of the use of Levine's conceptual model as the nursing curriculum guide at Allentown College of Saint Francis de Sales in Center Valley, Pennsylvania.

In addition, L. Zwanger (personal communication, June 4, 1982) reported that Levine's Conservation Model is used in nursing education programs sponsored by Kapat-Holim, the Health Insurance Institution of the General Federation of Labor in Israel, based in Tel-Aviv. Moreover, M. J. Stafford (personal communication, June 2, 1982) stated that she used the model "in teaching formal and informal classes such as the Critical Care Nursing course, Pacemaker Therapy, and The Nurse's Role in Electrocardiography" at the Hines Veterans Administration Hospital in Hines, Illinois.

Levine's Conservation Model has documented utility for nursing service administration. One role for administration was suggested by Levine (1969b) when she indicated that the person's perceptual system could serve as the basis for organization of hospital units. Levine explained that the patient's ability to receive information and interpret it must be taken into account, as well as territorial needs. Other rules have not yet been developed.

The utility of Levine's conceptual model for various administrative endeavors is evident. Taylor (1974) developed a form of evaluation of the quality of nursing care of patients with neurologic problems. The conservation principles served as the goals of nursing care and were used as the frame of reference for "defining commonly recurring nursing problems on the neurological service" (p. 342). In addition, M. J. Stafford (personal communication, June 2, 1982) commented that she used Levine's Conservation Model to identify process and outcome criteria in the nursing care of patients with cardiovascular problems. Furthermore, the utility of Levine's conceptual model for nursing administration is documented by its use at the Alverno Health Care Facility in Clinton, Iowa. Here, the conservation principles structure the format of the nursing care plan and provide guidelines for staff development. The nursing care plan contains an extensive summary of the patient's trophicognosis and care is organized according to the four conservation principles (Cox, 1985).

Contributions to Nursing Knowledge

Levine's Conservation Model makes a substantial contribution to nursing knowledge by focusing attention on the whole person. Levine moved beyond the idea of the total person to the concept of the person as a holistic being. Pointing to the limitations of the so-called total person approach, she noted (Levine, 1969b, p. 94):

> Nurses have long known that patients are complete persons, not groups of parts. It is out of this realization that the attempts toward "comprehensive care" and "total care" have come, and it is because we have been frustrated by failing to achieve the ideal of completion that the research for a more definitive approach to bedside care has continued.

This conceptual model is consistent in its approach to the person as a holistic being. Physiologic and behavioral responses are regarded as one and the same, and conservation principles are joined. Moreover, Levine's principles of conservation provide a framework for holistic nursing care. These principles focus attention on the patient as a unique individual.

The conservation model has a distinctive and extensive vocabulary that requires some study for mastery. However, Levine was careful to provide adequate definitions of most terms, so that there should be minimal confusion about the meaning of her ideas (see Glossary, Appendix C).

A hallmark of Levine's Conservation Model is the accurate use of knowledge from what Levine (1988a) called adjunctive disciplines. She has credited the scholars of other disciplines from whose works she has drawn for the development of her conceptual model, and she has used that knowledge appropriately.

Although documentation of the utility of Levine's conceptual model for nursing activities is increasing, its credibility must be established. More systematic evaluations of the use of the model in various clinical situations are needed, as are empirical studies that test theories directly derived from or linked with the conservation principles.

In conclusion, Levine's Conservation Model provides nursing with a logically congruent, holistic view of the person. Two theories related to the model have been formulated but require further development and empirical testing. The lack of major limitations suggests that this conceptual model may be an effective guide for nursing actions.

REFERENCES

Bates, M. (1967). A naturalist at large. Natural History, 76(6), 8–16.

Beland, I. (1971). Clinical nursing: Pathophysiological and psychosocial implications (2nd ed.). New York: Macmillan.

Blasage, M.C. (1987). Toward a general understanding of nursing education: A critical analysis of the work of Myra Estrin Levine. Dissertation Abstracts International, 47, 4457B.

Brunner, M. (1985). A conceptual approach to critical care. Focus on Critical Care, 12(2), 39–44.

Cannon, W.B. (1939). The wisdom of the body. New York: W.W. Norton & Co.

Cooper, D.M. (1989). Development and testing of an instrument to assess the visual characteristics of open, soft tissue wounds. Doctoral Dissertation, University of Pennsylvania.

Cox, B. (1988). Pregnancy, anxiety, and time perception. Dissertation Abstracts International, 48, 2260B.

Cox, R. (1985). Application of Levine's Conservation Model. Paper presented at conference on Nursing Theory in Action, Edmonton, Alberta, Canada. (Cassette recording)

Crawford-Gamble, P.E. (1986). An application of Levine's conceptual model. Perioperative Nursing Quarterly, 2(1), 64–70.

Dubos, R. (1961). Mirage of health. New York: Doubleday.
Dubos, R. (1965). Man adapting. New Haven: Yale University Press.
Erikson, E.H. (1964). Insight and responsibility. New York: W.W. Norton & Co.
Erikson, E.H. (1968). Identity: Youth and crisis. New York: W.W. Norton & Co.
Fawcett, J. (1989). Analysis and evaluation of conceptual models of nursing (2nd ed.). Philadelphia: F.A. Davis.
Fawcett, J., Cariello, F.P., Davis, D.A., Farley, J., Zimmaro, D.M., & Watts, R.J. (1987). Conceptual models of nursing: Application to critical care nursing practice. Dimensions of Critical Care Nursing, 6, 202–213.
Feynman, R. (1965). The character of physical law. Cambridge, MA: M.I.T. Press.
Fleming, N. (1988). Comparison of women with different perineal conditions after childbirth. Dissertation Abstracts International, 48, 2924B.
Foreman, M. (1988). The development of confusion in the hospitalized elderly. Dissertation Abstracts International, 48, 2261B–2262B.
Foreman, M. (1989). Confusion in the hospitalized elderly: Incidence, onset, and associated factors. Research in Nursing and Health, 12, 21–29.
Geden, E. (1982). Effects of lifting techniques on energy expenditure: A preliminary investigation. Nursing Research, 31, 214–218.
Geden, E. (1985). The relationship between self-care theory and empirical research. In J. Riehl-Sisca (Ed.), The science and art of self-care (pp. 265–270). Norwalk, CT: Appleton-Century-Crofts.
Gibson, J.E. (1966). The senses considered as perceptual systems. Boston: Houghton-Mifflin.
Goldstein, K. (1963). The organism. Boston: Beacon Press.
Hall, E. (1959). Silent language. Greenwich, CT: Fawcett.
Hall, E. (1966). The hidden dimension. Garden City, NY: Doubleday & Co.
Hall, K.V. (1979). Current trends in the use of conceptual frameworks in nursing education. Journal of Nursing Education, 18(4), 26–29.
Herbst, S. (1981). Impairments as a result of cancer. In N. Martin, N. Holt, & D. Hicks, (Eds.), Comprehensive rehabilitation nursing (pp. 553–578). New York: McGraw-Hill.
Hirschfeld, M.J. (1976). The cognitively impaired older adult. American Journal of Nursing, 76, 1981–1984.
Lathrop, V.G. (1982, May 5). Personal communication.
Levine, M.E. (1966a). Adaptation and assessment: A rationale for nursing intervention. American Journal of Nursing, 66, 2450–2453.
Levine, M.E. (1966b). Trophicognosis: An alternative to nursing diagnosis. In American Nurses' Association Regional Clinical Conference (Vol. 2, pp. 55–70). New York: American Nurses' Association.
Levine, M.E. (1967). The four conservation principles of nursing. Nursing Forum, 6, 454–59.
Levine, M.E. (1969a). Introduction to clinical nursing. Philadelphia: F.A. Davis.
Levine, M.E. (1969b). The pursuit of wholeness. American Journal of Nursing, 69, 93–98.
Levine, M.E. (1971). Holistic nursing. Nursing Clinics of North America, 6, 253–264.
Levine, M.E. (1973). Introduction to clinical nursing (2nd ed.). Philadelphia: F.A. Davis.
Levine, M.E. (1977). Nursing ethics and the ethical nurse. American Journal of Nursing, 77, 845–849.
Levine, M.E. (1978). The four conservation principles of nursing. Paper presented at Second Annual Nurse Educator Conference, New York. (Cassette recording)
Levine, M.E. (1982, February 2). Personal communication.
Levine, ME. (1984a, August). Myra Levine. Paper presented at the Nurse Theorist Conference, Edmonton, Alberta, Canada. (Cassette recording)
Levine, M.E. (1984b, August). Concurrent sessions. M. Levine. Discussion at the Nurse Theorist Conference, Edmonton, Alberta, Canada. (Cassette recording)
Levine, M.E. (1985, August). Myra Levine. Paper presented at conference on Nursing Theory in Action, Edmonton, Alberta, Canada. (Cassette recording)
Levine, M.E. (1986, August). Myra Levine. Paper presented at Nursing Theory Congress: Theoretical Pluralism: Direction for a Practice Discipline, Toronto, Ontario, Canada. (Cassette recording)
Levine, M.E. (1987). The Nurse Theorists: Portraits of Excellence. (Videotape)
Levine, M.E. (1987, July 15). Personal communication.
Levine, M.E. (1987, July 22). Personal communication to L. Criddle.
Levine, M.E. (1987, August 13). Personal communication.

Levine, M.E. (1988a). Antecedents from adjunctive disciplines: Creation of nursing theory. Nursing Science Quarterly, 1, 16–21.

Levine, M.E. (1988b). Myra Levine. In T.M. Schorr & A. Zimmerman (Eds.), Making choices. Taking changes. Nurse leaders tell their stories (pp. 215–228). St. Louis: C.V. Mosby.

Levine, M.E. (1989a). The conservation principles of nursing: Twenty years later. In J.P. Riehl (Ed.), Conceptual models for nursing practice (3rd ed., pp. 325–337). Norwalk, CT: Appleton & Lange.

Levine, M.E. (1989b). The ethics of nursing rhetoric. Image: Journal of Nursing Scholarship, 21, 4–6.

Levine, M.E. (1989c). Ration or rescue: The elderly patient in critical care. Critical Care Nursing Quarterly, 12(1), 82–89.

MacLean, S. (1988). Description of cues nurses use for diagnosing activity intolerance. Dissertation Abstracts International, 48, 2264B.

Marriner, A. (1986). Nursing theorists and their work. St. Louis: C.V. Mosby.

Meleis, A.I. (1985). Theoretical nursing: Development and progress. Philadelphia: J.B. Lippincott.

Mercer, M. (1983, December 10). Personal communication.

Newman, M.A. (1972). Nursing's theoretical evolution. Nursing Outlook, 20, 449–453.

Newport, M.A. (1984). Conserving thermal energy and social integrity in the newborn. Western Journal of Nursing Research, 6, 176–197.

Pond, J. (1985). Application of Levine's Conservation Model. Paper presented at conference on Nursing Theory in Action, Edmonton, Alberta, Canada (Cassette recording).

Riehl, J.P. (1980). Nursing models in current use. In J.P. Riehl & C. Roy (Eds.), Conceptual models for nursing practice (2nd ed., pp. 393–398). New York: Appleton-Century-Crofts.

Riehl-Sisca, J.P. (1989). Conceptual models for nursing practice (3rd ed.). Norwalk, CT: Appleton & Lange.

Savage, T.A., & Culbert, C. (1989). Early intervention: The unique role of nursing. Journal of Pediatric Nursing, 4, 339–345.

Selye, H. (1956). The stress of life. New York: McGraw-Hill.

Sherrington, A. (1906). Integrative function of the nervous system. New York: Scribner's.

Stafford, M.J. (1982, June 2). Personal communication.

Stevens, B.J. (1984). Nursing theory. Analysis, application, evaluation (2nd ed.). Boston: Little, Brown & Co.

Taylor, J.W. (1974). Measuring the outcomes of nursing care. Nursing Clinics of North America, 9, 337–348.

Tillich, P. (1961). The meaning of health. Perspectives in Biology and Medicine, 5, 92–100.

Tompkins, E.S. (1980). Effect of restricted mobility and dominance on perceived duration. Nursing Research, 29, 338–338.

Waddington, C.H. (Ed.). (1968). Towards a theoretical biology. I. Prolegomena. Chicago: Aldine.

Walker, L.O., & Nicholson, R. (1980). Criteria for evaluating nursing process models. Nurse Educator, 5(5), 8–9.

Winslow, E.H. (1982, October 6). Personal communication to M.E. Levine.

Winslow, E.H. (1983). Oxygen consumption and cardiovascular response in normal subjects and in acute myocardial infarction patients during basin bath, tub bath, and shower. Dissertation Abstracts International, 43, 2856B.

Winslow, E.H., Lane, L.D., & Gaffney, F.A. (1984). Oxygen consumption and cardiovascular response in patients and normal adults during in-bed and out-of-bed toileting. Journal of Cardiac Rehabilitation, 4, 348–354.

Winslow, E.H., Lane, L.D., & Gaffney, F.A. (1985). Oxygen consumption and cardiovascular response in control adults and acute myocardial infarction patients during bathing. Nursing Research, 34, 164–169.

Wolf, S. (1961). Disease as a way of life: Neural integration in systemic pathology. Perspectives in Biology and Medicine, 4, 288–305.

Yeates, D.A., & Roberts, J.E. (1984). A comparison of two bearing-down techniques during the second stage of labor. Journal of Nurse-Midwifery, 29, 3–11.

Zwanger, L. (1982, June 4). Personal communication.

THREE

Levine's Conservation Principles and Research

Karen Moore Schaefer, R.N., D.N.Sc.

Gathering information, formulating plans, and carrying out decisions based on these plans is a simple statement of the scientific method. Levine (1973) advocates the use of the scientific process to provide nursing care to the patient that will preserve wholeness and promote adaptation. The scientific process serves as the basis for selecting essential and prior data about the patient, which will structure the nature of nursing interventions.

Use of the scientific process at the bedside assumes that the nurse has a certain knowledge base from which to make observations and select relevant data to form diagnostic statements. This knowledge base makes the data, or what Levine (1969) calls provocative facts, meaningful. The nurse uses the provocative facts to make inferences about what changes are occurring in patients and where they will need help with adaptation. The nurse establishes a hypothesis that must be testable in order for the nurse to intervene. In essence the nurse is saying that "if this is true, then this must be true" (Levine, 1969, p. 28). This diagnostic decision is tested. The nurse observes for an organismic response, and if the patient responds, the hypothesis must be valid. If the patient does not respond, the hypothesis is not valid. The nurse goes back to the provocative facts and reformulates the hypothesis for further testing.

This account of the scientific process at the bedside provides some truth to the notion that nurses base decisions, in part, on scientific knowledge and, perhaps more important, are building that knowledge daily simply by caring for their patients. Nurses are constantly testing what they propose will work in their practice based on what they know. Critical to this process is what nurses know and have learned through experience. This prior knowledge places some limitations on the development of future knowledge (Winslow, 1976). However, if nurses continue to test alternative hypotheses in practice, they will continue to build that knowledge base. The ultimate outcome of this process will be knowledge expansion and improved patient care.

SIGNIFICANCE OF NURSING RESEARCH

Nursing research is the systematic study of phenomena of interest to nursing. Research is important to the profession of nursing for several reasons. Research on the phenomena over which nursing has control will help define the elements of nursing and what it is that nurses can offer to the recipients of their care. The mere fact that nurses engage in research keeps nursing in the mainstream of the professional arena. Most important, however, is the fact that research will expand old knowledge and identify new knowledge that is critical to the practice of nursing. With this knowledge, nurses will continue to improve nursing practice.

Keeping these goals in mind, Levine (1973) believes that the conservation principles offer an approach to nursing that is scientific, research oriented, and suitable for practice in many environments. The purpose of this chapter is to describe how to maintain wholeness in research, review and critique research that has used the conservation principles as a basis of study, discuss how research and wholeness can coexist, and make recommendations about the use of Levine's model and her conservation principles in research.

REVIEW OF EXISTING RESEARCH

Tompkins (1980) examined the effect of restricted mobility and dominance on perceived duration of time in 64 volunteer college students. This particular study was important to nursing because of the frequency with which nurses provide care to patients with restricted movement is associated with pathology and trauma. Usually loss of function of an extremity increases the amount of energy expended during movement. Tompkins found that one-joint restriction (ankle) and two-joint restriction (ankle and knee) of either leg significantly shortened perceived duration and significantly decreased cadence during walking. However, when comparing dominant side with nondominant side there was no significant difference. Although she did not identify a formalized framework for her study, Tompkins suggested that perceived duration changes may be part of successful coping when mobility is restricted, and could be indicative of maintenance of structural integrity. She referred to Levine's discussion of the notion that unity and integrity are axiomatic, and that nurses intervene with the hope of conserving the patient's energy. She suggested that when the perceptual input is altered through the haptic system, the organismic response to the perceptual stimuli is altered.

This alteration often requires nursing intervention during which the patient's perceptual input is filtered through the nurse's perceptual system in an attempt to maintain wholeness, the essence of all healing. Possibly the nurse would be more successful in mediating the patient's perceptual input in reference to time perception if consideration were given to the nurse's rate of subjective time, as well as to the *patient's*. The perceived duration of nurses working successfully in rehabilitative areas might be compared to that of nurses working successfully in critical care areas. If a difference should exist, its identification may be helpful in assigning nurses to the area in which they can be most effective. (pp. 337–338) (italics by the present author)

Geden (1982) examined the effects of a variety of lifting techniques (shoulder assist, rocking auxiliary, straight pull, self-lift, and mechanical lift) on energy expenditure of 14 student nurses. Argument for the study was grounded in the fact the nurses perform activities for the patients with the ultimate goal of expending the least amount of energy in the patient. Of importance is that nurses perform techniques to conserve patient energy with the least amount of potential for injury to the nurse. Hence, those lifting techniques that require the greatest amount of energy possibly place the nurse at the greatest amount of risk for injury. Although she did not use Levine's conservation principles as the basis of her study, she did refer to Levine as one of the theorists who includes energy as one of the components of patient status or nursing intervention. Energy expenditure in this study was operationalized as oxygen consumption, heart rate, respiratory rate, and blood pressure. She found that the mechanical lift required the greatest amount of energy but explained that this could have occurred because of the greater amount of manipulation of the patient prior to the lift. The self-lift technique expended the least amount of energy. She cautioned readers not to generalize the findings to the population until further study in this area is completed. No further studies comparing energy costs of patient lifts have been found in the nursing literature.

Winslow (1983) made some very important points about Geden's (1982) study based on Levine's conservation principles. She agreed that to conserve meant to keep together, however noted that Levine (1973) discusses energy conservation from the perspective of a proper disbursement of energy rather than one of simply limiting energy expenditure. Thus, encouraging ambulation and exercise, while not limiting energy expenditure, is balancing energy use with the patient's capabilities. Winslow (1983) also noted that proper attention to food intake was not considered in Geden's study. She argued that in order for food not to affect energy expenditure, the lifting measures should not have been taken until 2 hours after meals. Additionally she made the point that the actual amount of energy used with the mechanical lift is not outside the normal energy cost of any patient. Winslow recommended that since there were no clinically significant differences found when comparing lifts, patients should be able to choose the lift that is most comfortable for them. Finally, since the self-lift had the lowest energy cost, patients can move themselves very efficiently, and in fact the nurse's helping the patient may be costing the patient additional energy. It is important to note that patient energy cost was not measured in this study and was not intended to be the focus of the study. Comparing energy cost of the nurse with energy cost of the patient when the nurse is trying to conserve patient energy would be an important study to help the nurse select appropriate nursing interventions.

Yeates and Roberts (1984) studied the bearing-down phenomenon of the second stage of labor to contrast the effects of two learned approaches to parturient participation. The control group (n = 5) was taught the traditional sustained breath-holding technique, and the experimental group (n = 5) was taught to bear down only with involuntary urge. Levine's conservation principles were used as a basis of the study. Energy was operationalized as (1) the subjective rating of the amount of energy needed during the second stage of labor, (2) the duration of the second stage, (3) lactic acid measures in response to use of glucose stores, and (4) Apgar scores to reflect fetal distress. Structural integrity focused on the maternal perineum and included the incidence and extent of perineal lacerations and episiotomies. Personal integrity was the intervention of support versus direction. Supporting the women's involuntary urge involved being responsive to the women's behavioral cues, and conveying respect and confidence to them. Direction was more arbitrary and relied primarily on getting the woman to cooperate with sustained breath-holding. Social integrity referred to the active participation of the patient. It was operationalized as the nature of the support provided during the second stage of labor and the role of the parturient in accomplishing expulsion of her infant. No outcome measures were used for personal and social integrity. Although the sample size was small, placing limitations on the use of the findings of this study, the investigators found that the experimental group's perineal integrity was preserved when compared with the control group. There were no significant differences in Apgar score, duration of the second stage of labor, phases within the second stage of labor, and the maternal report of effort. The investigators suggested that further investigation be conducted into the common practice of encouraging women to bear down strenuously in the second stage of labor. This study supported the conclusion that responding to involuntary urges was as efficient as, and resulted in less perineal damage than, sustained breath-holding. Not measuring all the maternal organismic responses to the second stage of labor was another major limitation of this study in supporting the conservation principles identified by Levine.

Newport (1984) used Levine's conservation principles as a basis for organizing her study of the conservation of thermal energy and social integrity of the newborn infant. In general Newport proposed that supporting early bonding by placing the infant on the mother's chest after delivery would also conserve the infant's thermal energy. For the purpose of study, the 76 subjects were divided into an experimental group and a control group. The infants in both groups were dried after delivery and kept away from cooler surfaces. The experimental infants were wrapped with a blanket and placed close to their mother's chest. The control infants were placed on a heated surface in the Ohio Neonatal Unit. Infant temperatures were recorded prior to and 15 minutes after treatment, on admission to the nursery, and three more times thereafter. Additional measures of thermal energy were diarrhea, heart rate, respiratory rate, and the presence of ketoacidosis. The findings revealed no significant differences in all measures in the two groups, concluding that those mothers who wish to hold their infants immediately after birth can do so without compromising the conservation of thermal energy.

Diers (1984) provided an interesting critique of Newport's study with particular emphasis on the need for a model to do research. She said that Newport (1984) could have done the study without the help of Levine's model. She noted that Newport's (1984) clever linkage of two theories (thermal energy and bonding) was done previously by another researcher (reference to this researcher was not included in the critique). It is true that what makes research "nursing research" is that nurses have control over the phenomena being studied and that using nursing models in research does not necessarily add credence to the piece of work as nursing research. What the model does, however, is help the researcher focus on those things that are part of nursing according to that particular framework. It provides a consistent way for the researcher to present and explain her ideas. Models fall short of this task when the researcher introduces the conceptual premise in the beginning of the study and fails to explain the study's new findings within the context of the model. This happens with all models and theories, not just nursing models. Models and theories are meant to provide generalities from which specific ideas can be developed and tested. A number of hypotheses can be developed from a single model or theory, which help to make the model useful. Models help the nurses think in an organized fashion. Finally, Diers (1984) correctly criticized Newport for not including a single measure of bonding or social integrity. This forces one to wonder what the researcher was really trying to test. In the end Levine may not have been the correct model for analyzing these particular variables.

Winslow, Lane, and Gaffney (1984) examined physiologic responses before, during, and after three types of baths in 18 patients who were 5 to 17 days postinfarction and in 22 control patients. The physiologic measures showed that there were no significant differences in oxygen consumption, peak heart rate, and rate pressure product for the basin, tub, and shower bath. Although oxygen consumption during bathing was less than three times that for resting, the experimental group had a significantly lower oxygen consumption than the control group. Peak heart rates were higher than anticipated. However, peak heart rates were higher than anticipated. However, peak heart rate and dysrhythmia did not differ significantly among the three types of baths. Rate pressure product in women was significantly higher after tub bath than after basin and shower bath. The subjects had no cardiac symptoms during the baths and rated each bath as light exertion. The basin bath was disliked by most of the patients.

Winslow and associates' (1985) study supported the notion that the physiologic costs of the three types of baths are similar, and that the differences that do occur are more subject related than bath related. The patients in this study were able to safely select either type of bath without any cardiac sequelae. The investigators suggested that additional studies be conducted to determine those patients that might have exaggerated responses to the specific types of baths. Although the investigators did not state that they used Levine's model for their study, her principle of energy conservation is investigated. Essentially the investigators were able to support Winslow's (1983) previous point that energy use was not intended to be a negative principle but a guide based on the patient's capabilities and desires. If future research continues to support the notion that energy cost does not vary according to the type of bath the postinfarction patient takes, then the patients can take the type of baths that they prefer early after the infarction has occurred. If this particular study had included a dimension of social integrity such as cultural influence on the type of bath preferred by each participant, the study would have included all the integrities discussed by Levine (1973).

Foreman (1989) studied 71 nonsurgical patients over age 60 to obtain information about the incidence, onset, and variables associated with the onset of confusion. Twenty-seven of the patients in the study developed confusion. Ten psychosocial variables were significantly associated with the onset of confusion: hypernatremia, hypokalemia, hyperglycemia, hypotension, increased creatinine, increased urea nitrogen, receiving more medications, being more frequently perceived by nurses as confused, having more orienting objects in their immediate environment, and having fewer interactions with significant others. A combination of four variables (age, arterial pressure on bypass, and body temperature on the first and third postoperative days) best predicted delirious patients. This research is significant to the testing of Levine's Conservation Model because of the measurement of variables that represent all of the conservation principles. The findings reinforce the notion that for nursing interventions to be successful, they must be guided by all the conservation principles.

USING LEVINE'S CONSERVATION PRINCIPLES IN RESEARCH

Levine's Conservation Model is a theory of nursing. The theory provides a general approach to care (use of the conservation principles to provide therapeutic or supportive nursing interventions) and defines the nature (to promote adaptation and maintain wholeness) and the scope (for individuals in a variety of settings) of nursing (Tripp-Reimer, 1984). Levine (1966) stated that a theory of nursing must recognize the importance of unique detail of care for a single patient within an empiric framework that successfully describes the requirements of all patients. Theories must have clear-cut testable hypotheses. Consistent with Levine's premise related to the use of the scientific process at the bedside, nursing care plans should consist of testable hypotheses (e.g., cold compresses will reduce joint discomfort). All patients view themselves as whole. Further testing of the integrities is needed to determine if they successfully define the requirements in all patients. The discussion of the successful use of the model in a variety of patient populations in this book is, in part, a testament to the ability of a theory of nursing to describe the requirements of all patients.

From this theory of nursing, Levine is developing two theories for nursing: the theory of redundancy and the theory of therapeutic intention. The theory of therapeutic intention appears to extend the nursing process component of the conservation principles, but this relationship is purely speculative (Fawcett, 1989). The theory of redundancy has helped to redefine aging and everything else that has to do with human life. It may further operationalize the idea of adaptation and change (Fawcett, 1989). As these theories for nursing are further developed, nurses will have a better understanding of their unique contribution to patient care. Although there are limitations of Levine's theory of nursing, this does not mean that this will always be the case. In essence, theory is never complete but is always developing (Meleis, 1985). Based on these tentative truths, research using Levine's model will be proposed.

In order to ensure the holistic care of patients, research will need to include both qualitative and quantitative aspects of research. Sophisticated nursing assessment tools are probably the most reliable measures of the whole patient. However, the validity and reliability of tools to describe all of the requirements of a variety of patient populations using Levine's conservation principles must be tested. Tools have been developed (Taylor, 1987); however, there is no indication that they have been subjected to scientific testing.

Certain concepts associated with Levine's theory are known to nursing because they have been developed by other disciplines (adaptation, change, wholeness). What makes these concepts appropriate for nursing theory is that nursing has modified them to meet the specific goals and services of nurses and their patients (Meleis, 1985). Other concepts and commonplaces that are also known to other disciplines and help to operationalize the conservation principles are listed in Table 3–1.

Levine's conservation principles formulate the major propositions of the model and therefore serve as the basis of potential hypotheses for research in nursing (Meleis, 1985). Approaching nursing research from the perspective of the conservation principles is timely because the integrities are meant to be used by the nurse to plan and administer care and therefore provide an intervention focus for research. The expected outcome of the research, and hence the potential for prescription, is the promotion of adaptation and the maintenance of wholeness.

The energy conservation principle has been identified as the first principle to be considered by the nurse. Energy conservation involves the appropriate use of energy and the prevention of energy depletion. Some quantifiable measures of energy use include heart rate, respiratory rate, oxygen consumption, glucose levels, temperature, lactic acid accumulation, nitrogen balance, electrolyte levels (potassium, sodium), blood pressure, pulmonary artery pressures, pulmonary capillary wedge pressures, hemoglobin and hematocrit, vitamin deficiencies, and skin integrity. Physiologic alterations associated with illness will often be manifested as changes in some of these quantifiable measures. However, these measures, both necessary and valuable in the diagnostic statements of physicians, do not reveal how the patient is affected by these alterations. Understanding the qualitative portion of the illness is absolutely essential if the nurse is to promote adaptation and maintain wholeness of patients

TABLE 3-1. CONCEPTS AND COMMONPLACES OPERATIONALIZING
THE INTEGRITIES

Energy	Structural	Personal	Social
Anxiety	White blood cell count	Loneliness	Socialization
Oxygen saturation	Healing (granulation tissue)	Boredom	Moral development
Blood glucose	Skin integrity	Helplessness	Group process
Pulse	Sedimentation rate	Fear	Interaction
Temperature	Bone density	Self-esteem	Social isolation
Respirations	Muscle strength	Privacy	
Blood pressure	End organ damage (renal	Listening	
Hemoglobin	function, liver function)	Empathy	
Hematocrit		Control	
Skin turgor		Meaning	
Fluid and electrolytes		Teaching	
Heat		Learning	
Energy exchange		Role	
Diarrhea		Self-concept	
Blood loss			
Body weight			
Wound drainage			
Change*			
Wholeness*			
Adaptation*			

*Major concepts of all the integrities.

and their families. A simple question such as "How has this predicament (illness, life-style change, new baby, marriage, change in job) affected your normal life-style?" will help to identify those aspects of care that can be directed toward the whole person.

Some studies that focus on the conservation of energy might include the following:

1. Determine when fatigue is within the normal physiologic expectations or is indeed an indication of illness.
2. Determine whether the application of Bobath principles (exercises applied to the affected side) to the acutely ill patient who has suffered a cerebral vascular accident would conserve energy. The assumption is that the inability to use an extremity expends extra energy that may be needed for healing.
3. Determine whether restraints that are placed on patients against their will function as an external factor that depletes energy needed for healing. It is possible that restraints are more harmful than they are useful.
4. Determine how nutrition practices of different cultures and life styles affect individual energy levels and needs.
5. Study the effects of a variety of nursing interventions (music therapy, relaxation, visual imagery, breathing exercises) to determine the extent to which they conserve energy as measured by predetermined patient outcomes.

The conservation of structural integrity involves the process of healing. The body has a number of remarkable processes that come to its defense to protect it from things such as infection, lack of oxygen supply, lack of function, and movement away from dangerous objects (Levine, 1973). Levine (1973) noted that "structural integrity is the necessary defense of anatomical and physiological wholeness and is therefore the basis for a multitude of nursing interventions" (p. 16).

When a patient has a myocardial infarction, the area of the myocardial muscle that has been without oxygen (has been denied its natural energy supply) goes through a variety of cellular changes that eventually result in the formation of a scar. Although this scar cannot function as well as the original tissue, it serves to maintain the wholeness of the patient. Nurses play a major role in the preservation of the viable muscle; that is, they intervene to prevent extension of the damaged muscle. Although the outcome of the interventions is clearly related to the conservation of structural integrity, structural integrity is maintained by reducing energy demands on the myocardial muscle.

Winslow and colleagues (1984) have pioneered some very important research that has provided nurses with information about the energy use of a variety of interventions for the cardiac patient. Although they have cautioned nurses to complete more studies before implementing the findings, individual parameters could be used by the nurse to determine if patients are tolerating such activities as bath at the side of the bed and use of a bedside commode. Additional studies focusing on the ability of nursing interventions to promote healing and conserve structural integrity are needed. Suggestions for studies focusing on structural integrity might include the following:

1. Determine the effect of positioning on a variety of surgical incisions.
2. Work collaboratively to determine the effect of a variety of medications on healing, or, as in the case of heparin, the best way to administer heparin to reduce injury.
3. Determine the effects of nursing interventions on the ability of the immune system to function (appropriate patterns of rest and activity, guided imagery, music therapy).
4. Determine the frequency of passive-active exercises that prevents loss of function of an extremity.
5. Determine nursing interventions that can reduce the incidence of the phantom limb experience.
6. Determine the nursing interventions that preserve the function of vital organs in the premature infant based on long-term outcome measures that address both physiologic and psychologic parameters.
7. Determine the most effective way to maintain skin integrity in high-risk patients (paraplegic patients, bedridden patients).

The conservation of personal integrity involves the preservation of one's own sense of identity and self-worth. How one feels about himself or herself is affected by a variety of factors of such complexity (culture, religion, ethnic background, socioeconomic status, life experiences) that isolated variables are considered for the purpose of measurement only, with consideration as to how each variable fits into the larger whole. Examples of studies that focus on, but are not limited to, the conservation of personal integrity include:

1. Determine how nurses can best help to reduce the fear of acquired immune deficiency syndrome (AIDS).
2. Determine how pet therapy affects the feeling of loneliness in the aged patient.
3. Determine what types of nursing interventions reduce the boredom experienced by hospitalized patients of all ages.
4. Determine the relationship between control and self-esteem, and what nursing interventions can support that relationship to promote adaptation.
5. Determine the best way to organize information that will help the older patient learn.

Levine (1973) has said that "individual life has meaning only in the context of social life" (p. 17). People's lives take on meaning in relationship to the family, social contacts, community, job, and friends. Many studies have found that nurses need to consider how relationships affect illness or life-style changes, as well as how illness or life-style changes affect the relationships. Nursing research must continue to examine ways that nurses can support what is important and meaningful to the patient and identify what the patient may not have, but may need, to survive or adapt. One cannot help but consider how AIDS has affected the lives and relationships of those afflicted. They lose their jobs, their health insurance, their right to education, their loved ones, their homes, their desire to live, and their right to health care. Nurses must examine ways to preserve the social integrity of these people while conserving the energy, structural integrity, and personal integrity of both the patient and the caregiver. Of utmost importance is being able to work with other disciplines to find the most effective way to promote and maintain healthy life-styles without compromising what is important to the patient to the point that life no longer has meaning.

In summary, the application of Levine's conservation principles to research helps the researcher focus on nursing interventions that promote adaptation and maintain wholeness. Research that defines patient parameters according to the conservation principles is in direct opposition to the notion of wholeness; however, at times may be necessary for the purpose of measurement. When this does occur, the researcher should keep in mind the need to consider any aspect of the patient within the context of the larger whole. The latter is facilitated by combining the qualitative and quantitative approaches to research.

ACHIEVING THE GOAL OF WHOLENESS

According to Levine (1973), the goals of nursing are to promote adaptation and maintain wholeness. Nurses accomplish this through the use of the conservation principles. If the conservation principles provide a basis for nursing care, then they should provide a basis for the research that focuses on those things over which nurses have control. At the same time the research should accommodate or account for the whole patient, no matter how particular the research focus. For example, research that focuses on the energy expended when patients are restrained must consider how being restrained would affect the patients' skin integrity, perception of self, and ability to interact with other people. Knowledge of the energy used by patients when restrained is important to nursing practice but, in practice, must be considered within the framework of the total patient in order to maintain wholeness. Maintaining wholeness becomes the component that is unique to nursing.

Without careful thought, certain research methods available to nursing could place limitations on the ability to maintain wholeness. Although experimental designs may be the most scientific of research designs, the very characteristics that make experimental designs sound (control, manipulation, and randomization) also eliminate many of the variables that nurses will deal with on a daily basis. Because of these limitations it is difficult to consider the true nature of the whole person and to find situations in practice that would meet the specifications of a well-controlled study. Very few situations in nursing are typical or repeatable.

Qualitative research is rapidly gaining credibility in nursing for the very reason that it provides an approach that preserves the uniqueness of each situation with an attempt, at the same time, to identify similarities, if any, for the purpose of providing generalities to nursing practice. At the other end of the spectrum, experimental designs are so limited that the uniqueness of situations may be completely eliminated. Certainly combining qualitative and quantitative research methods is one way to maintain the wholeness perspective of the patient in research. This process is a form of triangulation that simply implies that the researcher uses more than one method to collect data, more than one data source, more than one tool to measure a single concept, or may even combine designs. The expectation is that the advantages of both approaches will outweigh the disadvantages of either approach.

Combining qualitative and quantitative methods also helps to preserve both the art and the science of nursing. Levine (1973) has expressed concern that the structure of nursing has not permitted the development of the creative portion of nursing—that is, the art of nursing. Nursing will always be an art and a science, but nurses, being so concerned about finding the best way to do a procedure, have failed to value and nurture their artistic talents. Encounters with patients are special, personal, and unique, probably never to be repeated again. Levine (1973, p. 18) stated:

> That kind of creativity has always been a part of nursing care. Nursing will be an art for as long as such creative acts continue to be a part of it. But they are not enough, these evanescent moments, and to bring them to many nurses and many patients, there must be a way to share them time and again. The nursing craft speaks in a language of its own—the silent language of human exchange which is eloquent and exciting without words.

The most nurses can hope for is that they will encounter similar situations in the future that will reinforce what they learned from these experiences. On one hand, if nurses would learn to record these experiences, at some point a collection of similar experiences may provide new insight to clinical experiences and be of such magnitude that it would be worth sharing with colleagues. On the other hand, including qualitative research methods in all research designs would help nurses formalize these experiences, which may help explain what the quantitative data suggest. The question of statistical versus clinical significance would perhaps be eliminated.

In summary, combining qualitative and quantitative research methods is one way to do research in which findings will ultimately help to promote adaptation and maintain wholeness of patients and their families. At the same time the combined approach will provide nurses with a mechanism to preserve the art, as well as develop the science, of nursing.

FATIGUE ASSOCIATED WITH CONGESTIVE HEART FAILURE: A CONCEPTUALIZATION AND RESEARCH APPLICATION

Everyone experiences fatigue at some point in life. Although acute fatigue may be adaptive in that it serves as a warning of more serious sequelae (muscle pain, viral infection, depression, stress, illnesses, anemia), chronic pain serves no purpose except to interfere with one's ability to function.

Understanding the fatigue experience, whether acute or chronic, is significant to nursing because it is one of the most common problems associated with all health-related disorders. Study of the phenomenon of fatigue in a variety of clinical populations is needed to determine appropriate and significant interventions.

Fatigue has many causes, appears in the healthy and the ill, can be acute or chronic, and can be muscle-specific or generalized in nature (Piper, 1986). From a nursing perspective, fatigue is conceptualized as an inability to continue in whatever situations people find themselves (Srivastava, 1986) and is often described as not having enough energy to do what they want to do. The North American Nursing Diagnoses Association (1988) defines fatigue as an overwhelming sustained sense of exhaustion and decreased capacity for physical and mental work.

Little research in nursing has addressed the systematic study of fatigue. Most references to fatigue are information articles or refer to the pathophysiology of fatigue. Some investigators have attempted to develop measures of fatigue, identify its significance, and describe its characteristic patterns.

Clinical research is beginning to provide practitioners with data about the fatigue experience. Most research suggests that fatigue is distressing and interferes with functional ability (Haylock & Hart, 1979; Krupp, Alvarez, LaRocca, & Scheinberg, 1988; McCorkle, 1981; Piper, 1988; Rhodes, Watson, & Hanson, 1988; Voith, Frank, & Pigg, 1987). It is not known whether fatigue is a universal experience or whether it is experienced in a similar manner transculturally. In order to determine the full nature of fatigue, its characteristics and patterns, one must study specific patient populations known to experience fatigue.

TABLE 3-2. FATIGUE SAMPLE QUESTIONS

1. When do you get fatigued?
2. What do you think causes you to be fatigued?
3. How do you feel about being fatigued?
4. What do you do to make the fatigue better?

According to Levine (1971) fatigue is a manifestation of the body's attempt to heal itself. Fatigue occurs when the energy supply is unable to meet the energy demand. Fatigue exacts a high toll in the emotional and physical well-being of the patient—particularly, those with congestive heart failure.

The sensation of fatigue is a perception of a complex interplay of somatic and psychologic factors (Piper, 1986). Fatigue is a multidimensional construct that includes temporal, severity, emotional, sensory, evaluative, and associated symptoms, and relief factors (Piper, 1988).

Using the integrities identified by Levine (1973), patients experiencing fatigue could manifest (a) rapid heart rate, elevated temperature, low hemoglobin, and elevated blood sugar (energy conservation); (b) physical injury (structural integrity); (c) reduced self-esteem (personal integrity); and (d) inability to socialize to the desired extent (social integrity). Consistent with Levine, the integrities are to be used by nurses to organize their care and not to compartmentalize the patient. The goal of nursing is to maintain wholeness. Although objective data (hemoglobin, hematocrit, blood glucose, blood gases, myocardial enzymes) representing energy use by the body will be collected to determine if there is a relationship between the subjective sensation of fatigue severity and energy depletion, the major focus is to describe the fatigue experience as perceived by the patient (Table 3–2). It is assumed that patients perceive themselves as integrated wholes.

This brief proposal provides the reader with an example of a beginning effort to maintain wholeness in research conceptualized according to Levine (1973). Other researchers have included both qualitative and quantitative approaches in their research for similar purposes, to obtain a complete picture of what is happening with the patients. What is unique to this proposal is the use of Levine's theory as a guide for developing the components of the study.

CONCLUSION

Levine's Conservation Model provides a pragmatic and scientific framework for the study of phenomena of interest to nursing and over which nursing has control. Although the concepts described by Levine are not unique to nursing, the conservation model operationalizes the concepts for use by nursing. To ensure accurate use of the model, nurses investigating variables within the model must consider the use of research techniques that will maintain the integrities or wholeness of the individual. I believe that the combined use of qualitative and quantitative methods will achieve that purpose. It is expected that with the continued effort of nurse researchers, the conservation principles will be operationalized in a manner that will describe a variety of patient populations, reinforcing the clinical utility of the model.

REFERENCES

Carroll-Johnson, R.M. (Ed.) (1989). Classification of nursing diagnosis: Proceedings of the eighth conference North American Nursing Diagnosis Association. Philadelphia: J.B. Lippincott.

Diers, D. (1984). Commentary. Western Journal of Nursing Research, 6(2), 193–194.

Fawcett, J. 1989. Analysis and evaluation of conceptual models of nursing (2nd ed.). Philadelphia: F.A. Davis.

Foreman, M.D. (1989). Confusion in the hospitalized elderly: Incidence, onset, and associated factors. Research in Health and Nursing, 12, 21–29.

Geden, E.A. (1982). Effects of lifting techniques on energy expenditure: A preliminary investigation. Nursing Research, 31(4), 214–218.

Haylock, P.J., & Hart, L.K. (1979). Fatigue in patients receiving localized radiation. Cancer Nursing, 2, 461–467.

Krupp, L.B., Alvarez, L.A., LaRocca, N.G., & Scheinberg, L.C. (1988). Fatigue in multiple sclerosis. Archives of Neurology, 45, 435–437.

Levine, M.E. (1966). Assessment and adaptation: A rationale for nursing intervention. American Journal of Nursing, (66)11, 2450–2453.

Levine, M.E. (1969). Introduction to clinical nursing (1st ed.). Philadelphia: F.A. Davis.

Levine, M.E. (1971). On creativity in nursing. Image, 3(3), 15–19.

Levine, M.E. (1973). Introduction to clinical nursing (2nd ed.). Philadelphia: F.A. Davis.

McCorkle, R. (1981). Social support and symptom distress in two samples with life-threatening diseases. Paper presented at the American Cancer Society Second Conference on Cancer Nursing Research, Seattle, Washington, August 17–19.

Meleis, A.I. (1985). Theoretical nursing: Development and progress. Philadelphia: J.B. Lippincott.

Newport, M.A. (1984). Conserving thermal energy and social integrity in the newborn. Western Journal of Nursing, 6(2), 175–197.

Piper, B. (1986). Fatigue. In V.K. Carrieri & A.M. Lindsey, Pathophysiological phenomena in nursing: Human response to illness. Philadelphia: W.B. Saunders.

Piper, B. (1988). Fatigue self-report scale developed. Reflections, 14(2), 11.

Rhodes, V.A., Watson, P.M., & Hanson, B. (1988). Patients' descriptions of the influence of tiredness and weakness on self-care abilities. Cancer Nursing, 11(3), 186–94.

Srivastava, R.H. (1986). Fatigue in the renal patient. American Neurological Nurses Association Journal, 13(5), 246–249.

Taylor, J.W. (1987). Organizing data for nursing diagnosis using conservation principles. In R.M. Carroll-Johnson (Ed.), Classification of nursing diagnosis: Proceedings of the eighth conference, North American Nursing Diagnosis Association, pp. 103–111. Philadelphia: J.B. Lippincott.

Tompkins, E.S. (1980). Effect of restricted mobility and dominance or perceived duration. Nursing Research, 29(6), 333–338.

Tripp-Reimer, T. (1984). Commentary. Western Journal of Nursing Research, 6(2), 195–197.

Winslow, E.H. (1976). The role of the nurse in patient education. Nursing Clinics of North America, 11(2), 213–222.

Winslow, E.H. (1983). Lifting techniques (letter to the editor. Nursing Research, 32(3), 188–189.

Winslow, E.H., Lane, L.D., & Gaffney, F.A. (1984). Oxygen consumption and cardiovascular response in patients and normal adults during in bed and out of bed toileting. Journal of Cardiac Rehabilitation, 4, 348–354.

Winslow, E.H., Lane, L.D., & Gaffney, F.A. (1985). Oxygen consumption and cardiovascular response in control adults and acute myocardial infarction patients during bathing. Nursing Research, 34, 164–169.

Voith, A.M., Frank, A.M. & Pigg, J. (1987). Validation of fatigue as a nursing diagnosis. In R.M. Carroll-Johnson (Ed.), Classifications of nursing diagnosis: Proceedings of the eighth conference, North American Nursing Diagnosis Association, pp. 453–458. Philadelphia: J.B. Lippincott.

Yeates, D.A., & Roberts, J.E. (1984). A comparison of two bearing-down techniques during the second stage of labor. Journal of Nurse Midwifery, 29(1), 3–11.

Chapter
FOUR

Perineal Integrity

Joyce E. Roberts, C.N.M., Ph.D
Nancy Fleming, C.N.M., Ph.D
Deborah (Yeates) Giese, C.N.M., M.S.

A major tenet in midwifery practice is the performance of an episiotomy upon specific indication for maternal or fetal well-being rather than as a routine or prophylactic procedure. Levine's conservation principles have provided the framework for addressing this issue in two research projects. The first project was conducted by Deborah (Yeates) Giese (Yeates, 1982), who compared the effects of two learned techniques of bearing down during the second stage of labor—sustained breath-holding or pushing only with the involuntary urge—on several birth outcomes (Yeates & Roberts, 1984). A control group (n = 5) was taught the traditional Lamaze pushing technique of sustained breath-holding and forceful bearing down upon recognition of complete cervical dilation. An experimental group (n = 5) was instructed in a less technique-oriented approach for the second stage of labor, in which they were taught to focus on spontaneous pushing and to coordinate their involuntary bearing-down efforts with touch relaxation. Compared with the control group, the experimental group received more discussion regarding the sensations experienced with second-stage labor contractions accompanied by the urge to bear down. Perineal integrity, as operationalized in the maintenance of an intact perineum versus the occurrence of an episiotomy or laceration, was one of the main dependent variables in this project.

The second project was conducted by Nancy Fleming (1987), who prospectively compared women (n = 102) with different perineal conditions after childbirth—episiotomies, intact perinea, sutured lacerations, unsutured lacerations, and cesareans. The women in the differing perineal outcome groups were compared in the areas of postpartum perineal pain, postpartum sexual function, prenatal and postpartum perineal muscle function, and perception of the perineal outlet.

The coauthors believe not only that clinical problems and research should be conceptualized within a nursing framework, but also that Levine's model could be operationalized within this specific aspect of midwifery practice. The four conservation principles that Levine identified in 1971 and 1973 seemed most suitable as a perspective from which to examine the issue of episiotomy and perineal condition within the context of nurse-midwifery practice and normal childbirth. While not all of Levine's interrelated concepts were operationalized within these two studies, together the four principles represent the context of childbirth within which nurse-midwifery practice occurs and the domains that should be considered in the provision of care.

The conceptualization of the two research projects within Levine's model enabled the identification of personal and social effects of receiving an episiotomy, as well as physical and physiologic consequences. The use of this conceptual framework provided an appropriate theoretical-conceptual basis for the variables being studied as they related to the goals and nature of this specialized practice in nursing (that is, midwifery and the

TABLE 4-1. VARIABLES ASSOCIATED WITH CHILDBIRTH CATEGORIZED BY LEVINE'S CONSERVATION PRINCIPLES

Conservation Principle	Variable	
	Conceptualized	Operationalized
Energy	Physical effort	Type of maternal bearing-down technique (Yeates); maternal report of effort used; duration of subphases of the second stage of labor
	Oxygen utilization	Newborn status, Apgar score
	Coping with pain and tissue damage	Level of pain and time required for healing of perineum; maternal self-report (Fleming)
Structural integrity	Perineal integrity	Incidence of intact perineum, episiotomy, first-degree sutured laceration, second- or third-degree unsutured laceration
	Vaginal muscle function/ integrity	Strength and endurance (vaginal myograph) (Fleming)
Personal integrity	Sense of achievement	Reliance on self-regulated involuntary bearing-down efforts (Yeates); caregiver's expression of confidence in women's own efforts and ability to give birth; women's report of achievement and of perineal condition; pain rating; "tightness" or "looseness"
Social integrity	Sexual relations	Time from birth to resumption of intercourse; incidence of dyspareunia; orgasmic pattern

performance of episiotomy versus efforts to preserve the structural integrity of the perineum). Additionally, as care is always transacted within a personal-social context, the use of Levine's model reflects midwiferys broad perspective and concern for women's varied needs, and facilitates the interpretation and application of research findings to the expectant or new mother to whom nurse-midwives provide care. Thus, Levine's conservation principles were conceptually operationalized for these two studies related to perineal condition and childbirth, and three of the principles were operationalized in measurable study variables (Table 4–1).

CONSERVATION OF ENERGY

Conservation of energy, when applied to the process of birth, dictates that nurses or other caregivers structure their activities in order to conserve the parturient's energy. Considering this principle in regard to perineal condition, the nurse-midwife's activities should be directed toward helping women to conserve their energy expenditure that accompanies birth and assist them to utilize their energy or mobilize appropriate reserves to meet their needs and avoid excessive fatigue. In Yeates' studies (1982, 1984), energy expenditure was operationalized as the type of physical effort reflected in the type of bearing-down technique taught and used during the second stage of labor as well as in reference to specific maternal and newborn outcomes. As indicated earlier, the control group of women who attended childbirth education classes was instructed in sustained forceful bearing down, which has been the traditional type of "pushing" technique taught. Women in the experimental group were instructed to bear down only in response to an involuntary urge, to focus their attention on the sensations that accompany the expulsive phase of labor, and to continue to use relaxation strategies. Pushing primarily in response to the involuntary urge is considered to be more congruent with the normal progression of the second stage of labor and with maternal self-regulatory efforts, that is, efforts that coordinate breathing and involuntary bearing down with the strong uterine contractions and accomplish fetal descent that normally occurs during this expulsive phase of labor. Thus, pushing primarily in response to the involuntary urge was hypothesized by Yeates (1982, 1984) to be less physiologically stressful than the sustained, forceful bearing-down technique and to result in less maternal fatigue, fetal hypoxic stress, and perineal trauma.

As an outcome measure in Yeates' study, energy expenditure for the mother was conceptualized in reference to the level of fatigue that occurred as a result of the type of bearing-down technique used. The amount of fatigue or effort exerted was assessed by asking the women immediately after the birth to rate the amount of effort or energy they thought had been required during the second stage of their labor. The amount of effort required was also assessed by measuring the duration of the second stage and specific subphase in relation to observable fetal descent. Second-stage labor was defined as the period of time from complete cervical dilation to the birth of the baby; the period of bearing down was the time from the initial involuntary bearing-down effort to the birth. The other time intervals were the time from head on view to delivery, the time from head on view to distention of the perineum, and the time from the head distending the perineum until the birth. These time intervals were assessed by a nonparticipant nurse-observer, rather than the nurse-researcher or birth attendant.

The conceptualization of energy conservation was extended to the use of oxygen and glucose by the fetus for its basic metabolic needs and also by the mother for completion of her expulsive efforts. The frequent, intense uterine contractions that usually accompany second-stage labor reduce the flow of oxygenated blood to the fetus. Additionally, the maternal muscular activity normally involved in expulsive efforts and coping with pain during birth, further consume maternal supplies of oxygen and glucose. Many authors raise the concern that strenuous pushing done in a sustained, breath-holding manner may result in additional physiologic stresses for the mother or baby, or both (Beynon, 1957; Caldeyro-Barcia, 1979; Noble, 1981; McKay & Roberts, 1985; Simkin, 1984). Not only do the sustained, breath-holding type of bearing-down efforts exhaust the parturient, but, when compared with spontaneous bearing down in response to an involuntary urge or bearing down that is accompanied by air release (exhalation pushing), the sustained, breath-holding pushes have been shown to contribute to fetal and newborn hypoxia. This hypoxia is manifested in fetal heart rate (FHR) decelerations or bradycardia and lower (more acidotic) cord blood pH at birth (Barnett & Humenick, 1982; Caldeyro-Barcia, 1979; Caldeyro-Barcia, Giussi, Storch, Poseiro, Lafaurie, Kettenhuber & Ballejo, 1981). If the fetus becomes hypoxic, it then relies on anaerobic metabolic pathways as the source of metabolic energy. Prolonged reliance on anaerobic metabolic pathways depletes glycogen stores and results in an accumulation of lactic acid, which is reflected in the lower fetal and newborn pH. Lower Apgar scores at birth have been correlated with lower (more acidotic) pH and are considered an indirect assessment of fetal condition.

Therefore, in the context of the second stage of labor in the study of Yeates and Roberts (1984), energy expenditure was operationalized in one independent variable—technique of bearing down—and in three dependent variables: (1) the duration of effort or energy exerted by the mother as measured by the duration of observable phases of the second stage of labor, (2) the amount of fatigue experienced by the mother as measured by her immediate postpartum report of the amount of effort she exerted, and (3) the Apgar score as an indirect outcome measure of the metabolic status of the infant.

In the study by Fleming (1987), conservation of energy was conceptualized in reference to the energy required to deal with postpartum perineal pain and for tissue healing. Fleming maintains that if episiotomies are not medically indicated, the nurse-midwife or physician should attempt to spare women the expenditure of energy for healing and coping with additional pain during the postpartum period. She operationalized and assessed the conservation of energy by quantifying postpartum levels of perineal pain and examining the length of time for perineal healing after birth. She also obtained newborn Apgar scores to determine if there was any difference in fetal or newborn condition for mothers with five different perineal outcomes—episiotomies, intact perinea, sutured lacerations, unsutured laceration, or nonemergency cesarean births.

CONSERVATION OF STRUCTURAL INTEGRITY

Conservation of structural integrity pertains to a person's physical condition. The goal of nursing is to assist individuals to maintain or restore the body's structural and functional integrity, to prevent physical breakdown, and to promote healing. In both Yeates's (1982, 1984) and Fleming's (1987) studies, structural integrity was conceptualized and operationalized as the condition of the maternal perineum. An earlier study by Beynon (1957) associated a higher incidence of episiotomy and forceps deliveries with directed, sustained bearing down. Accordingly, Yeates hypothesized that women who were instructed in and used the traditional sustained, strenuous bearing-down technique would have a higher incidence of perineal lacerations or episiotomies than the women who pushed primarily in response to the involuntary urge. Fleming sought to assess the consequences of different perineal outcomes in an obstetric practice that has a philosophy of care that includes the avoidance of unnecessary obstetric intervention, including the avoidance of episiotomy. Perineal integrity in Yeates's study was assessed by the incidence and extent of perineal lacerations and episiotomies. Fleming considered the consequences of episiotomy, sutured laceration, unsutured laceration, no episiotomy or laceration (intact perineum), or a cesarean birth on several subjective and objective maternal birth outcomes.

The general incidence of episiotomy in obstetric practice is 60 to 98 percent, reflecting the belief that subjecting the perineum to short-term damage from an episiotomy prevents long-term reproductive structural damage. Documentation for this allegation is lacking, resulting in an episiotomy rate of 0 to 30 percent in nurse-midwifery practices. Nurse-midwifery practice thus reflects a commitment to the principle of preserving structural integrity in the conduct of birth. Fleming's (1987) analysis of outcomes related to perineal outcome was intended to provide a basis for performing or not performing an episiotomy for birth. She operationalized structural integrity by collecting data on the frequency and severity of lacerations occurring when delivery is attempted over an intact perineum and noting the frequency of medically indicated episiotomies (i.e., those done when there was evidence of fetal compromise such as repeated late FHR decelerations, or sustained bradycardia [FHR 80 or less], or a rigid maternal perineum that would not allow the advance of the fetal head after a period of effective maternal bearing down). The incidence of episiotomy in the practice Fleming studied was 11 percent. In addition to the incidence of sutured and unsutured lacerations or episiotomies, Fleming measured perineal muscle function using a vaginal myograph to directly assess the functional integrity of the perineal muscles in both the antepartum and postpartum periods. In these ways, both the structural and functional integrity of the maternal perineum were assessed.

CONSERVATION OF PERSONAL INTEGRITY

Conservation of personal integrity in maternity care relates to the nurse or midwife's role in assisting parturients to have an optimal birth experience, including enhancement of their sense of achievement and self-esteem. Birth is an intensely personal and highly emotionally charged event. It is often considered the fulfillment of womanhood, and the ability to be "successful" with birth increases a woman's self-esteem. The perineum has strong sexual associations as well, so that a "damaged" perineum can be a threat to a woman's perception of wholeness. Gynecologic problems experienced later in life as the result of perineal outcome at birth can undoubtedly detract from the woman's personal integrity.

In Yeates's (1982) study personal integrity was viewed as the intervention of support of involuntary bearing-down efforts versus direction to bear down in a strenuous fashion. In primarily supporting the women's spontaneous efforts to bear down with her involuntary urge, the nurse or midwife not only had to be responsive to the parturient's behavior and recognize her behavioral cues, but also sought to foster the parturient's respect and confidence in her own body's sensations. Arbitrarily directing a woman to bear down upon complete cervical dilation is a more controlling approach that relies primarily on evoking the woman's cooperation. While there was no operational measure of this interpretation of preserving the woman's personal integrity as it related to the caregiver's intent, a nonparticipating nurse-observer rated the kind of direction or support that the nurse-researcher offered to the women in the control group (taught and provided with direction to bear down forcefully) and in the experimental group (taught to push in response to their involuntary urge and to continue to use relaxation techniques). Thus, there was documentation that the two different techniques were actually carried out in order to verify the internal validity of the study intervention (Yeates & Roberts, 1984). Therefore, in this study the principle of conservation of personal integrity was operationalized in the bearing-down techniques offered as care interventions, that is, operationalized as an aspect of the independent variable studied.

Fleming (1987) operationalized the personal integrity principle by asking the women in her study about their perception of their perineal condition in both the antepartum and postpartum periods. Additionally, a terminal interview asked the women about their feelings related to the presence or absence of a sense of achievement and enhanced self-esteem related to perineal condition after birth. Thus, preservation of personal integrity was assessed both through the implementation of a bearing-down technique that was responsive to the individual woman's personal sensations with the intent to enhance her own efforts, and through an assessment of her own perception of her perineal condition and birth experience with an emphasis on the unique perspective of the woman as opposed to arbitrary caregiver actions or unshared intentions.

CONSERVATION OF SOCIAL INTEGRITY

Conservation of social integrity is an extension of the principle of personal integrity. It further requires that the caregiver balance her active intervention with the patient as well as her family, assisting them to be active participants, as they are able or desire. This principle directs the nurse's attention to the importance of each person's ability for human interaction, including those with whom the patient has significant relationships. Related to birthing, this principle requires consideration of how a woman's perineal condition influences her relationships with others, especially those with her newborn and her partner.

Several sources (Goodlin, 1983; Hanley, 1980; Kitzinger, 1981; Willmott, 1979) have asserted that pain from episiotomy is great enough in the immediate postpartum period to interfere with maternal-infant bonding and lactation. These most immediate disruptions in interpersonal adjustments were not assessed in either study. However, Fleming (1987) assessed the potential for postpartum disturbances in the women's sexual relationships with their husbands based on the reports in the literature that there is a significant rate of dyspareunia following episiotomy that is often prolonged. Her assessment explored both dyspareunia and orgasmic changes following the birth. In these ways, social integrity was incorporated in Fleming's study design.

STUDY RESULTS

Although 40 couples agreed to participate in Yeates's study (1982), only 10 were able to be included in the final sample due to obstetric conditions that developed that excluded them from the study, such as need for medication during labor, a persistent posterior fetal position, pregnancy-induced hypertension, or need for a cesarean birth. There were five subjects in both the control and the experimental groups. Although there were no differences between the groups in the duration of second stage, the duration of subphases of second stage, infant Apgar scores, or mothers' perception of the amount of energy required during the bearing-down period, there was a significant difference in the incidence of episiotomy and lacerations. The control group that used the sustained, strenuous bearing-down technique had a significantly higher incidence of these disruptions in perineal integrity. Therefore, this study found support for relying on involuntary maternal bearing-down efforts as a strategy for preserving perineal or structural integrity.

It should be pointed out that the intervention in Yeates's (1982) study—type of bearing-down technique—represents the operationalization of two of Levine's conservation principles: conservation of energy and conservation of personal integrity. Nursing care is often a "package" of activities that includes specific actions (type of breathing, muscular effort, and possible positioning) and intentions (expressions of care, respect, confidence, kindness, and hope). It may be difficult to distinguish among the several factors that are operating to achieve the desired care outcomes because they become mixed in this collection of actions as well as mixed with the multiple maternal variables and personal antecedents that are brought to the birth experience. While the independent variable may be fairly explicit and operationalized to an observable extent, as it was in these studies, it is not possible to account for all the factors that may have explained the observable outcomes.

Fleming (1987) attempted to bring the objectivity and systematic nature of clinical research methods into an area of practice that has been guided by assumption, supposition, tradition, and habit (that of the routine performance of episiotomy for birth). In comparing the results of five different categories of perineal outcome, no support could be found for any of the maternal or fetal advantages attributed to this procedure. There was no difference in the infant Apgar scores at birth, indicating that the infants of mothers who did not have an episiotomy in this study (79 of 89) were not compromised by the avoidance of a procedure that might have hastened their infants' birth.

The groups of women who sustained either an episiotomy or a sutured laceration had more negative experiences in the categories of person and social integrity, as well as the disruption in structural integrity, than did women with intact perinea. Women with perineal tissue damage (either an episiotomy or a laceration) had more pronounced and prolonged perineal pain after birth. Women who had an episiotomy had the highest pain scores and reported a significantly longer period of time prior to resuming intercourse and more long-term dyspareunia. Women who had an episiotomy resumed intercourse more than 1 week later (6.4 weeks postpartum) than the sutured laceration group (who resumed intercourse at an average of 5.1 weeks postpartum), and more than 2 weeks later than the unsutured group (who resumed intercourse at an average of 4.2 weeks postpartum). Women with an episiotomy also reported three times as much dyspareunia as women with sutured lacerations. Thirty-three percent of the women with episiotomies also indicated continued discomfort during intercourse at 6 months postpartum, which they related to their sutures, as compared with 11 percent of women in the sutured laceration groups.

While women did not attribute changes in orgasmic pattern to perineal outcome, more than twice the percentage of women with episiotomies expressed orgasmic decline at 6 months postpartum as compared with any other perineal outcome group. The perineal muscle strength and endurance scores obtained with a vaginal myograph did not differ statistically during either the antepartum or postpartum periods, except in the group of women who eventually sustained second- or third-degree lacerations, whose mean myograph scores were significantly lower postpartally than the mean scores of the other groups. Fleming (1987) interpreted the lower scores in this subgroup as suggesting an inherent difference in their tissue and muscle integrity that may have predisposed them to this disruption in perineal integrity with birth. Compared with their antepartum scores, all groups experienced increased muscle strength and endurance scores postpartally, except for the episiotomy group, in which a significant decrease occurred. Therefore, rather than preserving vaginal or perineal muscle tone, episiotomy was associated with a decrease in muscle function. Additionally, performance of an episiotomy did not forestall either disadvanta-geous tears or rectal tears. Women with episiotomies had approximately the same percentage of labial tears and perineal extensions away from the midline as did women without episiotomies. Women with episiotomies, however, were five to eight times more likely to experience a rectal exten-sion as women without an episiotomy.

When viewed in light of Levine's conservation principles, it is evident that the current biases in favor of routine or prophylactic episiotomies are not consistent with optimal nursing practice which, from Levine's perspec-tive, is intended to conserve structural, personal, and social integrity, as these concepts were operationalized in these studies. It appears that the normal adaptations of the birth process provide the most physically, emo-tionally, and socially beneficial means for this physiologic function. Re-sults from Fleming's (1987) study support the conclusion that interventions that are employed as a course of routine rather than based on individual need actually increase the physiologic burden of healing following birth and act as a significant threat to the psychosocial adjustments of the post-partum period. The data from the several dependent variables of her re-search support the underlying conservation principle that the naturally occurring adaptations to physiologic events form the body's most expedi-tious response. The data, in fact, suggest the possibility that more favor-able outcomes in the areas of pain, sexuality, and muscle function result when a laceration separates tissue, possibly along the planes of natural tis-sue weakness, as opposed to when an episiotomy is cut through the tissue. If this is true, the intervention of episiotomy is an assault of the body's nat-urally adaptive energy-sparing mechanisms and structural integrity. Episi-otomy is not indicated as a routine or prophylactic procedure because it does not appear to be protective and it should be reserved for specific occa-sions when intervention is warranted.

Both Fleming's (1987) and Yeates's (1982) studies do not support the need for iatrogenically introducing arbitrary direction in the form of en-couraging sustained, strenuous bearing-down efforts or for iatrogenically producing perineal tissue disruption with an episiotomy unless there are indications that either of these interventions is necessary. Fleming identi-fied the occasions in which an episiotomy is indicated: when there is con-cern for fetal compromise and birth can be hastened with an episiotomy or when the maternal perineum seems unyielding after a period of effective bearing down. It is less clear from Yeates's results when direction in stren-uous bearing down is indicated. Both studies, however, indicate that such arbitrary direction is not accompanied by optimal birth outcomes with re-gard to perineal, personal, and social integrity. Support and encourage-ment for primarily involuntary bearing down does not necessarily prolong the second stage of labor, as indicated by the absence of differences in the duration of phases of the second stage in Yeates, study. However, the small sample size requires that the type of direction or support offered to women during the expulsive phase of labor be studied further.

The results of these studies support the investigation of care practices within a conceptual framework that considers at least these four dimen-sions of the human experience—the structural, personal, social, and energy expenditure aspects. Additionally, the overall goal of preserving the integrity of the whole is consistent with the context of nursing practice, which must regard patients and their needs within the social context of family and life situation.

REFERENCES

Barnett, M., & Humenick, S. (1982). Infant outcome in relation to second stage labor pushing method. Birth, 9, 221–228.

Beynon, C.L. (1957). The normal second stage of labor: A plea for reform in its conduct. Journal of Obstetrics and Gynecology of the British Empire, 64, 815–820.

Caldeyro-Barcia, R. (1979). The influence of maternal bearing-down during second stage on fetal well-being. Birth, 6, 17–21.

Caldeyro-Barcia, R., Giussi, G., Storch, E., Poseiro, J.J., Lafaurie, N., Kettenhuber, K., & Ballejo, G. (1981). The bearing-down effects on fetal heart rate, oxygenation, and acid-base balance. Journal of Perinatal Medicine, 9(1), 63–67.

Fleming, N. (1987). Comparison of women with different perineal conditions after childbirth (Doctoral dissertation, University of Illinois at Chicago, Health Sciences Center, 1987). Dissertation Abstracts International, No. 8728762.

Goodlin, R.C. (1983). After office hours. Obstetrics and Gynecology, 82:393–394.

Hanley, J. (1980). Opinion: Conflicting theories. Midwives Chronicle and Nursing Notes, 93, 48–49.

Kitzinger, S. (1981). Emotional aspects of episiotomy and postnatal sexual adjustment. In S. Kitzinger (Ed.). Episiotomy: Physical and emotional aspects (pp. 45–53). London: National Childbirth Trust.

Levine, M.E. (1971). Holistic nursing. Nursing Clinics of North America, 6, 253–264.

Levine, M.E. (1973). Introduction to clinical nursing. Philadelphia: F.A. Davis.

McKay, S., & Roberts, J. (1985). Second stage labor: What is normal? Journal of Obstetric, Gynecologic and Neonatal Nursing, 14, 101–106.

Noble, E. (1981). Controversies in maternal effort during labor and delivery. Journal of Nurse-Midwifery, 26(2), 16.

Simkin, P. (Ed.) (1984). Episiotomy and the second stage of labor. Seattle: Pennypress.

Wilmott, J. (1979). Community nursing: No need to flaw the pelvic floor. Nursing Mirror, 148(13), 131.

Yeates, D. (1982). A comparison of two bearing-down techniques during the second stage of labor. Master's thesis, University of Illinois at the Medical Center, Graduate College, Department of Nursign Sciences, Chicago.

Yeates, D.A., & Roberts, J.E. (1984). A comparison of two bearing-down techniques during the second stage of labor. Journal of Nurse-Midwifery, 29(1), 3–11.

Chapter
F I V E

Care of Children

Maureen Dever, R.N., M.S.N., C.R.N.P.

Hospitalization or any other health care contact can be a dehumanizing experience for patients. They have clothing and personal belongings exchanged for hospital gowns that gape open in the back. They have strangers attending to previously private activities and are often treated as though they are incapable of making appropriate decisions about their life. Imagine for a moment that you have been placed in this position. Embarrassment, fear, anger, and frustration are just a few of the sensations you may experience. Let us suppose that, additionally, you are not even consulted when your treatment is planned, and it does not matter if you protest against having a certain procedure performed because the staff will do it anyway? Scary? Definitely. Could these things really occur? They routinely do if the patient is a child. Now consider that you believe the hospitalization is a punishment for sneaking a cookie yesterday. Or that everyone in uniform will hurt you in some way. Or that when the people you trust most in the world walk out of your hospital room, they no longer exist. Silly? Not really. A child's age and development level allow for an entirely different perspective as a patient than that of an adult. The health care experience moves from the merely dehumanizing to the truly traumatic. As a pediatric nurse practitioner and a pediatric instructor, these facts required that I develop an approach in my nursing practice that considered many different aspects of a patient's life and still maintained a focus on the patient's uniqueness. The problem was how to accomplish this.

Nursing generally adopts a patient-centered approach to care, and many conceptual models have integrated this idea into their frameworks. In the past, I had used a systems orientation that focused on stressors and the patient's unique response to them. Somehow I felt that I was overlooking the totality of the situation by looking only at pieces of the patient's life. It was at this point I began to teach at a college whose nursing curriculum was based upon Levine's conservation principles. As I became more familiar with Levine's model, I was impressed with its focus on the influences and responses of the individual on an organismic level, considering the entire person at all times. I further identified with the emphasis placed on maintaining the integrity of the individual in terms of relationships: environmental and experiential, and through application of four conservation principles. Balance was based on "the private resources of (one's) own body" and on the interactions that take place with the environment (Levine, 1969, p. 94). Through the principles of conservation of energy, structural integrity, personal integrity, and social integrity, I found a framework that was appropriate for the pediatric patient.

THE CHILD AS PATIENT

Children have an amazing personal capacity to adapt. They are also marvelously matter-of-fact in the process of adaptation. This means that most of the contacts a child has with the health care system are wellness oriented. Patients receive routine health maintenance examinations and immunizations. Health problems are usually self-limiting, episodic, easily managed at home, and of minor inconvenience to the child (but perhaps more disrupting for the parents). The unusual cases in which a child requires greater professional intervention or hospitalization may indicate serious health concerns. This is when most nurses become involved in the care of the child.

Whereas infectious illness once dominated the serious health concerns, today's pediatric nurse is likely to find patients dealing with anything from chronic illnesses resulting from treatment for prematurity and birth defects to critical illnesses associated with trauma and surgery. Patient acuity is higher and contacts may be long-term and/or repeated. Parents and other family members are required to assume a greater role in hospitalization and care, often involving high-tech equipment and a variety of procedures. Nurses must provide direct care, discharge planning, patient and parent education, counseling, emotional support, and coordination of any number of social services. How is it possible to facilitate the meeting of all these needs in a holistic manner?

USE OF LEVINE'S CONSERVATION PRINCIPLES

The integral concept in Levine's conservation principles is adaptation. According to Levine (1989), adaptation is an interaction process that occurs between the individual and the environment, both internal and external, in which the individual maintains his or her integrity. As such, the environment is "not a passive backdrop against which the individual acts out life experiences," but rather is open, active, and mobile (Levine, 1989, p. 326). This is a particularly appropriate view to consider in pediatrics, in which a developing child's dependence on and interaction with the environment change over time in situation and perception.

The internal environment of a child consists of multiple adaptive and regulating mechanisms that are largely physiologic or behavioral in nature.

The younger the child, the greater the potential for less than optimal functioning of these mechanisms. For example, a newborn will not have a well-developed inflammatory response due to immaturity of the immune system (Marlow & Redding, 1988). Other mechanisms, such as the stress response, may result in readiness similar to that of an adult. However, the behavioral component may require alternative or unique external environment interaction to result in a desired activity (i.e., assistance of a parent initiated by the crying of the child).

The external environment can be explored through the examination of three aspects that affect the individual. These are operational, perceptual, and conceptual factors.

The operational environment consists of those factors that "interact with living things even though the individual does not possess sensory organs that record their presence" (Levine, 1989, p. 326). In a pediatric population, microorganisms pose a considerable threat. Aside from increased susceptibility, children often do not have sufficient awareness to avoid the threat through such simple activities as hand washing or covering their mouths when coughing. Other operational factors, which affect all humans but seem to be of greater danger to the very old or very young, include pollutants such as smoke and industrial waste and radiation such as ultraviolet rays from the sun. Again, protective mechanisms against these factors are not adequately functioning, or experience in protection is lacking.

Perceptual factors involve the recognition and processing of information through the sensory system. Children are very involved in their perceptual environment because it is the source of much of their knowledge and learning in the early years (Marlow & Redding, 1988). Children may also be more sensory aware than adults because they usually have greater freedom to concentrate in this area. Unfortunately, this sensory involvement may result in as many hazards as growth opportunities. For example, young children will taste most objects regardless of whether it is appropriate to do so or not. Adolescents may enjoy the sound and vibration of rock music to the detriment of their hearing. In the health care world, the strange and unfamiliar stimuli of white uniforms, antiseptic smells, painful procedures, and large equipment may prove overwhelming to a child. Personnel must be reminded that their *nonverbal* behavior is frequently recalled more readily than words by pediatric patients. Misinterpretation often leads to unnecessary stress for the child.

The conceptual environment of a pediatric patient is constantly growing and refining as the child develops intellectually, socially, and emotionally. Language and understanding are limited initially, then expand rapidly between 2 and 5 years of age (Marlow & Redding, 1988). Concepts such as object permanence, magical thinking, cause-and-effect thinking, reversibility, logical thought processes, and finally, abstract thinking have an impact on the attitudes and feelings of a child (Foster, Hunsberger, & Anderson, 1989). This allows for the preschool child to believe that an immunization injection is given as punishment and the adolescent to grasp the need for the same injection to stimulate immunity and prevent disease. Imagine the differing attitudes of these children toward the same nurse administering both injections. Cultural and spiritual ideation also influence the conceptual environment of a child. Cultural and spiritual beliefs are conveyed to the child through family and friends. As a child grows, he or she may similarly embrace, reject, or alter such concepts as illness caused by body imbalances, demons, or punishment from God, or the restoration of health through strong faith.

As may be apparent, the internal and external environments are irrevocably linked to each other and to the individual. The goal—in terms of health and, ultimately, survival—is to constantly balance or obtain a "best fit" (Levine, 1989). This adaptation should "cost the least to the individual in expense of effort and demand on well-being" (Levine, 1989, p. 329). In other words, adaptation retains or *conserves* the integrity of the individual in a unique, personal, and cost-effective manner. The nurse recognizes those adaptive patterns through observation and then assists the individual to maintain his or her unity and integrity. This may be accomplished through the guidelines of four conservation principles.

Conservation of *energy* is concerned with the balance of resources and expenditures of energy. "The ability of any person to function is predicated on his energy potential and the specific patterns of energy exchange available to him" (Levine, 1967, p. 47). Natural conservation of energy is readily apparent in the pediatric patient. Young children, when left to their own devices, will often eat when hungry, sleep when tired, and tone down activity when not feeling well. They "listen" to what their bodies are saying and may require adult assistance only for the best choices or for facilities to meet their needs. Problems arise when body messages are ignored or greater assistance at adaptation is necessary.

Children do have some age-associated characteristics that influence their available resources and subsequent expenditures of energy. Young children have higher metabolic rates—expressed through higher pulse rate, respiratory rate, and body temperature—than adults. This also means that a growing child needs more calories to meet normal energy demands. At the same time, febrile illnesses, which further increase pulse and respiration rates, quickly deplete energy and require higher replacement intake. The ill child requires more frequent feedings, actually having to be fed or to receive an altered diet to decrease the work of feeding (i.e., tube feeding, liquid diet, higher calorie concentration per ounce amount). Periods of uninterrupted rest corresponding to natural body rhythms will conserve energy. Obviously, decreasing the body temperature can also dramatically affect energy balance.

As a source of energy, diet is important in terms of both content and calories. Infants 6 months to 1 year old and adolescents have a tendency toward diet-related anemia. Maternal iron stores transmitted to an infant are depleted by about 6 months of age. Usually the addition of solid foods or use of iron-fortified feedings minimizes the impact on the child. Long-term illness at this time interferes with the re-establishment of balance. Adolescents, especially females, develop a tendency toward iron-deficiency anemia at puberty. Often it is exacerbated by poor dietary habits related to weight loss or dieting. Nutritional counseling initiated at an earlier age may prevent these difficulties (Marlow & Redding, 1988).

When children become ill, they automatically become less active than normal, decreasing energy use. In long-term or chronic conditions, however, some consideration must be made to maintain a level of activity that is beneficial for the normal growth and development of a child but does not seriously deplete energy resources. Scheduling a time for school and for play or fun activities is just as necessary as planning any care-related procedures. Usually modifications are possible to allow for a variety of opportunities for different ages and interests. Nurses must continually assess for signs of early fatigue, such as increased irritability or lack of attention, and intervene to promote energy balance.

A last pediatric difference that can influence conservation of energy is related to the infants' tendency toward generalized body system response to illness (Foster et al., 1989). For example, a child with an upper respiratory infection may also have vomiting, diarrhea, and sleep disturbances. Sleep disturbances have an obvious drain on energy resources at any age. Vomiting and diarrhea are of greater concern in the child less than 2 years of age because of the increased risk for dehydration. At this age, children have less ability to concentrate urine, greater body water content, and increased insensible loss through larger body surface area (Marlow & Redding, 1988). Dehydration acts as an additional energy drain as it interferes with normal body chemistry and the adaptation processes at a cellular level. Net results can range from an increased temperature to inability of the body to function due to electrolyte disturbances.

Conservation of energy requires an initial and ongoing observation and assessment of the individual's response to nursing action. A child's condition can rapidly change, either positively or negatively. Failure to conserve energy may ultimately result in respiratory arrest (Foster et al., 1989).

Conservation of *structural integrity* is concerned with the maintenance of structure and function as well as with healing as the "defense of wholeness" (Levine, 1989, p. 333). Children, despite starting life with some immature systems, develop remarkable reparative ability. Scrapes, cuts, and broken bones heal rapidly as do surgical incisions or manipulations. This is fortunate because the pediatric population is particularly prone to dermatologic disruptions in the form of fungal, viral, or bacterial infections and trauma related to poor judgments and accidents. Problems may arise when the child with a disruption in structural integrity is exposed to additional insults in the hospital. For example, children may develop nosocomial gastroenteritis or upper respiratory infection when originally hospitalized with appendicitis.

A unique pediatric influence on structural integrity results from birth defects or injuries. The resultant impairment of functioning may be temporary or permanent and includes such conditions as heart defects, microcephaly, and facial paralysis related to difficult vaginal delivery. Permanent alteration in structural integrity requires incorporation of changes into body image and long-term treatment involving a variety of health care personnel.

Finally, a continual reminder as to the importance of structural integrity is found in the preschool population. Any nurse caring for children of this age knows the necessity of placing a bandage over the offending break to prevent "insides" from leaking out. Obvious defects in integrity are feared and often exaggerated in the minds of these children.

The conservation of *personal integrity* is involved with the patient's sense of identity and self-esteem. True conservation of this integrity requires that the nurse be accepting of the patients regardless of how they may present or behave (Levine, 1967). Although nurses frequently relate to patients in an intimate or personal manner, Levine (1989) emphasizes that "it is simply impossible for one individual to surrender his or her privacy to another, no matter how much the individual must depend on the good offices of the caregiver" (p. 334). These statements are often forgotten when the patient is a child. Adults often relate to children as their superiors and, by doing so, automatically negate the child's autonomy or input into decision making. Likewise, children's personal feelings or wishes may not be taken seriously. To some degree, this may be essential for the well-being of the child. After all, 4-year-olds with limited knowledge and experience can hardly be expected to properly feed, clean, and clothe themselves. Unfortunately, this attitude also can lead to blanket disregard of *any* input when the child *is* able to contribute. Levine (1989) states that "all individuals must participate freely in decisions that affect them" (p. 335). As human beings, children have equal rights to personal consideration. Can 4-year-olds refuse a necessary injection? Probably not, but they should have a say as to whether Mom or Dad stays in the room, or perhaps should expect some acknowledgment of their discomfort, bravery, and fears related to the procedure.

Aside from issues of privacy, pediatric patients have special aspects of personal integrity that need to be noted. Developmental and intellectual level is quite influential in a child's expression of "self." Maturation is accompanied by changes in self-concept and body image. The relative importance of both also change at different ages. A newborn infant is felt to have extensive personal body "boundaries" that often incorporate caregivers and objects. Children may be uncertain as to where their own boundaries "stop" and others "begin" (Marlow & Redding, 1988). Adolescents are much more particular about their personal space and are often acutely aware of the most minute body changes. Independence is a related function of development. Toddlers strongly assert their preferences by repeated and intense use of the word *no*. School-aged children are more quiet and less concerned with direct confrontation, but by adolescence independence is a major issue once again (Marlow & Redding, 1988).

A child's coping and communication patterns are also, in part, a function of age. The toddler, who has limited ability to articulate, will often cry and respond to stress through temper tantrums or physical expression. School-aged children may cope by being "brave" and following staff instructions to the letter. Frequently the child is "better behaved" with staff than with family or significant others. Many nurses misinterpret this response as a result of parental "spoiling." More accurately, children feel safe enough with family to express themselves and work to conserve personal integrity. "Frequently the success of a coping pattern rests on the support and encouragement of a group that shares the concerns of the individual" (Levine, 1989, p. 336).

The aforementioned notable observation leads to the fourth principle, conservation of *social integrity*. "The human being knows himself in his reflection from others. The essence of his humanity is the result of his dynamic relationship with other human beings" (Levine, 1967, p. 56). The need to view a patient in the context of his or her family and community is perhaps most essential in the case of a pediatric patient, where there is tremendous overlap in personal and social integrity. The younger the child, the more likely that the true patient is the family.

The social world of the pediatric patient is becoming increasingly more complex. Parents may or may not be married or living together. Divorces result in single-parent families, or, with remarriage, blended families. The realities of finances may require extended-family living arrangements, with grandparents having a range of child-rearing responsibilities. As the child grows, relationships with peers also take on greater importance in maintaining social integrity. To an adolescent, visits from peers may even be an essential requirement for health if hospitalization is necessary.

Cultural beliefs also influence relationships. Individual as well as family roles and responsibilities differ from group to group. Parenting style may range from permissive to authoritarian. Perhaps the mother may have sole child care responsibility but the father must make all the decisions as the "head of the family." A shift in roles due to a contact with the health care system can prove unsettling to the child and family members.

Finally, some mention must be made of the nurse-patient relationship and its impact on the social integrity of a child. In many instances, the nurse may easily adopt a "surrogate mother" role. This is especially true in situations of child neglect or abuse and may have a positive or negative impact on the child and family. The child may initially feel secure in response to the nurse's perceived love and profession but may later experience disruption and confusion regarding the true parent (Foster et al., 1989). It is imperative that nurses recognize their long-range role in the child's life in maintaining a supportive versus distorted relationship. Observations and interventions must be adjusted accordingly.

As part of a holistic model, the conservation principles work in an integrated and interrelated manner with adaptation as a goal. They serve as a framework for nursing assessment and intervention that is therapeutic, positively influencing adaptation, or supportive, maintaining the status quo. Use of the conservation principles requires knowledge of each patient's "individual pattern of adaptive response" (Levine, 1971, p. 258) and an ability to focus interventions toward enhancement of these responses.

Case Presentation 5-1: Daniel

ASSESSMENT

I first saw Daniel (the name of the patient has been changed to protect the individual's identity) the morning after he had been admitted to the hospital with a diagnosis of respiratory distress secondary to pneumonia. Daniel is a 4½-month-old-child who had had symptoms of coughing, wheezing, rhinorrhea, and congestion for 3 weeks. He had been seen twice in the emergency room for subcutaneous epinephrine treatments, which provided some improvement through bronchodilation, but each time symptoms returned. During the previous night, symptoms had increased and included crackles and rhonchi, retractions, tachypnea, and poor feeding. At this point, he was admitted to the hospital. Initial assessment of Daniel, using the conservation principles, demonstrated a number of threats.

In terms of *energy*, Daniel had moderate to severe respiratory distress. His respiratory rate fluctuated from 40 to 70 breaths per minute. He had bilateral rhonchi and scattered crackles with the greater adventitious sounds in the right upper lobe and right middle lobe. Additionally, there were moderate intercostal and substernal retractions. Resting oximetry readings were 97 to 98 percent of normal but decreased to 80 to 85 percent of normal during coughing spasms. Daniel was tachycardic with apical pulse readings from 145 to 200, and was febrile to 102°F. His skin color and turgor were adequate. He had an intravenous infusion of 5 percent dextrose, quarter-strength normal saline, and 10 mEq of potassium chloride already infusing at 35 ml per hr with a theophylline drip piggybacked at 7 mg per hr. His theophylline level was 15.2 mg per kg and all electrolytes were within normal limits. The head of the bed was elevated and a croupette had been set up in the crib. There were a number of staff members around the crib or working with Daniel. He cried loudly when disturbed, frequently stopping only due to coughing spasms. At all other periods, he would fall immediately to sleep only to awaken shortly due to monitor alarms or the taking of vital signs. By history, he had not slept well in 3 days. When offered a bottle of clear liquids or a pacifier, Daniel would suck weakly and then cry. He had no oral intake for 6 hours.

Structurally, Daniel's chest x-ray indicated that he had a right upper lobe pneumonia. His white blood count was 14.5/mm^3 with an increase in neutrophils indicating acute infection. Daniel did have a moderate diaper rash that appeared to be related to irritants and was not fungal or bacterial in origin. He was 16 pounds, 14 ounces (birth weight 8 pounds, 3 ounces), and appeared to be well hydrated and well nourished. He had received his first oral polio vaccine (OPV) and diphtheria, pertussis, and tetanus (DPT) immunizations at age 2 months, but no others. While tachycardic, he had no murmurs and peripheral pulses were easily palpated. Daniel had three to four wet diapers a shift but no stools. His muscle tone was good, as was his flexibility and range of motion. The anterior fontanelle was open and flat, without bulging or depression. Neurologic activity appeared intact, although Daniel did appear fatigued. No other obvious structural deficits were noted.

At 4½ months of age, Daniel's *personal* integrity was difficult to validate. He should have been aware of his body boundaries and, indeed, seemed threatened only by actual body touching. Although he tended to cry when disturbed, he calmed when spoken to softly or perhaps when he realized the touch was not meant to cause pain. When calm, Daniel did open his eyes and make contact with staff. At one point, despite the distress, he offered a most beautiful smile in response to placement of a mobile and conversation. Communication was limited to nonverbal means and crying. Daniel's cries did differ in expression of pain, fear, or exhaustion.

He did respond positively to a soft voice and gentle stroking of arms or cheeks.

Daniel was dependent on staff to meet his needs. He did, however, communicate his displeasure or disagreement through crying or protest. According to Erikson (cited in Marlow & Redding, 1988), Daniel should have been in the trust versus mistrust stage where the meeting of his needs would foster security and a sense of belonging. Inherent in this stage is the need for closeness and cuddling, preferably with the mother. Sucking, which can also provide some security for the infant, was not possible with the respiratory distress.

Daniel's *social* integrity had several actual and potential threats. Daniel's mother was 16 years old, unmarried, and still in high school. She was maintaining a relationship with Daniel's father, 17 years old and also in school, but had become distanced from her own parents. After leaving the baby with the nurses, and despite requests to remain for further history, the child's mother had left. Attempts to reach her by phone were unsuccessful. Daniel's grandfather, however, was contacted and came to the hospital. The grandfather was visibly distressed by the equipment surrounding the child and by the child's obvious respiratory distress. He did not know where his daughter was living but planned to find her.

The family was white and Roman Catholic, although Daniel's parents were no longer active in the church. Because both were high school students, there was no income and no medical insurance. The grandfather was concerned about Daniel but did not wish to hold or touch the child.

Halfway through the shift, Daniel's mother did come to the hospital. She was accompanied by a girlfriend. After spending a few moments with Daniel, she stated she had to leave. Attempts to persuade her to stay were not successful. She did state that she and Daniel were "temporarily" living at the apartment of this same friend and provided a phone number. Both women were laughing and joking boisterously as they left, seemingly unaware of the serious nature of Daniel's problem. While distressing to staff, such a reaction (i.e., denial, lack of knowledge, withdrawal) is not uncommon in adolescents, especially in stressful or crisis situations (Foster et al., 1989).

NURSING JUDGMENTS, INTERVENTIONS, AND PATIENT RESPONSE

It was evident from the assessment that Daniel's greatest immediate threat was to his energy integrity and, as such, was the priority for therapeutic intervention. Aside from the theophylline ethylenediamine drip, Daniel was receiving metaproterenol sulfate aerosol treatments every 4 hours. Chest physiotherapy was performed after the aerosol treatments for maximal effect. As these procedures resulted in a high degree of agitation and crying, a schedule was made to ensure that Daniel was rested prior to beginning. All other procedures were grouped into times that allowed for uninterrupted sleep periods or positive interaction. Coordination with physicians ordering tests, laboratory technicians drawing blood, assessment activities, and routine vital signs or care procedures was accomplished through a primary nurse. Anxiety was also decreased by clearing the room of extraneous personnel, drawing the curtains around the bed (in a three-patient ward room), closing window blinds, and decreasing unfamiliar noises whenever possible. Those people who needed to interact with Daniel were told to approach him gently and talk quietly prior to any physical contact. Because Daniel was in a croupette, care was taken to maintain core temperature and avoid shivering by dressing him in heavy pajamas and frequently changing damp linens.

The replenishment of energy stores created several problems. Until his respiratory distress was controlled, Daniel would not be able to take a bottle because of the risk of formula aspiration. Furthermore, the work of a feeding could serve as an additional drain on energy resources. Some calories were obtained through the intravenous solution, minimal as they might be. Since Daniel's hydration status and weight were stable at that time, oral feedings were delayed until his repiratory status improved.

Within 8 hours, Daniel had improved significantly. His respiratory rate ranged from 30 to 60 breaths per minute, with an average of 40. His pulse decreased to 100 to 140 per minute and temperature stabilized at 100°F. He still had minor to moderate substernal and intercostal retractions but appeared to be more comfortable. Instead of dropping off to sleep immediately, Daniel now looked around the room or at his fingers. While still initially crying with contact, he quickly calmed to voice and positive verbal or physical interaction. Unfortunately, he still had 5- to 10-minute coughing spells two to three times an hour. Oximetry readings during coughing now remained in the upper 90s. The next day the croupette was discontinued. Within 24 hours, the coughing stopped. During the next 48 hours, half-strength formula feedings of 2 to 3 ounces were successfully attempted. Daniel was not to be awakened for feedings, but was offered formula every 2 to 3 hours if he seemed interested. The small amount appeared to satisfy him yet did not tire him. This was gauged by his behavior after feedings (i.e., whether he was playful, content, fairly active). His weight remained stable, indicating that therapeutic interventions were supportive.

The initial primary intervention toward conservation of structural integrity was the administration of a broad-spectrum antibiotic, cefuroxime. However, laboratory results in the next few days showed the most likely cause of Daniel's difficulty was influenza B, a potentially serious viral infection. All other cultures—blood, urine, respiratory syncytial virus, and pertussis—were negative. At this point, the antibiotic was discontinued. The chest x-ray showed a partial resolution of the pneumonia 5 days after admission. This corresponded with Daniel's improved clinical conditions.

Daniel's diaper rash was easily managed with exposure to air and careful cleaning with soap and water, followed by application of a protective zinc oxide ointment. When the croupette was discontinued, the length of time his buttocks were exposed to air was increased without concern for chilling and the hazards of a moist environment promoting bacterial growth.

As Daniel improved, his behavior showed the uniqueness of his personality. Interventions were individualized to conserve his personal integrity and to promote security. Daniel liked to be held, but early in the hospitalization his condition did not allow him to be out of the croupette for any extended period of time. Fortunately, he responded well to having his bottom patted, his head and back stroked, or the offer of a finger to grasp. When touching him, every effort was made to be in close physical proximity (i.e., putting one's head and arms into the croupette). He preferred hearing a human voice to any music or mobile noise, so attempts were unsuccessfully made to arrange for his mother's voice to be tape-recorded to supplement the "live" voices of nurses. In addition to sound and touch, Daniel was tightly wrapped in a blanket to increase a sense of boundary and security. Sucking, a favorite activity of infants that provides comfort and security, was also difficult to provide initially. As energy integrity was re-established, Daniel was allowed a pacifier, which was used in conjunction with the previous interventions. He also was allowed play time. Mobiles, brightly colored toys, and people were his favorite diversions. He smiled easily and frequently, occasionally even laughing at staff antics. Once stabilized, Daniel was a remarkably easy baby who was curious, enjoyed whatever activity he was involved with, and bounced back to a happy state rapidly after procedures or unpleasant interruptions, especially if he was allowed to suck on the pacifier afterward.

Conservation of Daniel's social integrity was perhaps the most difficult to accomplish. Social service was contacted to handle financial arrangements because Daniel's parents did not have insurance or jobs. Nursing interventions were directed toward Daniel's parents and their relationship toward him. His mother was the only parent who had been to the hospital, and her visits had been brief. Consequently, assessment of the social situation was very incomplete. Daniel's mother was contacted by phone and an interview attempted. It became apparent that she was concerned for her son but overwhelmed by his illness and hospitalization. She felt inadequate as a caregiver and responsible for the pneumonia. She was willing to come to the hospital to talk face to face with the primary nurse. Upon arrival, it was learned that Daniel's grandparents were not happy about their daughter's pregnancy. Since his birth, tensions had been very high, culminating in an argument 5 days ago that resulted in Daniel and his mother moving in with a friend. The living arrangements could only be temporary, so housing was a worry. Daniel's mother was rather surprised that her father had been to the hospital but seemed to think that his concern was a good sign.

Time was spent explaining equipment and procedures associated with Daniel's care. His mother, upon seeing him after this discussion, was more relaxed as she touched and held him. When he responded positively, she laughed and hugged him. She was encouraged to call the father and inform him of the hospitalization. Arrangements were also made for her to stay with Daniel and speak with the social worker. Later that evening the grandparents visited and, with mediation from the social worker, began reconciliation with their daughter. Plans were made for follow-up with a community agency to help the family work through their problems.

Seven days after admission, Daniel was discharged to his mother's care and his grandparent's home. He was happy and playful. Levine's conservation principles were valuable as an organizing framework for assessment and nursing care, but more important, the conservation principles allowed for Daniel and his family to be viewed humanistically. In a time of increasingly complex living, this holistic attitude is an essential component of nursing. Unfortunately, that does not often make it an easy thing to accomplish. Assessments are not complete with the first patient encounter, and care plans must be continually adjusted. Preset categories frequently do not fit patients, and loose ends rarely are neatly tied up. Fortunately, the intelligent nurse realizes that working with people requires an open exchange of thoughts, feelings, and ideas, which are often unpredictable. Levine's conservation principles are one way of accepting this concept and working with it to provide the best nursing care possible.

REFERENCES

Foster, R., Hunsberger, M., & Anderson, J. (1989). Family centered nursing care of children. Philadelphia: W.B. Saunders.

Levine, M.E. (1967). The four conservation principles of nursing. Nursing Forum, 6(1), 45–59.

Levine, M.E. (1969). The pursuit of wholeness. American Journal of Nursing, 69(1), 93–98.

Levine, M.E. (1971). Holistic nursing. Nursing Clinics of North America, 6(2), 253–263.

Levine, M.E. (1989). The conservation principles of nursing: Twenty years later. In J. Riehl-Sisca (Ed.), Conceptual models for nursing practice (pp. 325–37). Norwalk, CT: Appleton & Lange.

Marlow, D., & Redding, B. (1988). Textbook of pediatric nursing (6th ed.). Philadelphia: W.B. Saunders.

Chapter
S I X

Neurological Intensive Monitoring System

Unit Assessment Tool

Barbara H. McCall, R.N., B.S.N.

Nursing theories and conceptual models were not an integral part of my nursing practice until I returned to school to obtain my Bachelor of Science degree. I was aware of the existence of conceptual models and nursing theories but had not attempted to use them during my 4 years of practice. My limited knowledge of and familiarity with the nursing models were in theory only, and I did not believe that one could actually use them to guide and direct nursing care in a medical-surgical setting. This unfounded belief was changed while I was a student at Thomas Jefferson University in Philadelphia.

As a student I was introduced to Levine's Conservation Model and was challenged to explore the use of the model in practice. This personal challenge has been met and has led to the development of an assessment tool that facilitates the identification of the nursing care needs of patients with epilepsy.

THE EPILEPSY PATIENT IN THE NEUROLOGICAL INTENSIVE MONITORING SYSTEM UNIT

Epilepsy is a chronic neurologic disorder that is defined by the repeated occurrence of seizures, which are symptomatic of cerebral dysfunction (Dieter, 1989; Santilli & Sierzvant, 1987). It affects approximately 2 million Americans, or an estimated 1 percent of the U.S. population (Dieter, 1989; Santilli & Sierzvant, 1987). More than 60 percent of individuals with epilepsy have been able to control their disorder using anticonvulsant medication (Friedman, 1988). The remaining 40 percent continue to have seizures and remain refractory to anticonvulsant medication.

The Neurological Intensive Monitoring System (NIMS) Unit at Graduate Hospital in Philadelphia is a five-bed unit that was designed specifically to monitor and evaluate seizure activity of epileptic patients. The ultimate goal of the NIMS Unit is to provide a definitive diagnosis of epilepsy and prescribe various treatments, including surgical intervention.

Many of the patients who are admitted to the NIMS Unit have had a history of refractory seizures for 2 or more years, with seizures occurring at least once a month. Our youngest patient was 5 years old, and the oldest close to 50. Many come from the Philadelphia area, and some come from as far as Virginia, Maine, and Michigan, seeking assistance in the management and control of their seizure disorders. Some of the patients are either unemployed or underemployed, while others are successful in their respective occupations and careers. They are the children of concerned parents, significant others of loving partners, and employees of interested employers, whose quality of life has been affected by epilepsy. Several of the patients have sustained significant physical injuries and experienced humiliating social embarrassments as a result of their continued seizure activity. The following case studies provide an expanded profile of the complex histories of patients with epilepsy admitted to the NIMS Unit. The names and other identifying data have been changed to protect the identity of the actual patient.

Case Presentation 6–1: Cornelius

Cornelius, a 42-year-old man with a history of medullary refractory epilepsy since age 8, was admitted to the NIMS Unit for a presurgical evaluation. Cornelius's first generalized seizure occurred at the age of 8 months, with recurrent convulsions at ages 8, 12, 15, and 16. He was treated with phenobarbital and primidone during his teenage years and was seizure free between ages 16 and 25. Recurring seizures began with either a déjà vu aura or no warning at all and quickly progressed to clonic-tonic activity and occasional tongue biting. His most recent seizures began without an aura, in these, he lost consciousness and had prolonged periods of blank staring. Often he engaged in complex acts such as walking around in circles, disrobing, crossing streets, and eventually finding himself in unfamiliar surroundings. Cornelius injured himself on many occasions, secondary to falls during seizures. Injuries included scalp lacerations, broken teeth, a broken wrist, and several rib fractures. Cornelius had no other significant medical history. He was single and had never married. He had moved to the Philadelphia area after completing college and had no close relatives in the immediate area. His significant others consisted of concerned neighbors and former coworkers, who often solicited medical attention when Cornelius had his seizures at home.

Cornelius is currently an unemployed computer operator who has lost several jobs due to the increased frequency and intensity of his seizures. His current medication schedule is 500 mg of valproic acid four times a day, and he is reported to be consistently compliant with his regimen. Most recently Cornelius has become involved in group activities with other epilepsy patients. As a result, he's had the opportunity to discuss his difficulties in maintaining employment and social relationships as a result of his epilepsy.

Case Presentation 6–2: Erika

Erika, a 33-year-old divorced housewife with three children, was referred to our unit by her children's school counselor because her increased seizure activity was interfering with her two school-age children's attendance at school. Erika began having seizures of unknown etiology in her early 20s. Her initial seizures began with a brief loss of consciousness and automatism of her hands and lips. Long postictal periods accompanied these seizures. Medical intervention and treatment with carbamazepine did not prevent her seizures from occurring. Erika's seizures began to increase in frequency and duration, such that hours elapsed, preventing her from performing her daily tasks of walking her children to school, assisting them with their homework assignments, and other parental tasks. Erika's children missed many days of school because of her epilepsy and because of their desire to stay at home to protect her and care for their younger sibling.

Erika was evaluated at the NIMS Unit and it was determined that she might benefit from a temporal lobectomy. It was hoped this would decrease the severity of her seizures and possibly eliminate their occurrences, thus improving Erika's and her children's quality of life. While Erika was admitted to our unit, her neighbors and church members cared for her children.

APPLICATION OF LEVINE'S CONSERVATION PRINCIPLES

Levine (1967, p. 13) defines a principle as a "fundamental concept that forms the basis for a chain of reasoning" and nursing principles as "fundamental assumptions which provide a unifying structure for understanding a wide variety of nursing activities." Levine's conservation principles have enabled me to understand my role as a nurse in the NIMS Unit and provided some theoretical reasoning for many of my nursing actions. Levine (1967) views the role of the nurse as a "keeping together function." The four conservation principles—(1) conservation of energy, (2) conservation of structural integrity, (3) conservation of personal integrity, and (4) conservation of social integrity—were developed to keep the biologic, personal, and social integrity of the patient in proper balance (Levine, 1967). They are guidelines to direct nursing actions and interventions.

The conservation principles were derived in part from adaptation theory. Levine (1971) views adaptation as a process of change and a method in which individuals can maintain their integrity in their own environment. In addition to "keeping together," nurses' functions also include the facilitation and promotion of adaptation (Fawcett, 1989). These functions are achieved by the provision of therapeutic or supportive nursing interventions. Therapeutic and supportive nursing interventions are respectively defined by Levine (1967) as actions that alter the course of adaptation and actions that cannot alter the course of adaptation but maintain the status quo.

Nursing plays a vital role in the evaluation and treatment of epilepsy. The nurses "keeping together function" is paramount in the NIMS Unit. A thorough nursing assessment is critical to the development and success of treatment plans.

Levine's (1967) conservation principles were used to develop a comprehensive assessment for the NIMS patient population. This tool was designed to obtain data crucial to meeting the physical and psychosocial needs of this specific population and facilitating successful adaptation (Table 6–1).

TABLE 6-1. ASSESSMENT TOOL

I Conservation of Energy
Nursing interventions are directed toward preserving and increasing one's energy potential.
  A Seizure Description
    1 How many seizures do you have per day, week, month?
    2 If you can, describe what you do before, during, and after a seizure?
    3 What medications are your currently taking to prevent and control your seizures?
    4 How often do you take your medication?
    5 When was the last time you took your medication?
  B Other Medical History
    1 Do you have a history of heart disease? Asthma? Diabetes?
    2 Do you take any other medication in addition to your seizure medication?
    3 Do you have any allergies to medicine, food, or the environment?
II Conservation of Structural Integrity
Nursing interventions are directed toward preserving and protecting the body from injury.
  A Safety Measures
    1 Have you sustained injuries as a result of a seizure?
    2 Do you lose consciousness during your seizures?
    3 Do you fall during your seizures?
    4 Do you wander during your seizures?
    5 Do you wear glasses?
    6 Do you smoke?
III Conservation of Personal Integrity
Nursing interventions are directed toward maintaining the patient's self-respect and dignity.
  A Personal History
    1 How old are you?
    2 How old were you when your first seizure occurred?
    3 How have seizures affected you (e.g., loss of job, loss of significant others, unable to drive, inability to bear children)?
    4 Have you lost control of your bowel or bladder during or after a seizure?
    5 How do you feel after you have had a seizure (tired, sleepy, embarrassed)?
    6 Is there any thing else you would like us to know about you or your seizures?

TABLE 6-1. *Continued*

IV Conservation of Social Integrity
  Nursing interventions should recognize and include significant others in the caring process.
  A Social History
    1 Who are your significant others?
    2 Who would you like us to call in case of an emergency?
    3 Do you expect to have visitors daily?
    4 Do you like being alone most of the time?
    5 Would you like to meet other patients who also have a history of seizures?

Conservation of Energy

Conservation of energy utilizes nursing interventions that are directed toward preserving and increasing one's energy potential. This enables the body to perform its functions and establish a natural defense against disease (Hirschfeld, 1976; Waterman-Taylor, 1989). In caring for an epilepsy patient, the nurse's primary goals are to prevent status epilepticus and maintain a patent airway. Status epilepticus (a state wherein continuous seizures occur) is a potential hazard for most NIMS patients. The patient's medications are methodically adjusted and lowered to achieve subtherapeutic blood levels that will eventually allow seizures to occur in this controlled setting. Respiratory distress, hypoxia, and aspiration of saliva are also potential hazards that are directly related to the occurrence of seizures. Knowing the frequency and type of seizures the patient has will allow the nurse to prevent these possible dangers. The assessment tool was also designed to ascertain other medical information that may contribute to the aforementioned dangers (Table 6-1).

One of the NIMS patients did not have seizures for a long period of time. After admission, her medications were eventually discontinued, and her phenytoin sodium level dropped to 5 μg per ml, at which point she began to have seizures. When the seizures occurred (four within a 12-hour period) the nurse notified the physician and recommended that her phenytoin sodium be reordered to prevent the potential occurrence of status epilepticus. Respiratory equipment, oxygen, and an oral airway were placed in the room in anticipation of respiratory distress. Nursing interventions in this particular situation were therapeutic. The nurse intervened to conserve energy for this patient by restoring her anticonvulsants and securing emergency respiratory equipment to prevent status epilepticus and respiratory distress.

Conservation of Structural Integrity

Conservation of structural integrity focuses upon the anatomic structure and physiologic function of the body. Nursing interventions are guided to preserve and protect the body from damage and injury. Therapeutic and supportive nursing actions that will maintain the structure of the body are primary. Protecting the patient from injury is foremost when working with patients who have seizures. Impairment or loss of consciousness occurs in most of our seizure patients, and many falls and bodily injuries have resulted. Caring for a NIMS patient requires that safety precautions be instituted at the time of admission to prevent or reduce the probability of injuries during hospitalization. Standard precautions include carpeted floors in the patient's rooms and the hallway, and padded side rails in an upright position at all times. Additional precautions may include a posey vest at all times and/or a 24-hour companion (usually a close relative or friend) (Table 6–1). Smoking is permissible in the NIMS Unit if it can be determined that the person will not be a potential threat to the safety of others and with the understanding that smoking occurs in the presence of a nurse.

Cornelius required a posey vest during his admission. His previous history of multiple falls, resulting in a fractured wrist and ribs, was the basis for this therapeutic intervention. He did not wear glasses and he was a nonsmoker, thus minimizing the potential for additional injuries.

Conservation of Personal Integrity

Conservation of personal integrity is primarily centered around retaining the individual's identity (Fawcett, 1989). It is important that nursing interventions are provided in a manner that maintains the self-respect and dignity of patients. This is especially important when caring for patients with epilepsy. Many patients have come to the unit with altered personal integrities and poor self-concepts as a result of the general public's misconceptions regarding epilepsy and their behaviors as a consequence of their misconceptions. The nurse can be instrumental in preserving the personal integrities of these individuals by closing the curtains and doors when the patient is having a seizure, covering exposed body parts, and assisting with personal care after the patient becomes fully conscious. Fecal and urinary incontinence is not an uncommon occurrence after generalized seizures and can contribute to the loss of self-respect and personal dignity if not attended to in a gingerly but expedient fashion. Persons who have complex partial seizures have been reported to do some unusual things such as disrobing and rearranging furniture (Epilepsy Foundation of America, 1981). This can result in a great deal of humiliation if carried out in public places.

Prior knowledge of these activities and how it affects the patient can assist the nurse in his or her interpersonal interactions, whereby the nurse can allow patients to talk about how they feel about their disorder and how it has affected them, and can help them begin to work on overcoming some of the prejudices associated with epilepsy. These nursing interventions are viewed as supportive, for they do not change outcomes. Nursing provides a sounding board for these individuals. Referring the individuals for counseling and therapy are deemed therapeutic, for they may eventually effect change. Both Erika and Cornelius came to the unit with altered personal integrities. Erika perceived that she was an unfit mother because she was unable to care for her children properly as a result of her epilepsy. Cornelius had had many social embarrassments at work. He now avoids social contacts and has become a social recluse.

TABLE 6-2. NURSING CARE PLAN

Integrity	Goal	Nursing Interventions
Conservation of energy		
Potential for alteration in neurologic status	To prevent status epilepticus	Alert physician of seizure occurrence (S*)
		Document movements, duration frequency (S)
		Administer anticonvulsants as ordered (T†)
		Monitor therapeutic laboratory values (S)
Potential for alteration in respiratory status	To establish/maintain a patent airway during seizure	Properly position patient in a side-lying position during seizure (T)
	To ensure adequate oxygenation during seizure	Maintain nasal oxygen set-up, breathing bag, and oral airway at bedside (S & T)
		Administer oxygen as ordered (T)
Conservation of structural integrity		
Potential for bodily injury and harm	To prevent bodily harm and injuries secondary to seizures	Lower patient to floor or bed during seizure (T)
		Do not restrain limbs (S)
		Maintain padded side rails (S)
		Apply posey vest if patient is known to fall during seizures (T)
		Supervise smoking (S)
Conservation of personal integrity		
Potential/actual altered self-concept secondary to diagnosis of epilepsy	Patient will discuss how seizures have affected him/her	Active listening (S)
		Refer to social worker, psychologist, counselor (T)
Potential/actual altered self-concept secondary to behaviors associated with seizures (i.e., incontinence, automation, loss of consciousness)	Maintenance of privacy and personal dignity during seizures	Close curtains/doors to exclude general hospital environment (T)
		Cover exposed body parts (T)
		Update/inform patients of activities (S)
Conservation of social integrity		
Potential/actual altered family dynamics during hospitalization	To maintain frequent family contact and support during hospitalization	Encourage family members to visit (S)
		Provide visiting hours for family (S)
		Be flexible with visiting hours and curfew (S)
Potential/actual alterations in social interactions during hospitalizations	To socialize with other patients	Introduce all patients to each other upon admission (S)
	To actually engage in therapeutics activities (i.e., card games, puzzles, handicrafts)	Establish time for group activities and interactions (S)
		Provide board games, puzzles, and handicrafts
		Document social interactions (S)

Note: Trophicognosis is defined by Levine as a nursing care judgment arrived at by the scientific method of data collection; commonly known as nursing diagnosis.
*S = Supportive nursing interventions.
†T = Therapeutic nursing interventions.

Conservation of Social Integrity

The last principle of *conservation* is concerned with the *social integrity* of the individual. Levine (1971) states that "every individual is defined by his social group and often the integrity of the patient is intimately intertwined in the fabric of his cultural, ethnic, religion and family relationships" (p. 260). Nursing actions should recognize and include the family in the caring process and promote social interactions in the hospital environment. The NIMS patient would view the application of this integrity as the most important. The extensive monitoring equipment limits the patient's mobility. In addition to limited mobility, the patient is always in a private room, and hospitalization can be extended up to 6 weeks. All of these can lead to behaviors that are directly related to this often isolated and confining setting. Without concerted efforts from the nursing staff to encourage family visitation and social interaction among admitted patients, the social integrity of the NIMS patient would be totally neglected. There are plans in the near future to have a recreation room with the video monitoring and electroencephalogram equipment added to the unit to facilitate socialization and fraternization among the epilepsy patients. This prevents the loss of vital information while enhancing the social integrity of the patients. The NIMS Unit staff has documented that the patients want to meet with others who have the same disorder. They do not like being isolated and need to have some therapeutic activities to keep them busy during this evaluation period. It is expected that this group interaction will strengthen patients' identity and self-concept.

Levine's holistic view of the individual provides a framework for nursing to render holistic and comprehensive care using the conservation principles (Fawcett, 1989). This assessment tool using Levine's Conservation Model helps the nursing staff collect data in a systematic and methodical manner, while planning the treatment and care plans for a specific patient population (Table 6–2).

REFERENCES

Dieter, D.C. (1989). Corpus colostomy: The role of the nurse in family decision-making. Journal of Neuroscience Nursing, 21(4), 234–239.

Epilepsy Foundation of America. (1981). How to recognize and classify seizures. Landover, MD: Epilepsy Foundation of America.

Fawcett, J. (1989). Analysis and evaluation of conceptual models of nursing (2nd ed.). Philadelphia: F.A. Davis.

Friedman, D. (1988). Controlling epilepsy with surgery. RN, 2, 52–53.

Hirschfeld, M.J. (1976). The cognitively impaired older adult. American Journal of Nursing, 12, 1981–1984.

Levine, M.E. (1967). The four conservation principles of nursing. Nursing Forum, 6(1), 45–59.

Levine, M.E. (1971). Holistic nursing. Nursing Clinics of North America, 6(2), 253–264.

Santilli, N., & Sierzvant, T.L. (1987). Advances in the treatment of epilepsy. Journal of Neuroscience Nursing, 19(3), 141–155.

Waterman-Taylor, J. (1989). Levine conservation principles using the model for nursing diagnosis in a neurological setting. In J.P. Riehl-Sisca (Ed.), Conceptual models for nursing practice (3rd ed.). Norwalk, CT: Appleton & Lange.

Chapter
SEVEN

Care of the Burn Patient

Elizabeth W. Bayley, R.N., Ph.D.

A burn injury is the most complex form of trauma. A catastrophic event, it challenges all those who of necessity or desire seek to become involved. A major burn wound ultimately affects all organ systems and has the potential to alter every facet of the person's being.

Because of the broad spectrum of responses to thermal trauma, a holistic approach to the individual incurring this injury seems imperative. Because the logic of all human experience tells us that health is defined by wholeness, the nurse's actions with regard to the burn patient must be guided by a conceptual model that respects the essential integrities of the human being. Levine's Conservation Model fulfills this requirement (Levine, 1973).

As a nurse concerned with the burn patient, and as part of a team engaged in returning that individual to health or wholeness, I have purposefully sought a nursing model that affords that holistic perspective and complements the models of medicine, physiology, psychology, sociology, and the many other disciplines involved in understanding and treating the burned individual. As a teacher, I believe that Levine's model is an excellent heuristic, affording a comprehensive perspective on the assessments, diagnoses, interventions, and evaluations that burn nurses must perform.

CURRENT PRACTICE SETTING

People with burn injuries are cared for in a wide variety of practice settings. Initial care is provided in the prehospital arena by mobile intensive care nurses, paramedics, and flight nurses, working adjacent to a burning house, amid the noise and debris of an industrial explosion, or out on a highway in the dark of night. Emergency nurses are responsible for assessing and triaging one or more victims from a single injury-producing scenario and beginning resuscitation and stabilization activities. They assist in providing immediate care and instruction to those with minor burns, and transfer more severely injured patients to the most appropriate definitive care setting.

The settings may include surgical intensive care units, medical surgical intermediate units, or regional burn units. These units are characterized by a high level of technology and may expose the burn patient to hemodynamic monitors, ventilators, fluid pumps, hydrotherapy tanks, operating suites, warming lamps, cooling blankets, and myriad paraphernalia to support life and limb. Adding to the complexity is a constant parade of care providers—primary nurses; plastic surgeons; pulmonary specialists; physical, occupational, and respiratory therapists; dietitians; social workers; psychologists; and distraught family members.

PATIENTS IN THE SETTING

The patients in burn care settings, with the exception of those who attempt self-immolation, are uniformly surprised that within minutes their lives have dramatically changed. What appear to be innocuous everyday events such as making an early morning cup of tea, watching television while smoking a cigarette in the evening, setting up a household repair project, hosting a barbecue, or going out to play with a classmate turn into major catastrophes with long-range implications.

Immediately, the patient's structural integrity is interrupted as the heat source sears the skin, causing an intense physiologic response involving inflammation, fluid shifts, visceral organ dysfunction, and perhaps shock. Body energy sources are summoned to provide for accelerated cellular processes, maintain body warmth despite loss of the protective skin covering, and thwart the invasion of microscopic pathogens.

Pain, the fear of death or disfigurement or both, and disruption of the activities that define the individual threaten personal integrity. Concern for family and coworkers and the ability to cope and carry out expected roles are uppermost in the patient's mind, undermining his or her social integrity. Further, the majority of patients (76 percent) are victims of their own actions (National Burn Information Exchange, 1983). This only adds to their burden of guilt, self-condemnation, and being blamed by others. As the burn impinges on each aspect of the individual's life, Levine's conservation principles become increasingly relevant in providing a framework for the nurse's assessment.

Case Presentation 7–1: Barbara

"An individual cannot be understood outside of the context of (her) predicament of time and place" (Levine, 1989, p. 326). Barbara's encounter with a severe burn injury occurred as the following scenario unfolded. She arrived at her grandparents' seashore trailer home for a summer vacation, shortly after completing her eighth-grade studies in a distant state. A bright, tall, obese 13-year-old, Barbara looked forward to attending a family wedding with her grandparents the following weekend. As she lounged in the living room in a long fleece housecoat, Barbara had no idea that within minutes her life would be in jeopardy and her plans for the future abruptly changed.

A sudden explosion of unknown cause occurred, and a flash of flames ignited Barbara's clothing. Within seconds, dense smoke filled the room. Sirens sounded and firemen quickly discovered Barbara on the floor of the trailer's front room. Before she realized what was happening, Barbara was placed in an ambulance and immediately transported to the local hospital's emergency room.

Signs of inhalation injury, including singed nasal hairs and labored breathing, were noted and oxygen was started en route. Upon admission to the emergency department, two intravenous lines were started; nurses began to deliver large volumes of lactated Ringer's solution to avert burn shock. A quick assessment revealed that at least 30 percent of Barbara's body was covered with partial- or full-thickness burns.

During these early postinjury moments, Barbara's operational environment was most threatening because of the presence of carbon monoxide and other toxic gases inhaled with each breath in the closed-space fire and because of the many microorganisms—on her own body and on the hands and equipment of her care providers—eager to invade her denuded integument. Perceptually, she was assaulted by the noise of sirens, the searing heat of open flames, the movement of air currents on raw nerve endings in her skin, and the noxious odors produced by the burning trailer. The air-conditioned ambulance and emergency department, examination lights, and sound of unfamiliar voices were additional sensory factors. Conceptually, Barbara's thoughts were clouded by the effects of carboxyhemoglobin, the inability to interpret hospital jargon, feeling alone with strangers, the invasion of her privacy, and a great deal of anxiety and fear.

USE OF LEVINE'S CONSERVATION PRINCIPLES

Conservation of Energy.   Although individuals conserve their energy, even at perfect rest, energy from life-sustaining activities, such as biochemical changes, is expended. Immediately after burn injury, the patient enters a severely catabolic state, manifested by elevated metabolic rate, increased protein mobilization, and gluconeogenesis. Up to 5000 calories per day may be needed to meet the body's energy requirements and even aggressive nutritional therapy may not forestall some degree of weight loss (Burdge, Conkright, & Ruberg, 1986). The body must move from anabolism, in which energy is stored, to catabolism, in which energy is used. "The resting metabolic expenditure increases linearly, until a burn of 40 to 50% of body surface area has a metabolic rate of about twice normal" (Burdge et al., 1986, p. 49).[1]

Hormonal alterations are thought to account for the hypermetabolic response to burn injury. An increase in catecholamines, an initial decrease and then an increase in insulin production, and an increase in glucagon production are known to occur. Also significant for energy utilization is a reset of the body's core temperature to 38° to 39°C.

The nursing assessment of parameters related to conservation of energy focuses initially on body temperature, body fluid balance, hemodynamic status, tissue oxygenation, and stressful stimuli. Barbara's rectal temperature was 36.6°C. Vital signs included a rapid pulse, rapid respirations, and a normal blood pressure. The urine output had been 30 ml for the past hour.

Because inhalation injury was suspected, blood gases were drawn. Results demonstrated acidemia and metabolic acidosis with compensation. The alveolar-arterial oxygen gradient was over 600. Barbara complained of pain in areas of partial-thickness burn.

Barbara's initial nursing care needs included providing for an adequate airway and tissue oxygenation, replacing body fluids, preventing hypothermia, and monitoring systemic responses to the burn injury. Initial nursing measures were oriented toward helping Barbara adapt to physiologic alterations and supporting her body's response to trauma.

On subsequent days, while Barbara was cared for in the surgical unit, additional assessments were made to determine nutritional status, muscle mass and muscle strength, patterns of rest and comfort, mobility, functional ability, and activity tolerance. Albumin and prealbumin levels, daily caloric intake, and daily weights were monitored. A gradual loss of muscle mass and strength were noted as Barbara's weight decreased by 10 percent of her preburn hefty 85 kg.

Nursing care was aimed at maintaining Barbara's body mass through enteral and parenteral protein, carbohydrate, and fat; maintaining joint function through range-of-motion exercises; and helping her adapt to increased energy needs by spacing stressful activities, providing for short periods of undisturbed rest, reducing pain, and gradually increasing her activity level.

Barbara's pain and general discomfort, both metabolic stressors, varied with peaks occurring at the time of dressing changes and exercise. Therapeutic interventions included providing a narcotic analgesic prior to wound care and teaching Barbara relaxation exercises. By concentrating on specific breathing patterns and visual images during wound care procedures Barbara was able to gain better control over her pain. She tolerated brief walks with assistance fairly well, but tired when sitting up for more than 45 minutes. Verbal encouragement from the staff was therapeutic in increasing Barbara's time out of bed, in small increments, each day.

Meanwhile, her ventilatory status improved and Pao$_2$ remained above 70 mm Hg with an oxygen flow rate of 40 percent. Following fluid resuscitation, titrated to keep pace with fluids lost into the interstitial spaces due to capillary leaking, Barbara diuresed large amounts of fluid for 2 days. This indicated that capillaries had regained their integrity and that cardiac and renal functions were adequate.

Conservation of Structural Integrity.   Wholeness implies structural continuity. The body strives to restore continuity to an injured part through the processes of healing. The adaptive ability to heal is fundamental to all nursing interventions in the care of the burn patient; however, the biologic priority placed on structural continuity may, in itself, create serious damage.

Assessment of the structural integrity of the burn patient begins with an evaluation of the depth and extent of burn surface area. Barbara's legs, her right foot, and portions of her back and right buttocks were covered with mixed partial-and full-thickness burns. Her wounds drained extensive amounts of plasma, indicative of cellular damage.

The uninterrupted continuity of the body surface is the best protection against invasion by microorganisms. When the continuity is compromised by a burn wound, nursing care must support the individual's immune defenses and provide therapeutic interventions to protect the person from infection. Barbara's nursing care, therefore, included careful asepsis (as when doing invasive procedures and changing dressings), application of topical antibacterials, administration of intravenous antibiotics, and attention to critical protective behaviors, including hand washing.

Of particular concern was the potential for invasive burn wound sepsis. The nurses frequently assessed the character of Barbara's wounds, including color, drainage, odor, presence of exudate, and quality of surrounding skin. These assessments were supplemented with wound cultures twice a week. Support of the depressed immune system were assisted with adequate protein and caloric intake to provide for the formation of red and white blood cells and immunoglobulins.

The human body maintains its structural integrity best when the individual is able to move freely. Restriction of musculoskeletal freedom due to such factors as constricting edema, pain, or bulky dressings can result in structural damage. The nursing goals that support physiologic and anatomic functioning are designed to conserve structural integrity and include the prevention of pressure sores, contractures, atelectasis, and other hazards of malposition and immobility.

Because she was found in a closed space, Barbara was examined closely for signs of disruption of her pulmonary system. Labored breathing and flaring of the nostrils were noted on admission. Observation of her oronasal passages and pharynx, auscultation of the lungs, evaluation of blood gases, fiberoptic bronchoscopy, and chest x-ray examination revealed that Barbara had sustained significant injury to her upper and lower airways from the toxic products of combustion. Barbara was put on a volume-cycled ventilator with a tidal volume of 1300 and a respiratory rate of 18 to ensure adequate ventilation and blood oxygenation.

Peripheral tissue perfusion was assessed every hour using a Doppler device to detect finger and toe pulses. Tissue pressure was measured in Barbara's right foot. As circumferential edema increased, tissue pressure decreased and circulation was compromised, necessitating an escharotomy of this limb.

A complete physical assessment and hematology studies indicated that Barbara was otherwise in good health. Her vital signs and urine output and her mental status indicated that her circulatory, renal, and brain functions were normal. Hematologic studies revealed a high hemoglobin and hematocrit and serum potassium, initially, with the usual decrease in these parameters once fluid resuscitation was underway. Therapeutic nursing interventions included providing blood component therapy and potassium supplements over the course of Barbara's hospitalization.

Conservation of Personal Integrity. Levine (1989) notes that people try to define their identity, both in the hidden, very private person who dwells within and in the public face assumed in relationships with others. Conservation of personal integrity involves preserving the patient's right to privacy, dignity, and honest responses. Assessment begins with learning as much as one can about the person, including age, race, religion, educational background, occupation, skills, and intellectual level. The nurse identifies how patients respond to and cope with their current situation and how they perceive themselves. Feelings such as anxiety and fear, health beliefs, loss of control, values related to physical appearance, and self-concept must be assessed. Further information on spiritual beliefs, aspirations for the future, knowledge of the burn injury and its consequences, and past ability to handle stress is also useful in planning nursing interventions.

Barbara was an honor roll student, but she had a rather poor self-image due to her obesity. She verbalized feeling grateful that her face and arms were not burned and recognized that she had attractive facial features. However, as with most burn victims, the results of her injury would be visually apparent and lifelong. This was reinforced when she went to the hydrotherapy tub each day and witnessed the extent to which the surface that enclosed her body had been destroyed.

The ways in which visible handicaps alter psychologic and social functioning are powerful and important (Bernstein, 1976). Our own beauty or ugliness figure in the image others build up about us, which will be taken back into ourselves (in forming our self-concept). Nursing interventions such as helping Barbara to wash and comb her hair, suggesting that she wear her own clothes during her intensive rehabilitation, and planning a surprise party and cake for her August birthday were all therapeutic measures designed to bolster Barbara's self-esteem and identity as a unique and worthy individual.

Despite being heavy, Barbara was fairly active and enjoyed field hockey and lacrosse, playing on her school teams. This facet of her personality was of major importance in helping Barbara work hard to accomplish an aggressive exercise regimen and accept the view that her future functional ability could be comparable to the past if she followed through with prescribed therapy. In efforts to assist Barbara adapt to her burn injury, the nurses were aware that the ultimate goal was self-acceptance (i.e., the extent to which self-concept is congruent with the individual's description of his or her ideal self).

As a young adolescent, Barbara was often moody and "into herself." She seemed to identify with and developed a very trusting relationship with a staff nurse and one of the physical therapists. She shared more of her private feelings with them than with other members of the staff. According to Levine (1989), the most generous psychologic approach is to "limit the recording of confidences to only those generalizations that actually make a difference in the choice of treatment plans" (p. 334). This suggestion, coupled with allowing her to make decisions whenever possible, were primary supportive nursing goals conserving her personal integrity.

Conservation of Social Integrity.   Conservation of social integrity recognizes each person as a social being involved in dependent relationships with others. The integrity of a burn patient such as Barbara is intimately interwoven in the fabric of her cultural, ethnic, religious, and family relationships. The nursing assessment related to this conservation principle included interviewing Barbara and her parents and grandparents about her extended family, her role in the family, her peer group, the family's roles in the community, and their employment situations. Barbara's mother is a homemaker, separated from Barbara's father, a high school math teacher. He is employed during the summer vacation as the recreation director for the township and rents a room from another family during that time.

Barbara has two older brothers, both married and living in other states. Barbara's mother and grandparents stayed in a small apartment during the weeks after the trailer fire and commuted over an hour to visit Barbara each day. Her father visited only on weekends. Additional assessment data revealed that there was adequate third-party hospitalization insurance for Barbara's illness but little coverage for outpatient rehabilitation and follow-up care.

Barbara had two close girlfriends who frequently sent cards to her. Once weaned from the ventilator she expressed a desire to see her friends, but because of distance this was not possible. To support her peer relationships, the nursing staff suggested that her friends make tape recordings for her, and whenever a tape arrived Barbara could send a short message back. Her athletic coach also wrote to her, assuring her of a place on the team when she was able.

As noted by Levine (cited in Fawcett, 1989), the patient's family may be deeply affected by the changes resulting from illness. Indeed, Barbara's grandparents, who were out shopping at the time of the explosion, blamed themselves for her injury, feeling that the electrical wiring that triggered the explosion should have been repaired earlier. As a result, they were very solicitous of her every whim and sometimes acted at cross purposes to the burn team's plan to help Barbara become more independent in her daily activities.

To help her family adapt to the burn injury, the nursing staff included Barbara's mother and grandparents in planning her care. They restated the reasons why it was better to let her struggle to do things independently, no matter how painful and slow her progress seemed. Helping the family define their role during Barbara's hospitalization and making them feel that they belonged at her bedside were important. Providing emotional support, learning about burn injury and long-term care, setting realistic expectations, providing positive reinforcement for accomplishments, keeping Barbara in touch with the outside world, and helping her with diversional activities were major roles for the family.

From the beginning of Barbara's hospitalization, Barbara's mother was given information on the usual healing process with burn wounds. Over time, she learned how to do the required wound care, apply pressure garments to areas at risk for hypertrophic scars, and to perform the necessary exercises for Barbara's legs. The nurses showed their concern for the mother by letting her know it was all right for her to take a break from the grueling daily visits and go home for several days. This was only possible when she trusted the nurses to call her if problems arose.

Barbara's father was also kept informed and involved to the extent possible. At the staff's suggestion, he brought Barbara her favorite fast-food milkshakes every weekend—a treat she looked forward to as her healing progressed. These milkshakes also drew approval from the dietitian due to their high-calorie, high-protein content, essentials for healing. Because he saw her only weekly, Barbara's father was also most instrumental in pointing out to her the progress she was making. He was able to bring Barbara news of school happenings, which linked her to her peer group. Her grandparents kept her supplied with colored markers and drawing paper, which Barbara used to make the cartoons she enjoyed drawing and putting on the wall at the head of her bed.

Community support systems and provision for follow-up care are important factors in the nursing assessment. A home care service was able to help Barbara with her continued exercise regimen for a short period after hospitalization. Arrangements were made for home-tutoring for the month of September, after which Barbara would be able to return to school. Burn center nurses planned with Barbara's school nurse to provide a videotape about burn prevention and care, to be shown to Barbara's classmates prior to her return to school. These therapeutic interventions were instrumental in influencing Barbara's adaptation to her injury in a positive way.

SUMMARY

The nursing interventions described earlier were just a few of the many activities that were planned to establish a stable internal environment and energy-sparing condition for Barbara. Therapeutic and supportive measures were planned to help equip this burned person to "confront, and often correct, a wide spectrum of environmental challenges" (Levine, 1989, p. 329). In addition, Barbara was able to select stimuli from the environment, including information, other people's responses to her injury, the burn teams' necessary but sometimes painful treatments, and the family's loving attention, and convert them into experiences that were meaningful and integrated with her adaptive abilities.

The rewards in caring for individuals with burn injury are fostered by viewing those persons from the perspective of Levine's model. The long-term relationship with one's patient allows ample opportunity to know each aspect of the person in great depth and to see the beauty of the integration of all facets of that individual's being. Levine (1989) states, "Reaching out to find the humanity of another person arises from the willful anticipation of both" (p. 336). When assessments are guided by the conservation principles and nursing interventions are planned to effect and support adaptation to the crisis presented by severe burns, both nurse and patient have the optimal opportunity for growth and success.

REFERENCES

Bernstein, N.R. (1976). Emotional care of the facially burned and disfigured. Boston: Little, Brown & Co.

Burdge, J.J., Conkright, J.M., & Ruberg, R.L. (1986). Nutritional and metabolic consequences of thermal injury. Clinics in Plastic Surgery, 13(1), 49–55.

Fawcett, J. (1989). Analysis and evaluation of conceptual models of nursing (2nd ed.). Philadelphia: F. A. Davis.

Levine, M.E. (1973). Introduction to clinical nursing (2nd ed.). Philadelphia: F.A. Davis.

Levine, M.E. (1989). The four conservation principles: Twenty years later. In J.P. Riehl-Sisca (Ed.), Conceptual models for nursing practice (3rd ed.) (pp. 325–338). Norwalk, CT: Appleton & Lange.

National Burn Information Exchange. (1983, August). Newsletter, 2(1). Ann Arbor, MI: National Institute for Burn Medicine.

NOTE

1. Thermal injury results in an increase in capillary permeability. This vascular change is limited to the burned area in smaller burns, but in burns over 30 percent of body surface area the change occurs throughout the body. Plasma, proteins, and electrolytes leak out of the vascular compartment into the interstitial tissues, producing edema and a decreased circulating blood volume. Cardiac output also decreases. There is some loss of red cell mass as a result of thermal injury. Because the loss of noncellular elements is, however, much more rapid, the red cell concentration increases proportionately, elevating the hematocrit and blood viscosity.

The extravasation of plasma peaks at about 12 hours postinjury; within 36 hours postinjury the capillaries usually regain their integrity, permitting plasma fluid to return to the vascular compartment from the interstitial tissues. Early fluid resuscitation with crystalloids, later supplemented with colloids, is essential to maintain vascular volume, increase cardiac output, and maintain blood pressure and the perfusion of vital organs. Several resuscitation formulas, based on body weight and percent of body surface area burned, are available to help estimate patient needs. However, the individual's response to fluid therapy is the most important indicator of fluid needs. Continuous assessment of vital signs, urine output, mentation, and pulmonary function are required. Serum sodium, potassium, urea, and osmolality and urinary sodium, potassium, and osmolality may also be followed. A urine output of 30 to 50 ml per hour usually indicates adequate fluid intake. Hemodynamic monitoring may be used, particularly in patients who are elderly or who appear to have cardiovascular or renal compromise.

E I G H T

Chronic Pain Management

Angela Pasco, R.N., M.S.N.
Debra Halupa, R.N., M.S.N.

The use of Levine's conservation principles (Levine, 1967) became a fact of clinical practice during graduate school experience. Full appreciation of the principles' versatility and adaptability in a variety of clinical patient care situations evolved with repeated successful application.

Our personal philosophy of nursing emphasized the importance of caring for the "whole" patient and reflected the basic concepts of Levine's model (1971). Concern for how the cancer patient's chronic pain would affect family dynamics and fulfillment of prescribed roles or how the arthritic patient could cope with the physical demands of a job necessitated a nursing approach that considered the patient in relation to his or her environment. Levine (1989) stated, "The environment necessarily completes the wholeness of the individual" (p. 325). Levine's conservation principles provided the rubrics of a framework for holistic practice. Incorporating the conservation principles into the philosophy behind practice provided structure for our nursing care and the basis for all therapeutic and supportive nursing interventions.

PRACTICE SETTING

The patient experiencing chronic pain can be found in many settings. Since the hospital is our current practice setting, nursing care must be planned to facilitate adaptation of these patients in this and other environments such as home or job. In our attempts to assist patients with chronic pain to conserve energy and structural, personal, and social integrities, we create an environment that enables the patients to deal with their pain on a daily basis.

CHRONIC PAIN

Pain is one of life's paradoxes. "It is real, regardless of its cause. It is whatever the person experiencing it says it is and exists whenever he says it does" (McCaffrey, 1979, p. 11). Pain is so personal and private that each person's experience is unique. It can affect the individual's perception of self and create a deficit in his or her personal integrity. Yet, no definition of pain is ever completely satisfactory. An understanding of the physiologic basis of pain can provide some insight to patient responses.[1] Formulation of interventions appropriate for chronic pain management can be based on an understanding of the differences in the physiologic nature of pain and the meaning that pain has for the patient.

Sternbach (1968) has recommended thinking of chronic pain as a pattern of responses that operate to protect the organism from harm. This pattern is a response of the whole organism to that which is harming or threatening harm.

Chronic pain associated with cancer and other debilitating chronic diseases such as arthritis elicits both physiologic and behavioral responses in the individual. In addition to sensory perceptions, the patient can experience apathy, withdrawal, hopelessness, helplessness, anxiety, fear, anger, depression, irritability, preoccupation with self, and lack of satisfaction with life, all of which can intensify the pain experience (Meinhart & McCaffrey, 1983). These responses represent deficits in energy and in structural, personal, and social integrity and can reduce the patient's ability to actively interpret and integrate internal and external environmental information associated with chronic pain. The interactions of all body systems may be disrupted and the quality of the patient's protective organismic responses diminished.

Chronic pain provokes action of all protective systems. The activation stage of the pain response implies a perceptual awareness that initiates the fight-or-flight sympathetic response. During the rebound stage, the organism attempts to modulate the effect of acute pain through a parasympathetic response. However, in chronic pain this cannot occur. After prolonged pain, an adaptation of sorts takes place. The body no longer exhibits sympathetic responses ("Nursing Now: Pain," 1985). Physiologic indicators such as blood pressure and heart rate appear normal, but the patient continues to experience pain (Foley, 1985). Gradual changes in structural integrity produce a loss of adaptive energy. Uncontrolled chronic pain stresses the patient's adaptive response, compromising the well-being of the patient.

Because chronic pain is an intensely personal experience, each patient's unique physiologic, psychologic, social, spiritual, and cultural attributes influence his or her pain experiences and responses. Whether arthritic patients perceive their pain as a punishment to be stoically endured or cancer patients relate their meaningless pain as an antecedent to death will affect how assessment data are interpreted and interventions implemented. Consideration of (1) the physical basis of the pain, (2) the meaning of the pain to the individual, (3) the context of the situation in which the pain is encountered, and (4) the individual's past experiences with pain will assist the nurse in understanding chronic pain as a pattern of individual responses. The pain behaviors are the result of the response of the whole organism (Benoliel & Crowley, 1974), influenced and shaped by all that is unique to the patient.

Yet preconceived notions, attitudes, and prejudices concerning how an individual should respond to pain can influence care and compromise adaptation. The physical, psychologic, and cognitive components of the chronic pain experience must be considered if conservation of the patient's energy and structural, personal, and social integrity is to be achieved.

USE OF LEVINE'S CONSERVATION PRINCIPLES

Collection of pain assessment data can be facilitated through the use of the chronic pain assessment tool developed by the authors (Table 8–1). Appropriate interventions based on the conservation principles (Levine, 1967) can be quickly implemented, using this structured framework.

Levine (1967) states that when "nursing intervention can alter the course of the adaptation so that it is a good one, the nurse is acting in a therapeutic sense" (p. 47). Adaptation for the patient suffering with chronic pain involves a series of responses influenced by past, present, and future circumstances. These responses are determined by the patient as favorable or unfavorable. The nurse intervenes, guided by the patient-interpreted response, to promote what Levine (1989) terms "a state of conservation or homeostasis" (p. 329).

The nursing act in pain management is conservation, and the patient act is adaptation. The goal of the professional nurse is to conserve energy; conserve structural, personal, and social integrity; and promote holism. Necessary interventions can be performed in relation to Levine's conservation principles that can alter the patient's adaptation to chronic pain. Nurses can, therefore, help break the cycle of chronic pain and anxiety.

Many patients interpret pain as suffering or a threat to their well-being. Chronic pain creates anxiety and fear of the unknown. The sympathetic responses associated with anxiety only serve to increase the pain experience and deplete energy sources. "Survival depends on the adaptive ability to use responses that cost the least to the individual in expense of effort and demand on his or her well-being" (Levine, 1989, p. 329). If the patient's expenditure of energy exceeds the available energy resources, physical and mental deterioration can ensue.

"Structural change results in a change of function, and pathophysiological processes present a threat to structural integrity" (Levine, 1967, p. 50). Chronic pain is an example of such a threat to structural integrity. Patients with chronic pain may not perceive an end to their pain. It may be interpreted as a sign of deterioration or poor prognosis; therefore, patients feel pain more intensely. This, in turn, intensifies physiologic and psychologic deterioration with a resultant increase of stress and associated anxiety. Pain becomes the patients' primary focus and overshadows all aspects of life. It can impede their ability to perform activities of daily living. The

TABLE 8-1. CHRONIC PAIN ASSESSMENT TOOL: SUBJECTIVE DATA GUIDE*

Assessment of altered energy levels

1. How long have you had this pain?
2. Does your pain cause you to have difficulty breathing?
3. Has this pain affected your normal eating habits?
   How many meals do you eat during the day?
   What are your meals composed of?
4. Does your pain affect your ability to carry out activities of daily living?
5. Are you able to walk unassisted?
   How far are you able to walk?
6. Are you able to get out of bed to use the toilet, or do you use a bedpan?
7. Does this pain affect your ability to sleep?
   How many hours of uninterrupted sleep are you able to get?
   Do you feel better or worse upon arising?
   Are you able to nap?
   Do you require medication or other therapeutic measures to sleep?
8. How does the pain affect your ability to concentrate?
9. Does this pain interfere with daily plans you have made?
10. Have you experienced fever or infection?

Assessment of altered structural integrity

1. Where is your pain?
2. How would you describe your pain?
3. When do you have pain?
   How long does your pain last?
   Is there any time during the day that your pain is less?
4. What makes your pain worse?
5. How do you rate the intensity of your pain (use visual analog scale)?
6. What do you do to relieve your pain (list medications and other modalities)?
   Do these methods relieve your pain?
7. Do prescribed treatments make your pain better or worse (e.g., radiation, chemotherapy, physical therapy, occupational therapy)?
8. Has this pain caused other symptoms to occur such as:

   Nausea
   Vomiting
   Constipation
   Diarrhea
   Excessive sweating
   Difficulty urinating
   Headache
   Fainting
   Rashes

9. Have you lost or gained weight since this pain began?
10. Has your pain caused decreased movement?
11. Has your pain ever caused you to injure yourself?

Assessment of altered personal integrity

1. Has your pain affected the way you feel about yourself?
2. Describe how this pain makes you feel?

*Tool developed by D. Halupa, R.N., M.S.N., and A. Pasco, R.N., M.S.N., 1989.

Table 8-1. *Continued*

Angry
Frustrated
Dependent
Sad
Worthless
Guilty
Burdensome
Lonely
Anxious
Fearful

3. Has your pain affected your ability to care for yourself and/or your family?
4. Do you feel you are able to fulfill your ideal role as a family member (e.g., spouse, parent, sibling, grandparent)?
5. Are you able to make independent decisions?
6. Are you able to carry out job responsibilities?
7. Has your pain created a financial burden?
8. Do you feel your masculinity or femininity has been affected by your pain experience?
9. Are you able to fulfill your personal sexual needs?
10. How do you cope with your pain?
11. Do you feel this pain will interfere with your plans for the future?

Assessment of altered social integrity

1. Is there someone who helps you to better cope with your pain?
   Who is it?
2. Do you consult significant others concerning willingness or ability to provide care and on-going support?
3. Have you ever sought help outside of family and friends to help manage your pain?
4. Have you required special living arrangements in your home?
5. Are you included in family activities?
6. Are you able to maintain relationships (e.g., social, sexual, personal)?

Conclusion

1. How do you think we can help you manage your pain?

pain is dehumanizing and seems endless and purposeless (Tartaglia, 1987). This, in turn, increases anxiety and can lead to marked personality changes such a apathy, withdrawal, helplessness, hopelessness, and lack of satisfaction in all areas of life. This alteration in personal integrity ultimately has a serious impact upon the patients' self-identity and self-respect. The physical and mental anguish of this experience leads to total preoccupation with pain and self. Social integrity is threatened because "individuals define themselves by their relationships" (Levine, 1989, p. 335). Relationships within the family and community are endangered as pain remains uncontrolled. The patients are less able to cope, thus increasing pain and suffering. This process can also occur in the reverse manner, altering social, personal, and structural integrity, respectively. As a result, the expenditure of energy exceeds the patient's reserve, thereby increasing the level of pain and suffering.

Levine (1969) identified four levels of organismic response: (1) fear, (2) inflammation, (3) stress, and (4) sensation or perceptual awareness. Patients with chronic pain use these responses as protective mechanisms so that adaptation can occur.

For the patient with chronic pain, the fear of increasing pain, coupled with fear of the unknown, elicits a vicious cycle of pain and anxiety. The cancer patient's fear of death, of the future, of abandonment by others, and that any pain is a signal of progressive deterioration is constantly present. Nursing intervention breaks this vicious cycle and promotes adaptation.

The inflammatory response affects the patient's energy level and the patient's ability to heal. For example, a patient with chronic arthritic pain resulting from inflammation uses considerable energy in an attempt to restore the body's integrity. Efforts directed at fighting the cause and limiting the involvement reduces the energy reserves. Prescribed therapies that suppress the inflammatory-immune response of the cancer patient also help to compromise the body's integrity. Both radiation and chemotherapy weaken the body to such a degree that the efficiency of the inflammatory-immune response becomes severely limited. The secondary infections that can occur further deplete the body's energy and adaptive ability. The use of the inflammatory response in conservation is severely restricted, and nursing interventions are necessary to conserve the patient's remaining energy and facilitate adaptation.

The response to stress is the third-level organismic response described by Levine (1969). The stress response theory, developed by Selye (1976) and described as the general adaptation syndrome, is a nonspecific three-phase response of the body to stressors. The physiologic coordination of the response occurs through the central and autonomic nervous systems, as well as the pituitary and adrenal glands. During the *alarm phase*, bodily changes occur that are characteristic of initial exposure to a stressor. Resistance is diminished and death can ensue if the stressor is sufficiently strong. In the *resistance phase* the adaptive hormones from the pituitary and adrenal glands mediate the body's responses in an attempt to bring balance. Following lengthy exposure to the same stressor, adaptation energy can become exhausted. During the *exhaustion phase*, alarm signs reappear but the body can no longer adapt because the stress hormones are depleted. Death results (Selye, 1974).

Patients with chronic pain are continually bombarded with myriad stressors of varying intensity. In addition to dealing with the unrelieved pain, the patient must deal too with a wide range of systemic, emotional, environmental, and familial stressors (Tartaglia, 1987). In order for this patient to progress therapeutically, adaptation with energy conservation must occur. As time goes on and intensity of pain increases, adaptation becomes more difficult for the patient with chronic pain because needed hormones are depleted. The nurse considers this high degree of stress while minimizing further complications and conserving energy when devising a plan of care to meet each patient's unique needs.

Sensory response, the fourth-level response, involves the patient as an active participant in the environment. Each individual uses energy to search for information from the environment to ensure his or her safety and to identify potential sources of harm. The all-encompassing experience of chronic pain can decrease a patient's environmental awareness, posing as a threat to the patient's well-being. Patients may be so completely absorbed by the pain or so depressed from their unsuccessful attempts to cope that routine activities such as cooking and driving can become an environmental threat. Likewise, heavy sedation causing drowsiness and lethargy further diminishes patients' sensory awareness. Safety is compromised and well-being threatened. Nurses ensure a safe environment for their patients, constantly reassuring them that they are protected, and assisting them to conserve their limited energy.

Nursing care for the patient with chronic pain in the acute care facility can be planned, implemented, and evaluated using Levine's conservation principles. Use of the principles facilitates adaptation of the patient to whatever environmental imbalances are experienced.

Case Presentation 8–1: Joe

Joe, a 60-year-old sales executive, was admitted to the oncology unit with metastatic adenocarcinoma of the prostate. Diagnosed 2½ years earlier, Joe's cancer had metastasized to his bones. He had received radiation treatment and various oral narcotic regimens, including morphine sulfate elixir, hydromorphone hydrochloride, methadone, and oxycodone. These had provided some relief for approximately 1 year. The staff had cared for Joe intermittently since his diagnosis and earlier treatment and were surprised at his decline since his last admission. Metastasis was now widespread, and recent at-home management with 15 mg of morphine sulfate given intramuscularly every 3 hours by his wife was ineffective. Until recently, Joe had been active and self-sufficient; he was now lethargic, anorexic, cachectic, and in almost constant pain. His skin had become sclerotic from the multiple injections, further increasing his pain. When awake, he requested more pain medication and looked drawn, tense, and totally preoccupied.

Joe's pain was out of control. Implantation of an epidural catheter and subcutaneous infusion device for administration of intraspinal narcotics was being considered. His one wish was to be more awake and alert with some pain relief. For what he was sure would be his last summer, he wanted to be able to sit in the sun by his pool and enjoy his two grandchildren. Comprehensive assessment of Joe's pain and its effective management were essential if the nurses were going to be able to help Joe get his wish.

ASSESSMENT

Energy Deficits.   Joe's respirations were rapid and shallow, indicating unrelieved severe pain. His blood pressure was 138/78, probably due to adaptation to the prolonged sympathetic stimulation of his pain (McCaffrey, 1979). Sleeping patterns had progressed from short 2- to 3-hour intervals to an almost constant state of drowsiness or lethargy over the past 2 weeks. Self-care and activities of daily living required the assistance of his wife or son, and sedation was necessary before and after care. During the past 2 weeks, he rarely got out of bed except to use the bathroom or bedside commode and could no longer tolerate sitting in his favorite recliner-rocker. Although he had always enjoyed the daily newspaper and television news, his concentration was now very short and he would often fall asleep. Joe's appetite was poor. He would eat three or four spoonfuls of food and would soon feel full or nauseated. He had lost more than 15 pounds since his last doctor's visit 5 weeks before, and had recently begun to vomit. No foods really tempted his appetite, although he did prefer cool, soft foods. Often he would sleep during the family's mealtime and felt little motivation to eat, even if his wife sat with him. During the past 6 to 8 weeks, Joe had progressed from working 3 to 4 hours daily in his office and attending some social functions to his present somnolent, lethargic state.

Structural Deficits. Joe's pain was all-consuming. He described it as a deep, never-ending pain in his legs, back, and hips, and rated it as nearly the "worst pain" on a visual analog scale (Levy, 1985). Fifteen milligrams of intramuscular morphine sulfate was not controlling his pain but was making him sluggish and anorexic. The skin of Joe's buttocks, legs, and hips was painful, sclerotic, and ecchymotic. Skin turgor was sluggish, secondary to his limited fluid intake, poor diet, and weight loss. Musculoskeletal function was diminished with some leg muscle wasting and poor muscle tone. He was weak and required assistance to walk even a short distance. Joe reported difficulty moving his bowels, a common side effect of the morphine sulfate. His urine was dark and concentrated and he voided only in small amounts. When awake, Joe was alert and oriented but his periods of wakefulness were decreasing in length and frequency. He was "disgusted" with his sleepiness, weakness, and lethargy and had begun to experience frequent headaches while awake.

Personal Integrity Deficits. Joe stated that the cancer and pain were "consuming" his life. He was "angry" and "frustrated" that he was out of control, a situation he was not accustomed to as a top executive. His facial expression was tense and often detached. He worried constantly that his pain was reaching the point where soon nothing would relieve it. Joe's wife described his withdrawal from family interaction and daily activities during the past 2 to 3 weeks, and his frustration with his weakness and limited ability to care completely for himself. Joe was quiet, answered questions slowly, and offered little additional information. When asked how the pain made him feel, Joe replied, "Damn mad! I'm angry that nothing works and angry that I can't work either. I feel like my body is shutting down and soon it will just stop. When I sleep there's no pain, but every time I close my eyes I think this is it. Sometimes I wish it would be." Joe appeared helpless, hopeless, and beyond coping. His life belonged to his pain.

Social Integrity Deficits. Joe's wife, son, and daughter were his major support systems. Business associates and friends rarely called or visited, probably due to Joe's weakened and lethargic state. Social and business engagements had stopped weeks before. Although financially quite comfortable, Joe's wife stated that he frequently voiced concerns about his ability to support his wife and their younger son, a college student. He frequently spoke with sadness and regret about his grandchildren. He felt that he should be able to take them places and play with them. They should not, he said, have to see him "sleep the days away."

INTERVENTIONS

Following the initial interview and assessment session with Joe and his wife, a plan of care was developed. Considering Joe's terminal state, conservation, based on Levine's principles, was the focus. This would occur primarily through supportive nursing interventions designed to maintain Joe at his present level of adaptation (Levine, 1966).

Energy Conservation. Continuous control of Joe's pain was planned through administration of 10 to 15 mg of morphine sulfate intravenously every 3 hours around the clock. Breakthrough pain was managed with 5 mg of methadone every 6 hours. The nursing team's goal was to control his pain and increase his comfort level until the epidural catheter and infusion device (Infusaid pump) could be implanted. To enhance the effects of the prescribed medication and to allay some of the anxiety related to anticipation of pain, both Joe and his wife were instructed in progressive relaxation. They would both work together whenever the pain started to return. A consultation with the psychiatric nurse clinical specialist was also ordered. Both Joe and his wife were to be taught techniques of guided imagery.[2]

When consulted as to his preferred time for care, Joe identified late morning as the time of day when he felt most comfortable and controlled. Self-care with minimal assistance was possible at this time, if followed by medication and a period of uninterrupted rest. It was decided to administer sedation at the conclusion of Joe's care because it would allow him the rest he needed following such an expenditure of energy.

A flexible visiting schedule for his family was also planned, to coincide with his more wakeful and pain-controlled periods. A regular schedule of "checking in" to talk with and listen to Joe was initiated by his primary nurse on all shifts. It was hoped that this too would relieve some of his anxiety and concern.

A consultation was arranged with the dietitian, who with Joe and his primary nurse planned a dietary regimen that would include a high-calorie, high-protein diet of small frequent meals. These included foods Joe had identified as his favorites in addition to supplemental between-meal snacks such as milkshakes. His wife and children were invited to dine with him whenever possible, and were encouraged to bring favorite cooked foods from home.

Through these supportive interventions, it was intended that Joe's pain would be more adequately controlled and the anticipatory anxiety and subsequent stress reduced. With improved pain management techniques, he could remain awake, alert, and able to carry out his own care, and he could communicate and concentrate better. His sleep would be more restful and, with a carefully tailored diet, his weight would be controlled.

Structural Integrity Conservation. Because of the condition of Joe's skin and ineffectiveness of the intramuscular route to adequately control pain, his medication route was changed to intravenous. A schedule of hourly turning while in bed was implemented, as were warm, moist soaks on his buttocks, hips, and thighs. A foam mattress was placed on his bed and a pad on his bedside chair. Back rubs and massage were incorporated and offered after position changes. Bedside physical therapy was recommended for range-of-motion and muscle-strengthening exercises. Ambulation with assistance was initiated whenever Joe was feeling well controlled and less tired. It was anticipated that following insertion of the epidural catheter, Joe would be consistently pain-controlled and able to resume some regular activities. Conservation of musculoskeletal function was therefore essential. Constipation was a continual problem, secondary to the high doses of morphine sulfate, poor diet, and inactivity. Suppositories were prescribed twice daily. Warm liquids were also recommended with all meals, as were fruits and vegetables to his level of tolerance. Oral fluid intake was encouraged, and Joe's wife and nurses offered fluids whenever they were with him. He preferred fruit punch, which was kept stocked in the unit kitchen and was always at his bedside. Initially supplemental intravenous fluids were ordered, but these were eventually discontinued as his oral intake improved. While Joe was awake, his wife or one of his children was usually at his bedside. They would talk quietly or listen to his favorite classical music, which he discovered to be both soothing and relaxing (Cook, 1986).

Nursing expectations for these interventions included prevention of further skin damage, muscle weakness, and wasting. Establishment of a more regular bowel pattern was also a priority. When Joe became constipated, his pain control was more difficult to achieve and periods of relief were shorter. Improvement of Joe's urinary output, however, could be achieved only through establishment of adequate fluid and electrolyte balance. Assisting Joe to stay awake, alert, and relaxed was contingent on the efficiency of pain management techniques and the degree of energy conservation achieved through other supportive interventions.

Personal Integrity Conservation. Helping Joe to re-establish his sense of hope and self-esteem was to be a major nursing goal. Establishing rapport and a trusting relationship were priorities. It was hoped that letting him know that someone was always there, that he was not alone, and that medication was available would help to decrease his anxiety and fear. Frequent nursing checks on the effectiveness of Joe's pain control were also initiated. Reassurance that pain could be controlled and that epidural morphine sulfate and other modalities were especially successful might also help to improve his coping abilities. The entire staff made an effort to involve Joe in as much planning and decision-making regarding his care as he was able to physically and emotionally tolerate. His family was encouraged to continue to discuss family problems and work-related issues with him. They asked his opinions and talked about the future, a topic that had previously been carefully avoided. The psychiatric nurse clinical specialist was also requested to talk with Joe in order to help him better cope with his anger and frustration.

Social Integrity Conservation. Joe's family was encouraged to visit whenever possible. His grandchildren were daily visitors. Their visits were planned to coincide with Joe's waking periods. Joe's priest, Father Mike, a close personal friend and golf buddy, increased his visits at the urging of the staff. To relieve his concern over tiring Joe, he was reassured that Joe needed his social as well as his spiritual presence and concern. Realizing Joe's need to maintain some communication with his business associates and still feel a part of the corporate scene, the staff discussed with his wife the possible benefits of having one or two close associates call periodically. Considering Joe's concern over his finances, the hospital social worker was asked to meet with Joe and his wife in order to reassure him. The staff and his family understood that his concerns were unwarranted and were a manifestation of his anxiety about his future and frustration with his inability to control the course of his disease and his life. Staff also introduced the topic of support care (hospice) services at home for both Joe and his family when they decided that the time was right.

When supportive interventions were planned for Joe, nursing goals focused on reinforcing his and his family's social support systems. Everyone wanted Joe to still feel a part of the family, business, and social scene he loved and on which he thrived. With careful planning, they were able to work with and around his pain and give him back some of his control, enjoyment, and hope in life.

These supportive nursing interventions were generally successful. Joe's physical and mental status did improve following more effective pain management and control. Prior to insertion of the epidural catheter, Joe was more relaxed and less anxious, and his appetite improved somewhat. Two weeks following admission, an epidural catheter and subcutaneous Infusaid pump were implanted for more long-term pain control (Paice, 1986). Shortly after the implantation, Joe experienced withdrawal symptoms from his previous high narcotic doses, but no bone pain. Slowly he recovered, and after several days of receiving 5 mg of epidural morphine sulfate daily, he was alert and pain free. He was able to return to his office for a few hours two to three times a week and spent the remaining time lounging in his garden or by his pool with his family. His pain medication was gradually increased, but he remained awake, alert, controlled, and relatively free of side effects. Eventually he had to use a wheelchair, but he was still able to enjoy his life. He continued to practice imagery and relaxation techniques, which he was convinced provided him with renewed energy as well as pain control. Joe died 10 months later from complications of his cancer.

Case Presentation 8–2: Joan

Joan, a 56-year-old former waitress, was diagnosed with arthritis 10 years ago. Complicated by the hormonal changes of menopause, the chronic pain Joan experienced in her extremities and joints spread to other areas of her body. Denial was used as an initial defense mechanism to cope with anxiety associated with her disease process and accompanying pain.

As the pain continued and threatened her occupation as a waitress, she was forced to make some changes in her life-style. The biggest change was the necessity to give up her job. No longer employed, she lost not only financial but social benefits as well.

Joan's condition also affected her husband and two children, ages 10 and 15. She was no longer able to completely fill the roles of housewife and mother. The majority of the housework had to be done by her husband and children, with Joan in a supervisory position. Their family activities were limited because of Joan's pain and the financial burden created by the loss of Joan's employment and her chronic use of medication. Nonsteroidal anti-inflammatory drugs were used to help control her pain, yet they played a significant part in irritating the mucosal lining of her stomach. These gastric complications created additional stress and greatly decreased the enjoyment of family meals and celebrations. As a result more pain ensued. Joan was subsequently admitted to the orthopedic service of the hospital for a total right hip replacement, anticipating decreased pain and improved walking endurance.

A brief summary of Joan's history and physical examination revealed the following problems:

1. Extreme pain, swelling, and stiffness in extremity joints
2. Inability to bear weight on right leg for past 6 months
3. Rheumatic deformity in both upper and lower limbs with nodule development over bony prominences
4. Slight anemia as revealed by blood tests
5. Weight loss of 10 pounds over the past 2 years
6. Malaise even upon awakening
7. Palpable spleen
8. Mental depression for which she has been seeing a psychologist for the past 10 years

Levine's conservation principles were used to guide the nursing assessment and ensure that interventions focused on preserving wholeness.

ASSESSMENT

Energy Deficits.   Joan rated her pain as "worst pain" on a visual analog scale (Levy, 1985). This pain accompanied by joint stiffness made it very difficult for her to sleep. She explained that the pain was a constant reminder of the disease process, with no remission in sight. The lack of sleep resulted in fatigue and made it very difficult for her to perform activities of daily living. This loss of independence created stress and anxiety for Joan, which only made the pain worse. An oxygen deficit created by the anemia, coupled with a low-grade fever contributed even more to her fatigue and discomfort. At times it was an effort to simply hold a book or rosary. Joan missed the enjoyment of eating with her family due to her loss of appetite and irritated stomach. As a result Joan experienced not only weight loss but also a constant desire for a return to the way things were prior to her illness.

Structural Deficits.   Joan's painful joints were warm, red, swollen, and deformed. Paresthesias were experienced whenever she would try to exert herself beyond her limitations. Weakened hand grasps necessitated the use of specially adapted crutches. Painful nodules were present over her bony prominences near both elbows. Her major complaint was extreme pain in her right hip, preventing weight bearing on that leg. Because of her extreme body pain, she stated that she had to endure the side effects of the battery of prescribed anti-inflammatory medication. Nausea, slight swelling, and symptoms of mild diabetes were what Joan had to tolerate in exchange for the mild analgesic effect of the drugs she was taking. "At this time these drugs are my life," she commented.

Personal Integrity Deficits.   Joan's husband stated that since the chronic pain of arthritis had put limitations on Joan's ability to care for herself and others, there was a profound change in Joan's mental health. She looked very sad when she spoke, and all gestures seemed to require much energy. Joan indicated that her husband was a major support person, encouraging her every step of the way. However, she felt guilty because he limited his activities to spend time with her. She also expressed concern that her relationship with her two sons was changing because of her inability to remain physically active with them. She could not attend her sons' athletic competitions or become involved in their school functions. She noted: "When I sit I have pain, when I walk I have pain, and sometimes family members' hugs, which were always so comforting, cause me to have even more pain. It is not fair that I must live like this. I pray that God will listen to my prayers."

Social Integrity Deficits.   Joan was receiving disability payments; however, the battery of medications and therapies prescribed consumed most of this money. She missed all her work friends, despite the frequent visits she and her husband made to the restaurant where she had worked. Her husband provided the care Joan could not accomplish independently, and when he was not present, Joan's sister was willing to assist with this care. Since Joan could not bear weight on her right leg, a bed was moved to the first floor of their home to avoid having her walk up a flight of stairs. She had not had sexual intercourse with her husband for 2 years; however, a loving relationship was evident by frequent touching and hand-holding during the assessment. Joan stated that she and her husband spent much time together talking, looking at pictures, or playing games. She received additional support from a psychologist and priest with whom she met once a week.

INTERVENTIONS

Alteration in musculoskeletal functioning, body image changes, depression, fatigue, and extreme pain were Joan's major problems that required appropriate therapeutic and supporting nursing interventions. After a critical analysis of data, a plan of care was structured according to Levine's conservation principles. Most of the interventions were supportive and focused on conserving energy, providing comfort, and maintaining integrity. The success of therapeutic nursing interventions related to the surgical process was dependent on Joan's ability to adapt to this changed state.

Energy Conservation. Joan was placed in a semiprivate room with a patient also having a total hip replacement. This provided an opportunity for both Joan and her roommate to share experiences and feelings and provide encouragement for each other. Scheduled pain medication was given promptly and was planned around times of greatest pain (physical therapy). Other interventions for relief of Joan's pain, such as an early morning shower and warm milk and blankets prior to bedtime, were incorporated into her plan of care. Joan indicated that these interventions were soothing to her joints and better allowed her to perform intended activities. Since lack of sleep was a problem for Joan, interruptions during the night were limited. Guided imagery was used to help decrease pain intensity, promote muscle relaxation, and decrease anxiety. Joan stated that her favorite image was her past experiences at the beach with her husband and children. She reminisced about their long walks on the beach, waves rolling over their bare feet, and her ability to keep pace with her two children as they desperately searched for seashells. Frequent rest periods during activities, and whenever else needed, were provided. The nutritionist was asked to speak with Joan regarding preferred foods for each meal to prevent weight loss and improve her appetite. Green leafy vegetables and dried fruits were recommended to supply iron to help reverse her anemia.

Structural Conservation. Joan's painful joints required protection by supporting the affected limbs when helping her with activities of daily living. Crutches were positioned so that they were within her reach. A consult was made to occupational therapy for introduction of newly developed adaptive devices used by arthritic patients. Analgesics were administered a half hour prior to physical therapy treatments so that the full benefits of this therapy could be obtained. Joan received reinforcement of information concerning her prescribed medication and measures to reduce possible side effects (eating prior to taking steroids). Unacceptable side effects noticed by Joan or staff members would be reported to the physician. Plenty of fluids were incorporated in her daily diet to help reduce the occasional low grade fever she experienced. In her debilitated condition Joan required adequate rest periods during the day, especially after prescribed treatments and therapies. This was accomplished by emphasizing the importance of rest to Joan, ensuring privacy, and providing the support needed to achieve this relaxation.

Personal Integrity Conservation. Joan was encouraged to help develop her plan of care since she knew what made her feel most comfortable (early morning baths or showers). She was permitted to wear a loose-fitting house dress that buttoned in the front instead of a nightgown. This was more comfortable and easier to put on than a nightgown that required manipulation of Joan's arms. She was not rushed when performing care, and the staff provided encouragement each step of the way. Perioperative teaching was done according to her identified needs. Joan was encouraged to continue seeing her psychologist and priest while in the hospital. A private room was arranged for those meetings.

Joan's twisted hands and feet were not her only identifiable traits. Her warm smile, friendly manner, and determination were complimented and valued as important aspects of her personal integrity.

Social Integrity Conservation. Disturbances such as routine vital signs were kept to a minimum when Joan's husband, children, sister, or acquaintances came to visit. Her family was encouraged to assist with care activities as they did at home. Precautions regarding total hip replacement were taught when all family members were present. Joan was comfortable discussing her sexual needs with her primary nurse. She and her husband were encouraged to talk to a sex therapist who was highly recommended by the orthopedic surgeons on staff.

Joan received a right total hip replacement and was able to again bear weight on her right leg with much less pain. Goals for her physical therapy at this time concentrated on her walking with a specially adapted walker. This ability to walk again without intense pain provided encouragement for Joan, which facilitated her adaptation to the life-long struggle with arthritis.

CONCLUSION

Pain is a fact of life that plagues everyone. As an admonition or as part of the healing process, it is acutely managed in a therapeutic effort to diminish its existence. When pain becomes a life-long process, however, its management involves supportive efforts to maintain the status quo at best. The patient with chronic pain experiences a multifaceted repertoire of physical and emotional events that require this supportive management. With carefully planned and individualized supportive interventions, use of Levine's conservation principles helped Joe and Joan adapt successfully.

REFERENCES

Benoliel, J.Q., & Crowley, D.M. (1974). The patient in pain: New concepts. American Cancer Society Publication, 3–11.

Cook, J.D. (1986). Music as an intervention in the oncology setting. Cancer Nursing, 9(1), 23–28.

Foley, K.M. (1985). The treatment of cancer pain. New England Journal of Medicine, 313(2), 84–93.

Guyton, A. (1986). Textbook of medical physiology (7th ed.). Philadelphia: W.B. Saunders.

Levine, M.E. (1966). Adaptation and assessment: A rationale for nursing intervention. American Journal of Nursing, 66(11), 2450–2453.

Levine, M.E. (1967). The four conservation principles of nursing. Nursing Forum, 6, 45–49.

Levine, M.E. (1969). The pursuit of wholeness. American Journal of Nursing, 69, 93–98.

Levine, M.E. (1971). Holistic nursing. Nursing Clinics of North America, 6(2), 253–264.

Levine, M.E. (1989). The conservation principles of nursing. In J. Riehl-Sisca (Ed.), Conceptual models for nursing practice (pp. 325–337). Norwalk, CT: Appleton & Lange.

Levy, M.H. (1985). Pain management in advanced cancer. Seminars in Oncology, 12(4), 394–410.

McCaffrey, M. (1979). Nursing management of the patient with pain (2nd ed.). Philadelphia, J.B. Lippincott.

Meinhart, N., & McCaffrey, M. (1983). Pain: A nursing approach to assessment and analysis. Norwalk, CT: Appleton & Lange.

Nursing now: Pain. (1985). Springhouse, PA: Springhouse Corp.
Paice, J. (1986). Intrathecal morphine infusion for intractable cancer pain: A new use for implanted pumps. Oncology Nursing Forum, 13(3), 41–47.
Selye, H. (1974). Stress without distress. Philadelphia: J.B. Lippincott.
Selye, H. (1976). The stress of life. New York: McGraw-Hill.
Sternbach, R.A. (1968). Pain: A psychophysiological analysis. New York: Academic Press.
Tartaglia, M. (1987). Managing chronic cancer pain effectively. Nursing Life, 4, 50–55.

NOTES

1. Pain impulses are initiated when sensory receptors or nociceptors that respond to temperature, electrical energy, and chemical changes are stimulated. Chemical substances released following tissue injury—for example, histamine, bradykinin, serotonin, and prostaglandins—lower the stimulation threshold of nociceptors and increase pain sensitivity. The stimulated nociceptor then generates a pain (afferent) impulse through the release of chemicals such as substance P and prostaglandins, which act as neurotransmitters. The impulse is carried to the dorsal horn of the spinal cord by specialized afferent sensory fibers. Myelinated A-delta fibers conduct pain impulses quickly, whereas unmyelinated, smaller C fibers conduct impulses slowly. Different pain sensations result. Those impulses conducted along A-delta fibers are perceived as sharp, localized, and acute, whereas those conducted along C fibers are perceived as aching, burning, diffuse, and persistent. This sensation tends to become more painful over a period of time and gives one the intolerable suffering of long-continued chronic pain (Guyton, 1986).

Only when the pain impulse is relayed to the brain can pain result. The impulse travels from the spinal cord to the brain (thalamus) through the ascending divisions of the lateral spinothalamic tract. The paleospinothalamic tract transmits the slow-chronic impulses and terminates the reticular formation of the brainstem and the thalamus. Because of the effect on the reticular activating system, this tract is involved in emotional responses to pain.

The neospinothalamic tract transmits impulses quickly and directly to the thalamus and to the somatic sensory cortex. Localization of the pain is probably the most important function of these signals (Guyton, 1986).

The brain relays its responses from the cerebral cortex and brainstem down the descending pathways of efferent fibers in the lateral and ventral pyramidal and extrapyramidal tracts.

Under certain circumstances pain impulses can be blocked at various levels in both the brain and the spinal cord. Endogenous opiatelike substances (endorphins and enkephalins) can be released in response to pain. They modulate pain by binding with opiate-receptor sites and may inhibit release of neurotransmitters or they may alter pain perception.

Pain relief therapies such as transelectrical nerve stimulation and acupuncture, found to be helpful in the management of chronic cancer pain, may stimulate release of these endogenous opioids. While research continues, the body's own "analgesia system" may serve as the basis for future efforts toward pain control (Guyton, 1986).

2. Guided imagery is a cognitive strategy that has had success in pain relief by making use of the mind's ability to affect physiologic response as well as pain perception. It allows the patient to use imagination to create sensory images that decrease pain intensity or that become a nonpainful substitute for pain (McCaffrey, 1979). Imagery also promotes muscle relaxation and decreases anxiety, which are helpful in conserving energy expenditures.

The imagery technique taught to Joe and his wife involved the following components:

a. Selection of the image of beach and ocean as experienced from his beach cottage at the New Jersey shore. Sitting on the deck overlooking the ocean at sunrise or walking the beach at sunset had always been pleasant and fulfilling experiences for Joe.

b. He was instructed to use all five senses to increase the vividness and effectiveness of his beach scene. He was asked to imagine feeling a cool ocean breeze as he walked barefoot along the warm, moist sand. Hearing the waves lap rhythmically onto the beach while experiencing the smell and taste of salt spray were also events that Joe recalled with pleasure. The reds, oranges, and pinks displayed by the sun as it seemed to sink into the ocean depths reminded Joe of the peace, relaxation, and solitude he felt as he sat on the beach staring out at the darkening ocean.

c. To prepare for this experience, Joe's wife would close the drapes and dim the lights to approximate sunset. Joe would attempt to find a comfortable position and times were selected when there would be little noise or interruption.

d. Deep breathing relaxation exercises were encouraged to prepare Joe to begin imagery.

e. Joe was then told to close his eyes and concentrate on his beach image. He was asked to describe all of the sensations that he had previously identified. With practice, these sensations were eventually easily evoked.

f. A 20-minute time period for each session was agreed on. At the conclusion, Joe was instructed to arouse himself by silently counting from one to three. On the last count he was to take a deep breath, open his eyes, and say "I feel refreshed and relaxed."

g. Joe and his wife were encouraged to practice the imagery techniques and, if desired, to use tape-recordings of ocean sounds to facilitate and heighten the effects.

Chapter
NINE

Care of the Patient with Congestive Heart Failure

Karen Moore Schaefer, R.N., D.N.Sc.

Earlier in the day, Jake became very warm and placed a portable fan in front of him to "cool off." Although there was no environmental reason for him to feel warm, his wife went about her work forgetting her initial thoughts of how strange this behavior seemed. It was unusual for Jake to be sitting around watching television, but he had been much less active since he had been in the hospital for unstable angina 3 months ago, and the physicians told him he should "take it easy." Normally he would walk a couple of miles a day, work in the garden, cook all the meals, and visit with neighbors. If he thought an activity would bring on an anginal attack, he would take a nitroglycerin (NTG) tablet prophylactically. His subtle change in activity over the months had not really been noticed, at least in a way that would cause his family concern.

Later that same day he experienced some chest pain while watching television and took some NTG. After taking six tablets without relief, he told his wife that he thought he had better go to the hospital. His daughter, a nurse, was summoned and she drove him to the hospital, during which time she was able to elicit that the pain was deep, radiating through the back, and that he had no nausea, was not sweating, and was not short of breath. She thought his breathing appeared somewhat labored, his skin was very pale, almost deathlike, and his facial expression was one of panic. When he arrived in the emergency room he was immediately placed in a semi-Fowler's position, oxygen was started at 6 liters per minute, an intravenous infusion was placed in his left forearm to keep the vein open, 2 mg of morphine sulfate was administered intravenously, and a battery of laboratory work and x-ray examinations was completed while both the nurse and the physician finished their assessments. The chest x-ray confirmed that he had "fluid in his lungs," and 40 mg of furosemide was administered intravenously with an almost immediate urinary response. An NTG drip was started at 5 µg per minute to control his chest pain (Gawlinski, 1989). Within 30 minutes he felt and looked much better. His chest pain was almost completely gone, his normal color had returned, and his breathing had become more relaxed. The provocative facts suggested that he may have had a heart attack, and he was to be admitted to the hospital. His wife and daughter remained with him until he was settled in the critical care unit.

CONGESTIVE HEART FAILURE

Congestive heart failure (CHF) occurs when the heart is no longer able to meet the needs of the body during exercise or rest. When this occurs the cardiac output is usually reduced and the body tissues are hypoperfused. Tissue hypoxia occurs secondary to a reduced oxygen supply, and the removal of waste products is slowed. Lactic acid and pyruvate accumulate and produce a variety of sensations in the patient. Early and subtle feelings of generalized discomfort and fatigue may occur (Hudak, Gallo, & Lohr, 1986). These nonspecific symptoms are frequently attributed to a myriad of causes usually related to activities of daily living (not enough sleep, too much exercise, not eating right) rather than to problems with the heart. Some patients may complain that they are always tired or are napping all the time (disturbed rest and sleep patterns). These sleep-rest disturbances are further aggravated by the fact that older people, often being the population of patients with CHF, are light sleepers.

Kellum (1986) suggests that CHF involves the systemic level of function and produces disorganization. Because the cardiovascular system is unable to effectively meet the nutritional needs of the tissues, the cardiovascular system is unable to act as an integrated and effective whole.

As the CHF worsens the patient has difficulty breathing. This respiratory discomfort often triggers anxiety. Anxiety precipitates a neuroendocrine response (increased catecholamines), which aggravates an already energy-depleted system. This energy expenditure is more dramatic when the body's normal compensatory mechanisms (increased pulse, myocardial hypertrophy) are stressed beyond their ability to function. If this process is allowed to continue, there is danger of system failure (Price & Wilson, 1986).

CHF → FATIGUE → ANXIETY → CHF → DYSPNEA →
ANXIETY → DYSPNEA → ANXIETY → FATIGUE → *FAILURE*

In Jake's case, assessments by the nurse and the physician resulted in rapid intervention. The nurses checked with Jake and his family frequently to offer continued reassurance and to assure Jake that his family physician would be in to see him soon. Jake's wife and daughter were relieved that he responded so quickly to therapy and remained with him in the emergency room, providing support for each other.

ANTECEDENTS TO CONGESTIVE HEART FAILURE

CHF is caused primarily by muscle, valvular, or rhythm disorders. The failure secondary to valvular disorder usually occurs in the heart chamber behind a stenosis or in the chamber in front of a regurgitation. For example, if the mitral valve is stenosed, the left atrium may experience some failure due to volume overload. On the other hand, if the mitral valve is regurgitant, the left ventricle would be overloaded with volume predisposing the left ventricle to failure. Rhythm disturbances alter the electrical stimulus initiating the mechanical response, interfering with the response needed for synchronous contraction and cardiac output (Price & Wilson, 1986).

Jake had had a myocardial infarction, which caused tissue anoxia and death to the anterior and lateral walls of his myocardial muscle, 18 months prior to this hospitalization. As a result of the damage, the muscle pump was weakened.

When failure occurs, the body attempts to compensate for the decreased blood supply by increasing the pulse to get more blood to the tissues, dilating the ventricle so it can handle more blood, and thickening the wall of the muscle to improve the contractile force (hypertrophy). These compensatory mechanisms work to a certain point, at which time Starling's law of energy and force is compromised and the volume of blood delivered to the myocardial muscle pump can no longer be handled.[1] The extra fluid tips into the tissues and lungs, causing the symptoms that Jake experienced the night he went to the emergency room. Although the CHF in this case had its origin at the cellular level (myocardial infarction), the effects of the failure are systemic (Table 9–1). CHF creates a situation whereby the body becomes energy-depleted and the patient experiences fatigue. The goal of nursing is to promote and maintain wholeness through the use of the four conservation principles.

TABLE 9-1. SYSTEMIC EFFECTS OF CONGESTIVE HEART FAILURE

Right-Sided Failure	Left-Sided Failure
Neck vein distention	Dyspnea
Ankle swelling	Crackles in the lungs
Enlarged liver	Coughing
Elevated venous pressure	S3
Nausea	Elevated capillary wedge pressure

SOURCE: Adapted from Kenner et al., 1985.

FATIGUE ASSOCIATED WITH CONGESTIVE HEART FAILURE

CHF is pathophysiologic such that the fatigue cannot be simply over-come by resting and adopting a change in life-style; the person's restor-ative ability is diminished. Experts agree that fatigue is a perceptual phenomenon (Kellum, 1986; Potempa, Lopex, Reid, & Lawson, 1986). The fatigue of CHF, a systemic somatic function, also has a psychologic dimen-sion. Although the basic physiologic process cannot be changed, function can be improved and the psychologic component can be modified.

The approach to care becomes more complex, however, when the nurse considers other factors that may be affecting the patient's response to failure. Patients may experience depression secondary to the chronic nature of the heart disease. Concomitantly patients may manifest a de-creased self-esteem, loss of interest in activities and reduced socialization. The initial reduced energy level that may actually be precipitating these psychologic responses becomes even worse. With the subsequent reduced activity level and sedentary life-style in the context of chronic illness, there is reduced aerobic capacity. In this case aerobic training will probably not be effective because of the disease state (Kellum, 1986). The patient be-comes less and less motivated to engage in the simplest of daily activities. The wholeness of the patient is threatened, requiring intervention by the nurse.

LEVINE'S CONSERVATION MODEL

According to Levine (1973) the individual responds in an integrated yet singular fashion to factors in both the internal and external environ-ments. The individuals have meaning only within the context of their envi-ronment. Health and disease are interpreted as patterns of adaptation. When the capacity to adapt is no longer functioning, the individual seeks nursing care. For example, Jake's chest pain continued despite the use of NTG (internal adaptation did not occur) and he sought health care.

Nursing care of the patient is organized according to the conservation principles with consideration of how the person adapts to threats in both the internal and external environments. The internal environment is com-posed of the physiologic and structural changes associated with the pro-cess of congestive heart failure. As discussed earlier, when the body's compensatory responses are stressed beyond a certain point, congestive heart failure occurs and the person usually seeks help. Mechanisms are provided to reduce the overload of fluids (preload and afterload reducers, angiotensin converting enzyme inhibitors), reduce energy requirements (balance activity and rest), improve cellular nutrition (oxygen), and reduce any associated pain (use of nitroglycerin, morphine sulfate). The nurse monitors the patient's response to these efforts to correct the failure by as-sessing blood pressure, pulse, respiratory rate and quality, temperature, arterial pressures, pulmonary capillary wedge pressures, fluid balance (intake and output), quality of peripheral pulses, cardiac rhythm, pain control, and electrolyte and blood gas measurements.

External environmental threats for the patient with CHF can be classified according to perceptual, operational, and conceptual factors (Levine, 1973). Perceptual factors are those that the patient responds to through the senses; for the patient with CHF these might include fatigue, pain, and dyspnea. Operational factors are those that pose a threat to the individual but cannot be perceived by the senses; for the patient with CHF this might include sudden changes in weather conditions (warm to extremely cold) and microorganisms from family members or colleagues that may be sick with colds or other illnesses. The conceptual environment includes the cultural and personal values about health care (when to go to the hospital), the meaning of health and illness to the individual (the importance of the heart to the function of the body and the fear of death associated with any malfunction of the heart), knowledge about health care (the symptoms that suggest the individual should seek health care), spiritual beliefs (relationships, beliefs in higher powers, ability to love, and ability to enjoy life), language (the ability to express their concerns), and education (knowing what questions to ask about self-care related to controlling the disease). Conceptually patients with CHF frequently fear the loss of control and are frustrated with the limitations that the disease places on their life-style.

The goal of nursing is to maintain or restore a person to a state of wholeness by conserving energy, structural integrity, personal integrity, and social integrity—to keep together via the conservation principles. Nursing interventions are successful only when all the conservation principles are used to deliver care (Foreman, 1989).

The *conservation of energy* involves a balancing of energy input and energy output to avoid excessive fatigue. Levine (1973) emphasizes a need for the proper dispersion of energy allowing for activity in the range of individual capability, safety, and comfort. When caring for the patient with cardiac problems this is particularly important. Life is supported in part by the continuous action of the heart; total rest for healing would result in death. Therefore, a balance of energy supply and demand on the heart must be achieved to promote healing. This balance is evaluated by observing the patient's organismic response to all supportive and therapeutic interventions. An adequate supply of nutrition and oxygen, as well as sufficient rest and sleep, will help to develop energy reserve to promote structural, personal, and social integrity.

The *conservation of structural integrity* involves maintaining or restoring the structure of the body such as preventing physical breakdown and promoting healing. For the patient with cardiac disease, this usually focuses on the prevention of further myocardial damage and maximizing the area of viable and functional cardiac muscle. These goals are met through observation of the patient for responses to medication therapy and increasing activity only within the safe limits of the particular patient.

The *conservation of personal integrity* involves the maintenance or restoration of the patient's sense of identity and self-worth. Damage to the heart poses a serious threat to a patient's sense of self. To ensure the patient's personal integrity, they must be a participant in their plan of care to the degree that they are capable. Hospitalization and the illness threaten a loss of control, such that every effort must be made to find ways for the patient to retain control. Loss of control creates emotional responses such as anxiety and denial that could deny the body energy needs for healing.

The *conservation of social integrity* involves the acknowledgment of the patient as a social being. The patient's life takes on meaning in the context of his or her social environment. Essential parts of the patients' lives are shared. The "victims" of critical illness cannot be understood without adequate attention to the family (Levine, 1973). Consideration must be given to the patient's life-style and whether any changes will be needed as a result of the insult to the patient's body. Teaching regarding these changes, such as risk factor modification, needs to be discussed with the patient and the family to be effective and to ensure mutual understanding and support as these frequently difficult changes are made.

Using the conservation principles and the knowledge of potential and actual internal and external threats to the individual, the nurse assists the patient and the family to adapt to changes that threaten the individual's integrity, thus maintaining wholeness.

ASSESSING THE PATIENT: USE OF LEVINE'S CONSERVATION MODEL

To establish an objective and scientific basis of nursing care, the nurse must have knowledge of the following: (1) the disease process, (2) the planned medical regimen, (3) the results of diagnostic studies, (4) the patient's response to medical therapy, (5) how to adapt nursing care to the needs of the patient and the principles of nursing science, (6) a mechanism whereby the nurse can record and review data about the patient, and (7) the ability to use information obtained from the family members and others concerned about the care of the patient (Levine, 1966). Using the conservation principles the nurse organizes the assessment to facilitate an accurate and thorough plan of care for the patient and the family.

Energy Conservation

Although Jake apparently had some trouble breathing prior to treatment in the emergency room, according to the blood gas results, his respirations were normal and effective on 6 liters of oxygen per minute. He had a history of atrial fibrillation controlled on digoxin. He was currently in normal sinus rhythm. Both his hemoglobin and hematocrit levels were normal for a man his age. He had a 15-year history of non–insulin-dependent diabetes mellitus controlled by glyburide and an 1800-calorie diet. When hospitalized he usually required supplemental insulin, and on arrival to the critical care unit his blood glucose level was 290, which was covered by 15 units of regular humulin insulin. Of importance was that his blood cholesterol level within the past 3 months was 158. His appetite was good; in fact, he said it was "too good." His wife felt that he ate too many "fatty foods."

He did most of the food shopping and the cooking. On further questioning, it was noted that he did not pay much attention to the food labels; he bought what he liked.

Jake insisted that his activity level had not really changed very much in the last few months, although he continued to remind us that he had had a heart attack 3 months ago. He denied feeling fatigued. His wife, however, said that he no longer walked into town as he had done before; he took the bus instead. He had also lost interest in taking care of the yard. She attributed this to the fact that he might be afraid that he would have chest pain. He was sleeping all the time. Further questioning of Jake and his wife revealed that he was taking a lot of NTG. He thought taking the NTG was appropriate since it was for anticipated pain rather than to relieve pain. He was also having up to six bouts of chest pain per day relieved by one to three NTG tablets. He had his NTG tablets refilled once a month. Examination of his old record indicated that he had 100 percent blockage of the circumflex artery and the right coronary artery, and about 75 percent blockage of the left anterior descending artery. Consequently, his cardiac muscle had limited blood supply. His ejection fraction was estimated to be 35 percent.[2]

Structural Integrity

Jake's skin was in good condition except for a callous on the left foot that was being treated by his physician. The day prior to admission to the hospital he had had the callous opened by the physician. About 10 years ago he had had one third of his right foot removed because of an infection that had invaded the bone and was not healing. He had no further problems since the amputation and wore specially made shoes that provide for good balance. He suspected that he had some neuropathy but it does not affect his ability to walk and maintain balance. He was also blind in his left eye and had been blind long before he was diagnosed with diabetes. He admitted to impotence for the past 10 years as a result of his diabetes but did not see this as a problem. Recently he had experienced amaurosis of the right eye, attributed to the 100 percent blockage of his right internal carotid artery. He was started on dipyridamole to complement the warfarin sodium that he was already taking. The rest of his senses were intact, and his muscle strength for his age was adequate.

Jake's bowel function was normal. According to his wife, he became very concerned if his bowels were not regular and would ask for a laxative such as milk of magnesia. He had a prostatectomy 5 years ago and had had no further urinary problems. He attributed frequent urination to his antihypertensive pills. This was confirmed by his physician. His weight (165 pounds) had not changed when he had been to the physician's office 1 week prior to admission, but he did not have a scale at home. (His weight dropped 5 pounds after 2 days of hospitalization.) His serum electrolytes were all within normal limits. Maintenance medications included 0.25 mg of digoxin daily, 90 mg of diltiazem three times daily, furosemide 40 mg daily, one potassium pill daily, 2.5 mg warfarin daily, 20 mg isosorbide dinitrate four times daily, and 2.5 mg glyburide daily.

Personal Integrity

Jake had no difficulty communicating. He was extremely jovial and loved to joke around with the nurses in a pleasant way. According to his wife and his daughter, this was the way he always was. He was totally independent. Data collected previously did indicate that his activity level had changed to the point that he was not doing what he normally did for the previous 3 months. He accepted this as part of getting old and having heart "trouble," but was frustrated with continued admissions to the hospital. This only further compromised his independence. He "seemed" to be very concerned about being in the hospital, but when asked if he was worried he said no. At a later point his wife indicated that he normally did not share his emotions. His daughter thought he was frustrated and frightened. She said that she and her father were talking about the fact that he might not pull through one of these angina attacks, and he responded by saying, "That's scary." Apparently this was the only time he shared how he felt about being "sick." Jake's wife said that, when upset he usually worked around the house, and also noted that he was very impatient. He was described as a man who believed in God but did not practice formalized religion, although recently he had been going to church with his wife.

Social Integrity

Jake was 71 years old and had been married for 49 years. He had two married daughters, one of whom was a nurse; one son; and one 18-month-old grandson. His family, including his only living brother, all lived nearby. His wife could not drive, so their children would take her to visit him in the hospital and helped her with food shopping. Her three sisters helped by arranging for transportation and taking her to church. His wife had non-insulin-dependent diabetes, currently being treated with low-dose NPH humulin insulin, and had to be very careful to monitor for hypoglycemic responses. She had a history of seizures, which were being controlled by 100 mg of phenytoin nightly. Because of his wife's chronic illnesses he had always prided himself in taking care of her, and now worried about her health.

Jake had been retired for 10 years and was financially secure. He and his wife spent their time traveling locally and taking care of their grandson whenever possible. They were a loving family.

NURSING JUDGMENTS AND CARE

Jake stabilized physically after therapeutic interventions in the emergency room. When he arrived in the intensive care unit, he wanted to relax and get some sleep. His wife and daughter left after reassuring him that they would be in to see him the next day. Levine's Conservation Model provides the basis for a comprehensive approach to the care of the hospitalized patient. His plan of care was initiated in the intensive care unit and continued when he was transferred to a regular medical-surgical unit a day after admission to the hospital.

Energy Conservation

Jake's history and assessment indicated that he was admitted into the hospital with actual energy depletion that had been symptomatically treated. Because of the structural and physiologic changes of his heart, he was at risk for energy imbalance. Nursing care focused on providing interventions that would promote a balance of energy supply and demand.

Jake received intravenous nitroglycerin to reduce afterload and preload, thus reducing the energy requirements of the myocardial muscle.[3] His vital signs and blood pressure were monitored closely; the goal to maintain the blood pressure at about 130/80 was achieved. His fluid intake and output were monitored, along with his weight, to ensure fluid balance as a response to the continued furosemide therapy.

Applying the findings of research that showed there were no significant differences in energy use between three methods of toileting and bathing, Jake's preferences for bathing and toileting were determined (Winslow, Lane, & Gaffney, 1984, 1985). When he was assisted to the bathroom and to the chair to eat his meals, his vital signs were monitored to ensure energy balance. He was queried for symptoms of weakness, dizziness, and chest and/or leg pain. His 1800-calorie diet was modified to include no added salt. Jake was not very happy about that but was hungry and ate almost everything. His blood sugar continued to be high, probably secondary to the stress of hospitalization and the cellular disorganization created by the failure (Kellum, 1986). He was given daily insulin based on his daily blood glucose levels. Three meals plus a snack in the evening prevented him from having any hypoglycemic reactions.

Jake's bed was kept in a semi-Fowler's position to prevent excessive cardiac workload due to recumbency. He took flurazepam hydrochloride nightly for sleep. He asked the nurses to wake him as little as possible during the night. The nursing staff planned to see to it that he got at least 6 hours of uninterrupted sleep whenever possible. Jake's room was changed midway through the hospitalization because of a very ill patient requiring frequent interventions, subsequently interrupting his sleep. In principle, the nurses preserved Jake's personal space, which contributed to his perception of himself as a healing patient (Levine, 1973).

A bottle of NTG tablets was left at the bedside. If he had chest pain, he was asked to take the NTG and immediately call the nurse. He remained pain free in the critical care unit.

Structural Integrity

Preventing further injury to Jake's left foot and preventing additional damage to the myocardial muscle were major goals of care. By maintaining energy balance further damage to the myocardial muscle was prevented. As his activity was increased, his organismic response was monitored by checking vital signs and asking him to report the occurrence of symptoms (chest pain, shortness of breath, pain in his legs). He was able to sit at the side of the bed and walk to the bathroom without difficulty. According to his electrocardiogram he remained in normal sinus rhythm with ST elevation consistent with muscle ischemia.

Jake's foot was cleansed daily with Betadine and wrapped with a sterile bandage. The skin remained pink and warm to touch. No bleeding was noted.

As indicated earlier, Jake's weight dropped to 160 pounds. This weight was maintained on 40 mg of furosemide daily and the no-added-salt diet. His electrolytes remained normal and his cardiac enzymes were not consistent with myocardiac damage.

Personal and Social Integrity

In retrospect there was a suggestion that Jake did not understand his health status as well as he should. There seemed to be a conflict between his current health and what he would like to be rather than what he was. He had definitely changed his life-style because of his disease. The goals were to provide Jake with the information he needed and wanted in order to make decisions about his health care and to help him find ways to maintain his independence without so much fear of chest pain.

Through very close work with the physicians and the family, the nurses were able to help Jake make some very important decisions. His daughter was extremely instrumental in helping Jake to understand what might lie ahead. The nurses were very aware that she was worried about her father and provided her with time to share her feelings and concerns.

Jake was doing well in the hospital but his recent unstable angina and the status of his coronary arteries made his future seem very tentative. He had been told previously that he was inoperable. It seemed as though there was nothing to do but accept the fact that Jake might die "the next time." His daughter asked to have a new cardiologist see her father, after discussing it with both Jake and his wife. The cardiologist reviewed his history and

---

TABLE 9–2. IMMEDIATE POST–CARDIAC CATHETERIZATION CARE—USING LEVINE'S CONSERVATION PRINCIPLES

Energy conservation

Take the patient's vital signs every 30 minutes for several hours.

Encourage the patient to drink plenty of fluids.

Check the patient's urinary output to ensure fluid balance.

Structural integrity

Check the catheter insertion site every 30 minutes for bleeding or swelling.

Encourage the patient to keep the access extremity immobile as ordered by the physician.

Assist the patient out of bed when ordered by the physician.

Encourage the patient to exercise the free extremities while in bed.

Encourage deep breathing every hour while in bed.

Personal integrity

Provide the patient with diversional activity according to interest (television, reading, music).

Social integrity

Reassure the patient that the physician will discuss the results of the study with the patient and the family.

explained that he had not had a second heart attack in June, as Jake had thought, but that he had been experiencing unstable angina, a very precarious situation. Usually the recommended therapy is a coronary artery bypass graft (CABG), and Jake thought that in his case this was definitely not an option. A repeat cardiac catheterization was recommended to reassess for therapeutic options; Jake consented.

The physician's explanation of Jake's cardiac status was reinforced. He underwent the cardiac catheterization without incident (Table 9–2).

His daughter and wife came to see him that evening and asked to speak to the cardiologist. The cardiologist recommended a CABG, explaining that his cardiac status was not as poor as had previously been assessed. His arteries were severely blocked with fairly good collateral circulation. His ejection fraction was 40 percent. Jake said, "Do what you have to do." His wife and daughter supported that decision. He was scheduled for surgery in 2 days.

Jake—the Whole Person

The subsequent 2 days were spent preparing Jake for surgery, most of which consisted of providing him and his family all the time they wanted to be together. At one point his children, grandchild, and wife were with him all at the same time. Jake said he was not scared; his niece, who worked on another unit of the hospital, said he cried when she hugged him; his daughter sensed he was afraid but felt very positive about the surgery. Jake began to have some chest pain at rest, confirming the urgency of his surgery. He was worried each time it happened, but he relaxed as soon as he took the NTG and the nurses reassured him of their presence. "Hug therapy" was initiated because he would kid all the nurses about giving him a hug, so they did, unsolicited.

Jake and his family talked about the surgery together. His daughter wanted to explain the experience to them, and just ask the nurses questions about what she thought might be unique to the hospital. Jake did not want to talk much about the procedure, but he was able to accurately answer the few questions asked in order to prompt any additional questions he might have. He spent the evening before surgery with his family and had a visit from his minister. Jake went to surgery with a good understanding of his health status, without additional muscle damage, and appropriately fearful of the outcome. Family members were told that they would be called early in the afternoon and were encouraged to go to work rather than "sitting around" waiting for a telephone call. They were reassured that they would be able to see Jake the day of the surgery, although he probably would never remember that first day. The outcome was up to God, the surgeon, and Jake.

CONCLUSION

Jake had chronic congestive heart failure but denied ever experiencing fatigue. It is probable that he had adapted to the changes taking place in his body and truly did not feel fatigued. He felt sick only when the body's compensatory mechanisms in response to the weakened cardiac muscle failed to accommodate the body's needs.

Levine's Conservation Model provided a workable framework for the assessment and implementation of care for Jake and his family. The model is pragmatic and parsimonious, and helps the nurse to focus on those phenomena that are important to nursing care as well as those needs that require collaborative interventions.

POSTSCRIPT

Jake is now home recovering and, in his words, "feels better every day." Jake and his family are back to life as usual, only modified by the chance to share life once again.

REFERENCES

Foreman, M.D. (1989). Confusion in the hospitalized elderly: Incidence, onset, and associated factors. Research in Nursing and Health, 12, 21–29.

Gawlinski, A. (1989). Nursing care after an AMI: A comprehensive review. Critical Care Nursing Quarterly, 12(2), 64–72.

Hudak, C.M., Gallo, B.M., & Lohr, T. (1986). Critical care nursing: A holistic approach (4th ed.). Philadelphia: J.B. Lippincott.

Kellum, M.D. (1986). Fatigue. In M.M. Jacobs & W. Geels (Eds.), Signs and symptoms in nursing: Interpretation and management. Philadelphia: J.B. Lippincott.

Kenner, C.V., Guzzetta, C.E., & Dossey, B.M. (1985). Critical care nursing: Body-mind-spirit. Boston: Little, Brown & Co.

Levine, M.E. (1966). Adaptation and assessment: A rationale for nursing intervention. American Journal of Nursing, 66(11), 2450–2454.

Levine, M.E. (1973). Introduction to clinical nursing (2nd ed.). Philadelphia: F.A. Davis.

Potempa, K., Lopex, M., Reid, C., & Lawson, L. (1986). Chronic fatigue. Image, 18(4), 165–169.

Price, S.A., & Wilson, L.M. (1986). Pathophysiology: Clinical concepts of disease processes. New York: McGraw-Hill.

Winslow, E.H., Lane, L.D., & Gaffney, F.A. (1984). Oxygen consumption and cardiovascular response in patients and normal adults during in bed and out of bed toileting. Journal of Cardiac Rehabilitation, 4, 3438–3454.

Winslow, E.H., Lane, L.D., & Gaffney, F.A. (1985). Oxygen consumption and cardiovascular response in control adults and acute myocardiac infarction patients during bathing. Nursing Research, 34, 164–169.

NOTES

1. Within limits, the more the heart is filled during diastole, the greater will be the force of contraction and the resulting stroke volume during systole. Essentially the striated cardiac muscle contracts with greater force when stretched. In failure the heart is operating at the upper end of the Starling curve and further dilation will reduce the stroke volume. The initial contractile force is reduced, decreasing ventricular filling (Andreoli, K.G., Aepis, D.P., Wallace, A.G., Kinney, M.R., & Fowlers, V.K. [1987]. Comprehensive cardiac care. St. Louis: C.V. Mosby).

2. The ejection fraction is the percentage of blood ejected from the ventricle with each cardiac cycle. Normal ejection fraction from the ventricle is greater than 55 percent. The ejection fraction is an indication of the degree of muscle damage. Clinically, an ejection fraction less than 30 percent often is manifested as severe fatigue (Mayberry-Toth, B., & Landon, S. [1989]. Complications associated with an acute myocardial infarction. Critical Care Nursing Quarterly, 12[2], 49–63).

3. Preload refers to Starling's law of the heart. Afterload is impedence to the left ventricle. It is likened to pushing against a door with the wind behind it (Hudak, C.M., Gallo, B.M., & Lohr, T. [1986]. Critical care nursing: A holistic approach [4th ed.]. Philadelphia: J.B. Lippincott).

Chapter

TEN

Conserving Cognitive Integrity of the Hospitalized Elderly*

Marquis D. Foreman, R.N., Ph.D.

An acute confusional state, a phenomenon also known as delirium, is a significant health problem for elderly acutely ill hospitalized patients. While hospitalized, 24 to 80 percent of elderly patients experience some degree of an acute confusional state (Cavanaugh, 1983; Foreman, 1989; Gillick, Serrell, & Gillick, 1982; Lipowski, 1983; Williams, Holloway, Winn, Wolanin, Lawer, Westwick, & Chin, 1979; Williams, Campbell, Raynor, Mlynarczyk, & Ward, 1985a). Although acute confusion has been described as benign and self-limited (Lipowski, 1983, 1987), it is associated with increased morbidity and mortality (Lipowski, 1983; Weddington, 1982), longer hospitalizations (Lipowski, 1983; Weddington, 1982), and an increased intensity of nursing care (Williams, Ward, & Campbell, 1986). All of these factors contribute to the increased daily hospital costs in providing care for acutely confused elders. Furthermore, it has been estimated that if the length of hospitalization could be reduced by just one day, the savings to Medicare would amount to $1 to $2 billion annually (Levkoff, Besdine, & Wetle, 1986).

Despite the importance of this health problem, 37 to 72 percent of elderly patients who become acutely confused are never recognized by physicians or nurses as suffering from an acute confusional state (Knights & Folstein, 1977; Palmateer & McCartney, 1985). Yet failure to diagnose and treat this condition is associated with the progression to a permanent state of cognitive impairment and a corresponding loss of the ability to care for oneself (Lipowski, 1983) or to maintain an independent life in the commu-

*The research was supported under a National Research Service Award, #5F31NU-05837-02, from the Division of Nursing, PHS, DHHS.

nity. Hence, elderly patients who become acutely confused in the hospital are more likely to be placed in a nursing home and to suffer the personal, social, and financial consequences of institutionalization (Levkoff et al., 1986; Zarit & Zarit, 1983).

In spite of the serious functional, psychologic, social, and economic sequelae, acute confusional states remain a neglected focus of scientific inquiry (Foreman, 1986; Levkoff et al., 1986). (Hence, the knowledge of this phenomenon is predominantly anecdotally based and is therefore limited.) Additionally, the research into acute confusional states is problematic in that it has been approached atheoretically (Foreman, in press; Roberts & Lincoln, 1988). As a result, the knowledge of acute confusional states consists of many unrelated facts, facts that are difficult, if not impossible, to integrate into a comprehensive body of knowledge (Foreman, 1986). Therefore, one aim of this exploratory study was to determine whether a clearer and more comprehensive understanding of acute confusional states could be obtained by examining it from the theoretical perspective of Levine's Conservation Model.

LEVINE'S CONSERVATION MODEL

The commonplaces of Levine's Conservation Model are person, environment, adaptation, and nursing. A description of these commonplaces and their underlying assumptions follows.

Person

A person is conceptualized as a holistic being who cherishes and defends that wholeness (Levine, 1969b). A person is thought of as an ever-changing being whose totality is greater than the sum of its parts (Levine, 1971). The assumptions upon which this conceptualization of the human organism is based are that a person (Levine, 1967a, 1967b, 1971) is multidimensional, exists within the context of and is in constant interaction with the environment, is constantly striving to maintain or to conserve his or her integrity, and responds to environmental demands in a singular yet integrated fashion to maintain that integrity.

Environment

The environment is both internal and external (Levine, 1969a). The internal environment equates with physiologic and pathophysiologic aspects of the organism (Foli, Johnson, Marriner, Poat, Poppa, & Zoretich, 1986), that is, structure and function. Conversely, there are three levels of the external environment (Bates, 1967): perceptual, operational, and conceptual. The perceptual environment comprises those aspects of the external environment obtained through sensory organs. Five sensory systems have been identified (Gibson, 1966): basic orienting, auditory, visual, taste-smell, and haptic. The operational environment comprises those aspects that affect a person physically. "All forms of radiation, micro-organisms, pollutants, which are odorless and colorless—every unseen, and unheard aspects of the individual's lifespace represents the impinging upon him of the operational environment" (Levine, 1986, p. 3). The conceptual environment comprises the symbolic and cultural aspects of the external environment—the environment of language, ideas, symbols, concepts, and invention (Levine, 1986). These notions about the environment are based on the assumption that the environment is the context in which a person lives; the environment provides meaning to the organism's existence as well as creates demands to which the organism must adapt if integrity is to be conserved.

Adaptation

Adaptation is the process of interaction between the organism and its environment by which integrity is conserved (Levine, 1973). Adaptation is hypothesized to be facilitated by four responses of the organism (Levine, 1969b). These organismic responses, considered predetermined and protective of integrity, are (1) fight or flight, (2) inflammatory, (3) response to stress, and (4) sensory response.

With respect to the process of adaptation, health and disease are conceptualized as multidimensional adaptive patterns (Levine, 1966). Disease is considered an unsuccessful adaptive process; illness represents a state in which organismic integrity has not been maintained. Conversely, health is considered a successful adaptive process; health represents a process that has maintained the wholeness of the organism.

Successful adaptive processes are those that best fit the organism in its environment. "A 'best fit' is accomplished with the least expenditure of effort, with sufficient protective devices built in so that the goal is achieved in as economic and expeditious a manner as possible" (Levine, 1986, p. 9). This "best fit," or the maintenance of organismic integrity, is achieved through the conservation of energy and structural, personal, and social integrity—the four conservation principles (Levine, 1967a).

The conservation of energy focuses on the balance between the supply of energy and the rate at which it is consumed, a balance without which organismic integrity cannot be maintained (Levine, 1986). The conservation of structural integrity is concerned with the process of healing, and has as its focus the maintenance of structure and function, that is anatomic and physiologic completeness (Levine, 1966, 1986). The conservation of personal integrity has as its focus the sense of personal identity, self-worth, and individual uniqueness, values, beliefs, and goals (Levine, 1967, 1971, 1986). Last, because a person must be viewed within the context of his or her social existence, the conservation of social integrity is concerned with the relationships of the individual with the community—those dynamic relationships of human beings—relationships through which life gains meaning (Foli et al., 1986). "The conservation principles do not operate singly or in isolation from each other. They are joined within the individual as a cascade of life events, churning and changing as the environmental challenge is confronted in each individual's unique way" (Levine, 1986, p. 21). Together, the four conservation principles provide a framework for the deduction of specific nursing actions from scientific principles (Levine, 1966).

Nursing

Nursing is a human interaction with the purpose of promoting and/or conserving the wholeness of the individual (Levine, 1966, 1969a), which is best accomplished by designing interventions that are based on the unique behavior of the individual's adaptive response and that facilitate the best fit between the individual and his or her environment (Levine, 1966, 1967a, 1986). Rubrics useful for designing nursing care that facilitate successful adaptation are the four conservation principles—the conservation of energy and of structural, personal, and social integrity (Levine, 1967, 1986).

Summary

Levine conceives the human being as a holistic, multidimensional organism whose predicament in life is the dynamic and enduring struggle to maintain the wholeness of his or her being. This struggle emanates from demands on the individual created by the environment, an element that is both internal and external to the individual. To maintain the wholeness of the being, the individual must adapt successfully to these environmental demands. Successful adaptive responses achieve the best fit between the individual and the environment, thereby maintaining the wholeness of the individual and attaining a state known as health. To facilitate the best fit between the environment and the individual—that is, to conserve the wholeness of the individual—is the purpose of nursing. Rubrics useful for designing nursing care that facilitate successful adaptation are the four conservation principles: the conservation of energy and of structural, personal, and social integrity.

Within the framework of Levine's Conservation Model, an acute confusional state is defined as a multidimensional adaptive pattern that occurs as a result of an actual or perceived alteration in the environment. However, this adaptive response is one that does not achieve a best fit between the individual and environment and, as a result, the wholeness of the individual is not conserved. This adaptive pattern, called acute confusion, is manifested by simultaneous disturbances in attention, thinking, consciousness, memory, perception, the sleep-wake cycle, psychomotor behavior, and orientation (American Psychiatric Association, 1987). These symptoms of confusion usually develop abruptly over a period of hours to days, and tend to fluctuate diurnally.

Therefore, the aims of this study were to (1) obtain information about the incidence, onset, and psychophysiologic variables associated with the onset of acute confusional states in elderly patients hospitalized for nonoperative reasons, and (2) determine whether a more clear and comprehensive understanding of acute confusion could be obtained by examining it within the framework of Levine's Conservation Model (Levine, 1967, 1971).

METHOD

Sample

The sample was selected from patients 60 years of age or older admitted within the previous 24 hours to the medical units of the critical care division of a university teaching hospital. To be considered eligible for inclusion in this study, patients also had to be able to speak and understand English and be willing to participate in the study. Patients were deemed ineligible if they (1) were admitted for any surgical procedure; (2) had changes in cognitive function due to alcoholism or a diagnosis of dementia, or had a score less than 24 on initial mental status testing; (3) had a primary neurologic diagnosis; (4) were unconscious; or (5) were unable to hear, see, or verbally communicate. On the basis of these criteria, 71 elderly patients became subjects in this study of acute confusional states. Once enrolled, no subject requested to withdraw.

Measures

To identify variables considered important in the development of confusion in the hospitalized elderly, an extensive and critical review of the literature about acute confusional states, delirium, cognitive impairment, and information-processing was conducted (Foreman, 1986). Numerous variables, both physiologic and nonphysiologic in nature, have been identified as being causally related to acute confusion in older patients. Because this list of causal variables is extensive and, therefore, impossible to examine within the context of one study, the variables critical for normal cell function, especially those well known to alter cerebral function, as well as those identified in previous studies of acute confusional states, were selected for examination in this study. Additionally, these variables were reduced in number by eliminating vague, imprecise, and/or redundant variables, and were categorized according to Levine's four conservation principles.

Because the four conservation principles are not mutually exclusive, categorization is somewhat arbitrary (Levine, personal communication, May, 1986). For example, the variable Po_2 can be used as information about respiratory physiology (conservation of structural integrity) or as an index of the energy available for the central nervous system (conservation of energy). As a result, the rationale for the categorization of variables is based on the intended use of the information represented by the variable (Levine, personal communication, May, 1986). These variables can be categorized (Table 10–1) as variables within the domain of (1) the conservation of energy, (2) the conservation of structural integrity, (3) the conservation of personal integrity, and (4) the conservation of social integrity.

TABLE 10-1. **VARIABLES ASSOCIATED WITH CONFUSION CATEGORIZED BY LEVINE'S FOUR CONSERVATION PRINCIPLES**

Conservation Principle	Variable
Energy	Serum albumin
	Serum glucose
	Leukocytes
	Body temperature
	Heart rate
	Mean arterial pressure
	pH
	Serum creatinine
Structural Integrity	Serum sodium
	Serum potassium
	Serum calcium
	Hemoglobin
	Blood urea nitrogen
	Po_2
Personal Integrity	Visual status
	Auditory status
	Medications
	Orienting objects
Social Integrity	Presence of significant others
	Nurse's perception of confusion

SOURCE: Foreman, M.D. (1989). Confusion in the hospitalized elderly: Incidence, onset, and associated factors. Research in Nursing & Health, 12:23, with permission.

CONSERVATION OF ENERGY

Variables categorized within this domain indirectly provided information about cerebral metabolism and included:

1. Short- and long-term nutritional indices of serum albumin, glucose, and leukocytes (Christensen & Kehlet, 1984; Kane, Ouslander, & Abrass, 1984; Shields, 1980). Blood levels of albumin were obtained only on admission as these values fluctuate little over time and were considered reliable indicators of preadmission nutritional status (Shields, 1980). Conversely, serum glucose and leukocytes are more variable and, therefore, were obtained as frequently as every four hours, as determined by the medical status of the patient.
2. Vital signs (blood pressure, respirations, heart rate, and temperature) for information about energy production and use (Hirschfeld, 1976; Levine, 1969). These measures were obtained at the time of each interview by the investigator and as documented in each patient's hospital record.
3. Information about factors influencing cerebral metabolism obtained from blood pH (Plum & Posner, 1982, pp. 185–188) and serum creatinine (Guyton, 1986, p. 454; Plum & Posner, 1982, pp. 226–230). Values of these factors were obtained at least daily, and more frequently, as determined by the medical status of the patient.

CONSERVATION OF STRUCTURAL INTEGRITY

Variables categorized within this domain indirectly provided information about structure and function, and included:

1. Information about respiratory function obtained via Po_2 (Guyton, 1986, pp. 481–492; Plum & Posner, 1982, pp. 230–233). Because 97 percent of the oxygen is transported in combination with hemoglobin (Guyton, 1986, pp. 497–499), an evaluation of oxygenation also included the hemoglobin content. These values were obtained daily and as warranted by the medical status of the patient.
2. Information about neural functioning obtained via sodium, potassium, and calcium values (Guyton, 1986, pp. 106–110; Plum & Posner, 1982, p. 179). Serum levels of these electrolytes were obtained at least daily.
3. Information about renal function, a determinant of the body's internal environment (Guyton, 1986, pp. 410–424; Kane et al., 1984, pp. 275–276; Plum & Posner, 1982, pp. 225–230). Daily evaluation of levels of blood urea nitrogen (BUN) were made.

CONSERVATION OF PERSONAL INTEGRITY

Variables categorized within this domain provided data about aspects of the individual that influence how information is perceived and interpreted. Variables categorized within the domain of personal integrity included:

1. Medications previously identified as adversely affecting cognitive function (Khan, 1986; Task Force of the NIA, 1980; Wolanin, 1981). Such medications included sedatives, hypnotics, analgesics, and anticholinergics. The frequency with which each medication was administered was noted and summed daily (Roberts & Lincoln, 1988).
2. The status of visual and auditory functioning. Assessment was made of the patient's ability to read newsprint, and the whispered voice test was used to assess hearing (Bates, 1979; Roberts & Lincoln, 1988). Sensory functioning was assessed at each interview by the investigator. The number of abnormal senses weighted by the degree of impairment were added for a total score of sensory deficits (Roberts & Lincoln, 1988).
3. Various aspects of the patient's immediate environment thought to be important in the maintenance of cognitive functioning (Foreman, 1984, 1986; Roberts & Lincoln, 1988; Williams, 1988; Williams et al., 1979, 1985a; Williams, Campbell, Raynor, Musholt, Mlynarczyk, & Crane, 1985b; Wolanin & Phillips, 1981). These aspects of the environment included objects that provide meaning and orientation (e.g., newspapers, timepieces, radios, televisions) and the presence of personal belongings. The number of these objects in the patient's immediate environment were noted and summed daily (Roberts & Lincoln, 1988).

CONSERVATION OF SOCIAL INTEGRITY

Variables categorized within this domain provided an assessment of the individual's social existence, and included:

1. Presence of significant others (Campbell, Williams, & Mlynarczyk, 1986; Hirschfeld, 1976). Each subject's nurse was requested to provide an estimate of the number of visitors and length of visit. The length of time each visitor spent with the patients was noted and summed daily.
2. Context of the nurse-patient relationship. Evaluation of context was determined by use of the Visual Analog Scale for Confusion (VAS-C) (Nagley, 1984; Vermeersch, 1986).

Instruments

MINI-MENTAL STATE EXAMINATION

The Mini-Mental State Examination (MMSE) (Folstein, Folstein, & McHugh, 1975) is commonly used in gerontologic research and clinical practice and has been demonstrated to be valid and reliable (Anthony, LeResche, Niaz, Von Korff, & Folstein, 1982; Foreman, 1987, 1989). It is a simplified scored form of 11 questions representing seven dimensions of acute confusion, and requiring 5 to 10 minutes to complete. Aspects of cognition assessed by the MMSE include (Foreman, 1987) orientation; memory; attention; constructional ability; general knowledge; use of language; and thought processes, content, and form. Each question is scored as either right or wrong; the total score ranges from 0 to 30 and is the number of corrected responses (Folstein et al., 1975). A score of less than 24, or having six or more errors, is considered evidence of confusion (Anthony et al., 1982).

CLINICAL ASSESSMENT OF CONFUSION

The Clinical Assessment of Confusion (CAC) is a checklist of 25 psychomotor behaviors representing seven dimensions of acute confusion. These behaviors are associated with varying degrees of confusion; the greater the number of behaviors observed, the more severe the confusion (Vermeersch, 1986). The observer is requested to evaluate each patient on the basis of the presence or absence of each behavior. The score, ranging from 0 to 25, is the total number of observed behaviors; the presence of any behavior is considered evidence of confusion (Vermeersch, 1986). Information about the psychometric properties of the CAC have been reported previously by Foreman (1989) and Vermeersch (1986).

VISUAL ANALOG SCALE FOR CONFUSION

The VAS-C (Nagley, 1984, 1986; Vermeersch, 1986) was used to obtain information about the context of the nurse-subject relationship (i.e., did the nurse perceive and, therefore, relate to the patient as if confused?).

The VAS-C is a 10-cm horizontal line with anchors of "No confusion" and "Severe confusion." Nurses were asked to place a slash through a line indicating their perception of the patient's degree of confusion, which was determined by measuring in centimeters the distance of the respondent's mark from the "No confusion" end of the scale. Psychometric properties of the VAS-C have been evaluated by Foreman (1989), Nagley (1984, 1986), and Vermeersch (1986), who have demonstrated the scale to be both valid and reliable in numerous samples of hospitalized elders.

VISUAL ANALOG SCALE FOR DEPRESSION

Because the cognitive deficits of depression are similar to those of acute confusion (Kane et al., 1984; Zarit & Zarit, 1983), a method for discriminating between acutely confused and depressed patients was used. A Visual Analog Scale for Depression (VAS-D) (Aitken, 1969), a 10-cm horizontal line representing an effective continuum, was used for that purpose. The VAS-D is anchored at the left end (0 cm) with "I am not depressed" and on the right (10 cm) with "I am as depressed as I can possibly imagine myself being." Subjects were instructed to place a slash through this line at the point that indicated their feelings at the moment. The degree of depression was determined by measuring in centimeters from the left end, that is, the "I am not depressed" end, to the respondent's slash. Results of reliability and validity testing were reported by Foreman (1987).

Procedure

The subjects, selected within 24 hours of admission to the hospital, were interviewed daily by the investigator for a maximum of 8 days, or until the patient was discharged or became acutely confused. This interview required approximately 20 to 30 minutes to complete the MMSE, CAC, and VAS-D. Information relative to sociodemographic and environmental characteristics considered relevant to the study of acute confusional states also were obtained during this interview. Additionally, data about medications and the results of selected laboratory tests were obtained from each patient's hospital record.

To ensure that all instances of acute confusion were detected, the nurses caring for the subjects completed a VAS-C and a CAC once per shift with their initial assessment of the subject. If a change was observed in the patient's level of alertness, psychomotor behavior, and/or orientation, the nurses again completed a VAS-C and a CAC, as well as an MMSE.

The classification of being acutely confused was made on the basis of the combined criteria of the MMSE and CAC administered by the investigator. Thus, to be considered acutely confused, subjects had to score less than 24 on the MMSE and exhibit four or more of the behaviors comprising the CAC.

For the purpose of analysis, the values of all variables were used from the day each subject developed acute confusion (range = day 2 to day 6;

mode = day 2). To ensure comparability, the values of all variables from day 2 were used for all subjects who did not become acutely confused.

RESULTS

Demographic characteristics of the 71 subjects are presented in Table 10-2. Of the 71 subjects, 38 percent (n = 27), became acutely confused within 6 days of admission to the hospital. Nineteen of these 27 patients developed an acute confusional state by the second day, an additional four patients did so by the fourth day, and another four patients by the sixth day of hospitalization. No new episodes of acute confusion were identified after the sixth day of hospitalization.

Because various aspects of cognition are influenced by gender, race, education, and effective status, these variables were examined to test if they were determinants of the acute confusional state. The acutely confused (n = 27) and not confused (n = 44) groups were homogeneous with respect to age, gender, race, and admission medical diagnoses. The two groups did, however, differ significantly with respect to educational preparation, $t(69) = 3.09$, $p = .003$, and depression $t(69) = -6.02$, $p = .001$. In other words, the patients who developed an acute confusional state while hospitalized were less educated and reported higher levels of depression. Thus, data were analyzed, when appropriate, with educational preparation and depression as covariates; however, no statistically significant ($p < .05$) interactive effects, either separately or in combination, were observed. Multivariate analysis of variance (MANOVA) was used to examine the dif-

TABLE 10-2. **CHARACTERISTICS OF THE SAMPLE**

Characteristic	Not Confused Subjects (n = 44)		Confused Subjects (n = 27)		All Subjects (n = 71)	
	n	%	n	%	n	%
Sex						
Female	26	59.1	19	70.4	45	63.4
Male	18	40.9	8	29.6	26	36.6
Race						
Caucasian	20	45.5	11	40.7	31	43.7
Black	24	54.5	13	48.1	37	52.1
Hispanic			3	11.1	3	4.2
	M	**(SD)**	**M**	**(SD)**	**M**	**(SD)**
Age	72.93	(7.35)	74.78	(8.13)	73.63	(7.65)
Education	11.43	(2.96)	9.33	(2.45)	10.63	(2.94)
Depression	0.03	(0.15)	0.89	(0.93)	0.36	(0.72)

SOURCE: Foreman, M.D. (1989). Confusion in the hospitalized elderly: Incidence, onset, and associated factors. Research in Nursing & Health, 12:25, with permission.

TABLE 10-3. CLASSIFICATION OF SUBJECTS[a] AS CONFUSED OR NOT
CONFUSED ON THE BASIS OF THE DISCRIMINANT EQUATION

| | Predicted Group Membership | | | |
| | Not Confused | | Confused | |
Actual Group Membership[b]	n	(%)	n	(%)
Not Confused (n = 40)	38	(95.0)	2[c]	(5.0)
Confused (n = 27)	2[d]	(7.4)	25	(92.6)
Total (n = 67)	40		27	

[a]Four cases were excluded from this analysis as a result of at least one missing discriminant variable.
[b]As determined by the Mini-Mental State Examination and Clinical Assessment of Confusion
[c]False-positive misclassifications
[d]False-negative misclassifications
SOURCE: Foreman, M.D. (1989). Confusion in the hospitalized elderly: Incidence, onset, and associated factors. Research in Nursing & Health, 12:26, with permission.

ferences between acutely confused and not confused subjects with respect to the multiple variables categorized within Levine's conservation principles (see Table 10–1). The overall MANOVA was significant, multivariate $F(14,48) = 37.88$, $p < .0001$. To determine the combination of variables and the status of these variables best describing the differences between patients who became acutely confused and those in whom cognitive integrity was maintained, a stepwise discriminant function analysis was performed. The resulting discriminant equation was significant, $\chi^2(13) = 137.61$, $p = .0001$:

$$D = 0.91 \text{ (sodium)} - 1.41 \text{ (potassium)} + 1.08 \text{ (glucose)} + 2.13 \text{ (creatinine)} - 0.30 \text{ (mean arterial pressure)} + 2.03 \text{ (nurse ratings of confusion)} + 0.90 \text{ (blood urea nitrogen)} + 0.45 \text{ (medications)} + 1.50 \text{ (orienting objects)} - 0.63 \text{ (interaction with significant others)}$$

Because statistical significance is necessary but not sufficient for meaningful discrimination, the adequacy of the discrimination of the equation was evaluated. On the basis of the discriminant equation, 94 percent of the subjects were correctly identified as either acutely confused or not confused. Although there was an equivalent number of false-positive and false-negative misclassifications (Table 10–3), there was slightly greater bias in identifying more accurately patients who did not develop an acute confusional state (85 percent) than in identifying those who did become acutely confused (93 percent).

DISCUSSION

The first aim of this study was to obtain information about the incidence, onset, and psychophysiologic variables associated with the onset of acute confusional states in elderly hospitalized patients. Slightly more than one third of the patients in this study developed confusion within 6 days of admission to the hospital; that is, approximately one in every three patients experienced an episode of acute confusion while hospitalized. Although the 38 percent incidence of acute confusion is alarming, it is low in comparison to the 30 to 80 percent rate reported in the literature (Cavanaugh, 1983; Gillick et al., 1982; Kral, 1975; Liston, 1982; Sadler, 1979, 1981; Williams et al., 1985b). This lower rate of incidence could have resulted from the exclusion of patients who were deemed acutely confused upon admission to the hospital, or exclusion of those in whom the acute confusional state was superimposed on a chronic form of cognitive impairment—patients who have not been excluded in previous studies (Cavanaugh, 1983; Chisholm, Deniston, Ingrisan, & Barbus, 1982; Williams et al., 1979). Or, it could indicate that the incidence of acute confusion is lower in patients who are admitted to the hospital for nonoperative reasons. Nonetheless, a 38 percent rate of incidence supports the notion that confusion is a major health problem for the hospitalized elderly. For this reason, nurses are obligated to carefully and systematically assess the patient's physical and cognitive status at the time of admission (Foreman, Gillies, & Wagner, 1989). This assessment should be performed routinely (i.e., at least every 8 hours) throughout hospitalization for the timely detection of any cognitive problem, for without detecting this problem there can be no attempts to intervene. Recommended guidelines for systematically and routinely assessing an elder's cognitive status have been described in detail by Foreman et al. (1989).

The findings of this study relative to the onset of acute confusion during hospitalization provide direction as to when to assess for this health problem. The rather precipitous onset of an acute confusional state, on day 2 of hospitalization in this study, could result from current health care policy and reimbursement regulations that favor delayed and emergent hospitalization of acutely or critically ill patients. The time of onset also may reflect the etiology of the cognitive impairment. For instance, cognitive impairment occurring rather precipitously after hospitalization may indicate the problem to be an acute confusional state with an etiology of some combination of the stresses related to the hospitalization and psychophysiologic alterations associated with the underlying physical illness. Manifestations of cognitive impairment occurring later in the course of hospitalization—for example, after the sixth day—may indicate the etiology to be iatrogenic or nosocomial or that the phenomenon is a condition other than an acute confusional state (e.g., depression). Nonetheless, having knowledge about when a patient is more likely to become acutely confused can be useful for targeting more appropriately and effectively the surveillance efforts for acute confusional states. Thus, it is more likely that an acute confusional state would be detected and interventions initiated.

The onset of confusion was reported in the literature (Chisholm et al., 1982; Hogue, 1986; Williams et al., 1979, 1985b) as equally likely across the first 7 days of hospitalization. The difference in the time of onset between that of this study and that reported in the literature could be a function of the patient populations studied (i.e., medical versus surgical patients). Onset of confusion also could have been influenced by the change in health care policy that favors earlier discharge of sicker patients. In either event, knowing when confusion is more likely to occur can assist in focusing more appropriate and effective efforts at detection, thereby reducing or eliminating the sequelae associated with confusion. Furthermore, the time of onset of cognitive problems may facilitate differentiating among the various types of cognitive impairment that hospitalized elderly patients experience (e.g., between delirium and depression).

Ten psychophysiologic variables were associated significantly with the onset of confusion; it is impossible to conclude whether these variables are causes, effects, or just simply correlates of confusion. Nonetheless, a profile of the confused elderly patient is derived from the discriminant function equation. Specifically, confused patients were hypernatremic, hypokalemic, hyperglycemic, and hypotensive; had elevated blood levels of creatinine and urea nitrogen; received more medications; were more frequently perceived by nurses as confused; had more orienting objects in their immediate environment; and had fewer interactions with significant others.

The relationships between the 10 variables and confusion are all logical except one: acutely confused patients had more orienting objects in their immediate environment than did nonconfused patients. This unexpected relationship may have been a function of the measurement of the variable. The assumption was that the mere presence of orienting objects, (e.g., timepieces, calendars, newspapers, televisions, radios, and personal possessions) would orient the patient to time and space. However, this presumes that all objects have the same meaning and function for all persons and that these orienting objects function actively (i.e., orienting objects would achieve their purpose whether or not these objects are used as such), assumptions that may not be reasonable. If this conclusion is true, it necessitates the rethinking of the current operationalization of orienting objects with respect to the nursing research and care of patients experiencing an episode of acute confusion.

Another more plausible and optimistic explanation is that the greater number of orienting objects in the immediate environment of the acutely confused reflected nurses' attempts to intervene. This seems reasonable to conclude, since nurses are universally taught to include such objects as a means for ameliorating confused behavior in hospitalized patients.

There are similarities between the profile of acutely confused elderly patients in this study and those found in studies of surgical patients (Budd & Brown, 1974; Sadler, 1981; Williams et al., 1979, 1985a, 1985b). Acutely confused postcardiotomy patients differed significantly from those who did not become confused, in that acutely confused patients had lower cardiac output and higher temperatures (Budd & Brown, 1974). Sadler (1981) also studied postcardiotomy patients and reported a combination of four variables that best predicted acute confusion: age, arterial pressure on bypass, and body temperature on the first and third postoperative days. Williams et al. (1979), after studying postsurgical hip-fractured patients, described the composite confused patient as "the very aged person who had been on tranquilizers, was male, had urinary problems, and who, for whatever reason, was more immobilized than patients with similar injury and surgery" (p. 35). More recently, Williams et al. (1985b) found combinations of age, prehospital level of activity, previous episodes of confusion, and urine elimination problems to best predict the presence of confusion. Given the differences in populations sampled, it is difficult to determine which of these variables linked to confusion are specific to confusion and which are specific to the underlying medical condition for which the patients were hospitalized. In either event, it is clear that further study of the causes of acute confusional states is warranted.

Despite the fact that the knowledge of acute confusional states is incomplete, implications for the nursing care of acutely confused patients can be extrapolated from the findings of this study. It is suggested that the approach for the nursing care of confused patients be holistic, that is, conserve the wholeness of the individual, by conserving:

1. Energy. Foster cerebral metabolism by maintaining the balance between the supply of energy and the rate at which it is consumed. Specific factors to monitor and maintain within normal limits include mean arterial pressure and serum creatinine and glucose.
2. Structural integrity. Ensure that the internal environment of the body supports normal neural functioning. To promptly detect and correct any deviations before structural integrity is compromised, monitor blood values of sodium, potassium, and urea nitrogen.
3. Personal integrity. Create an environment that promotes orientation through active use of orienting objects (e.g., timepieces, calendars). Additionally, facilitate the accurate interpretation of environmental information via the judicious administration of medications.
4. Social integrity. Include significant others in the care of the patient.

Collectively, from these nursing actions, the "best fit" can be obtained and, thus, the integrity of the individual conserved.

The second aim of this study was to determine whether a clearer, more comprehensive understanding of acute confusion could be obtained by examining it within the framework of Levine's Conservation Model. Several models have been developed for explaining or predicting the development of acute confusional states in hospitalized elders (Williams et al., 1985b; Roberts & Lincoln, 1988). However, these models have failed to view the problem holistically and/or theoretically, thus limiting the abilities of the respective models. Williams et al. (1985b) developed three models for predicting acute confusional states in hospitalized elderly patients. These models accurately predicted acute confusion in 54 to 65.5 percent of the cases, a predictive ability that is not much better than chance. Additionally, the variables found most useful in predicting acute confusion provided little direction for preventing or intervening in such instances. The model developed by Roberts and Lincoln (1988) is an improvement in that the model was theoretically based and provides direction for clinical care; however, the model explained only 39 percent of the variance. The model developed here is a further improvement because (1) it is parsimonious in that it incorporates a few variables that can be realistically assessed in a real clinical setting; (2) it is more accurate in identifying acute confusion than previously developed models; and (3) it provides direction for nursing strategies for preventing and intervening in cases of acute confusion in the hospitalized elderly. Nonetheless, examining the findings of all three investigations indicates that our knowledge of the causes of acute confusional states remains incomplete (Foreman, in press).

Of additional interest was the support of a fundamental premise upon which the conservation model was based. Specifically, the theoretical notion that the conservation principles do not operate singly or in isolation of one another (Levine, 1966, 1986) is supported. Acutely confused patients were differentiated best from those not confused by 10 variables representing all four conservation principles (see Table 10–1). This solution supports the contention that for nursing interventions to be successful, they must be guided by all four conservation principles. According to Levine (1966), to consider less than all four conservation principles is to consider less than the whole person. As such, interventions are incomplete, cannot achieve the best fit between the organism and its environment, and, therefore, cannot be effective. This notion may explain why previous nursing measures intended for reducing confusion were relatively unsuccessful, since these interventions conserved only aspects of personal and/or social integrity (Budd & Brown, 1974; Chatham, 1978; Williams et al., 1985a).

With respect to the conduct of scientific inquiry into confusion, the understanding of this complex, dynamic, and multifaceted phenomenon is embryonic, and much investigation is needed. Specifically, studies are needed that (1) provide definitive evidence linking specific psychophysiologic disturbances to the onset of confusion, (2) describe the evolution and resolution of confusion, (3) confirm the defining characteristics of the phenomenon of confusion, (4) examine confusion across multiple medical diagnostic categories to identify which characteristics are specific to the phenomenon and which are specific to the medical diagnostic category, and (5) delineate protocols for the effective nursing care of acutely confused patients. Of additional importance is that these studies be conducted from a theoretical stance, such as that obtained from Levine's Conservation Model, to enable the integration and synthesis of this information into a comprehensive body of knowledge.

REFERENCES

Aitken, R.C.B. (1969). Measurement of feelings using visual analogue scales. Proceedings of the Royal Society of Medicine, 67, 989–993.

American Psychiatric Association. (1987). Diagnostic and statistical manual of mental disorders (3rd ed., rev.). Washington, DC: American Psychiatric Association.

Anthony, J.C., LeResche, L., Niaz, U., Von Korff, M.R., & Folstein, M.F. (1982). Limits of the "mini-mental state" as a screening test for dementia and delirium among hospitalized patients. Psychological Medicine, 12, 396–408.

Bates, B. (1967). A guide to physical examination (1st ed.). Philadelphia: J.B. Lippincott.

Bates, B. (1979). A guide to physical examination (2nd ed.). Philadelphia: J.B. Lippincott.

Budd, S., & Brown, W. (1974). Effect of a reorientation technique on postcardiotomy delirium. Nursing Research, 23, 314–348.

Campbell, E.B., Williams, M.A., & Mlynarczyk, S.M. (1986). After the fall—Confusion. American Journal of Nursing, 86, 151–154.

Cavanaugh, S. (1983). The prevalence of emotional and cognitive dysfunction in a general medical population: Using the MMSE, GHQ, and BDI. General Hospital Psychiatry, 5, 115–124.

Chatham, M.A. (1978). The effect of family involvement on patients' manifestations of post-cardiotomy psychosis. Heart & Lung, 7, 995–999.

Chisholm, S.E., Deniston, O.L., Ingrisan, R.M., & Barbus, A.J. (1982). Prevalence of confusion in elderly hospitalized patients. Journal of Gerontological Nursing, 8, 87–96.

Christensen, T., & Kehlet, H. (1984). Postoperative fatigue and changes in nutritional status. British Journal of Surgery, 71, 473–476.

Foli, K.J., Johnson, T., Marriner, A., Poat, M.C., Poppa, L., & Zoretich, S.T. (1986). Myra Estrin Levine: Four conservation principles. In A. Marriner (Ed.), Nursing theorists and their work (pp. 335–344). St. Louis: C.V. Mosby.

Folstein, M.F., Folstein, S.E., & McHugh, P.R. (1975). "Mini-mental state": A practical guide for grading the cognitive state of patients for clinicians. Journal of Psychiatric Research, 12, 189–198.

Foreman, M.D. (1984). Acute confusional states in the elderly: An algorithm. Dimensions of Critical Care Nursing, 3, 207–215.

Foreman, M.D. (1986). Acute confusional states in the hospitalized elderly: A research dilemma. Nursing Research, 35, 34–38.

Foreman, M.D. (1987). Reliability and validity of mental status questionnaires in elderly hospitalized patients. Nursing Research, 36, 216–220.

Foreman, M.D. (1989). Confusion in the hospitalized elderly: Incidence, onset, and associated factors. Research in Nursing & Health, 12, 21–29.

Foreman, M.D. (in press). The cognitive and behavioral nature of acute confusional states. Scholarly Inquiry for Nursing Practice.

Foreman, M.D., Gillies, D.A., & Wagner, D. (1989). Impaired cognition in the critically ill elderly patients: Clinical implications. Critical Care Nursing Quarterly, 12(1), 61–73.

Gibson, J.E. (1966). The senses considered as perceptual systems. Boston: Houghton-Mifflin.

Gillick, M.R., Serrell, N.A., & Gillick, L.S. (1982). Adverse consequences of hospitalization in the elderly. Social Science and Medicine, 16, 1033–1038.

Guyton, A.C. (1986). Textbook of medical physiology (7th ed.). Philadelphia: W.B. Saunders.

Hirschfeld, M.J. (1976). The cognitively impaired older adult. American Journal of Nursing, 76, 1981–1984.

Hogue, C.C. (1986). Delirium in elderly surgical patients (abstract). In S.M. Stinson, J.C. Kerr, P. Giovanetti, P.A. Field, & J. MacPhail (Eds.), New frontiers in nursing research (p. 182). Edmonton: University of Alberta.

Kane, R.L., Ouslander, J.G., & Abrass, I.B. (1984). Essentials of clinical geriatrics. New York: McGraw-Hill.

Khan, A.U. (1986). Clinical disorders of memory. New York: Plenum.

Knights, E.B., & Folstein, M.F. (1977). Unsuspected emotional and cognitive disturbance in medical patients. Annals of Internal Medicine, 87, 723–724.

Kral, V.A. (1975). Confusional states: Description and management. In J.G. Howels (Ed.), Modern perspectives in the psychiatry of old age, (pp. 296–331). New York: Brunner/Mazel.

Levine, M.E. (1966). Adaptation and assessment: A rationale for nursing intervention. American Journal of Nursing, 66, 2450–2454.

Levine, M.E. (1967a). The four conservation principles of nursing. Nursing Forum, VI(1), 45–59.

Levine, M.E. (1967b). This I believe . . . About patient centered care. Nursing Outlook, 15, 53–55.

Levine, M.E. (1969a). The pursuit of wholeness. American Journal of Nursing, 69, 253–264.

Levine, M.E. (1969b). Introduction to clinical nursing. Philadelphia: F.A. Davis.

Levine, M.E. (1971). Holistic nursing. Nursing Clinics of North America, 6, 253–264.

Levine, M.E. (1973). Introduction to clinical nursing (2nd ed.). Philadelphia: F.A. Davis.

Levine, M.E. (1986, May). Personal communication.

Levine, M.E. (1986, August). The four conservation principles of nursing: Twenty years later. Paper presented at the Nursing Theory Congress, Toronto.

Levkoff, S.E., Besdine, R.W., & Wetle, T. (1986). Acute confusional states (delirium) in the hospitalized elderly. In C. Eisdorfer (Ed.), Annual Review of Gerontology and Geriatrics: Vol. 6 (pp. 1–26). New York: Springer.

Lipowski, Z.J. (1983). Transient cognitive disorders (delirium, acute confusional state in the elderly). American Journal of Psychiatry, 140, 1426–1436.

Lipowski, Z.J. (1987). Delirium (acute confusional states). Journal of the American Medical Association, 258, 1789–1792.

Liston, E.H. (1982). Delirium in the aged. Psychiatric Clinics of North America, 5(1), 49–66.

Nagley, S.J. (1984). Prevention of confusion in hospitalized elderly persons. Unpublished doctoral dissertation. Case Western Reserve University, Cleveland.

Nagley, S.J. (1986). Predicting and preventing confusion in your patients. Journal of Gerontological Nursing, 12(3), 27–31.

Palmateer, L.M., & McCartney, J.R. (1985). Do nurses know when patients have cognitive deficits? Journal of Gerontological Nursing, 11, 6–16.

Plum, F., & Posner, J.B. (1982). Diagnosis of stupor and coma (3rd ed.). Philadelphia: F.A. Davis.

Roberts, B.L., & Lincoln, R.E. (1988). Cognitive disturbance in hospitalized and institutionalized elders. Research in Nursing & Health, 11, 309–319.

Sadler, D.P. (1979). Nursing assessment of postcardiotomy delirium. Heart & Lung, 8, 745–750.

Sadler, D.P. (1981). Incidence, degree, and duration of postcardiotomy delirium. Heart & Lung, 10, 1084–1092.

Shields, H. (1980). Nutritional therapy. In J.J. Frietag & L.W. Miller (Eds.), Manual of medical therapeutics (2nd ed.) pp. 221–238. Boston: Little, Brown & Co.

Task Force of the National Institute on Aging. (1980). Senility reconsidered: Treatment possibilities for the mental impairment in the elderly. Journal of the American Medical Association, 244, 259–262.

Vermeersch, P.E.H. (1986). Development of a scale to measure confusion in hospitalized adults. Unpublished doctoral dissertation. Case Western Reserve University, Cleveland.

Weddington, W.W., Jr. (1982). The mortality of delirium: An underappreciated problem. Psychosomatics, 23, 1232–1235.

Williams, M.A. (1988). The physical environment and patient care. In J.J. Fitzpatric & R.L. Taunton (Eds.), Annual Review of Nursing Research, Vol. 6 (pp. 61–84). New York: Springer.

Williams, M.A., Campbell, E.B., Raynor, W.J., Jr., Mlynarczyk, S.M., & Ward, S.E. (1985a). Reduction in incidence of acute confusional states in elderly patients by nursing measures. Research in Nursing & Health, 8, 329–337.

Williams, M.A., Campbell, E.B., Raynor, W.J., Jr., Musholt, M.A., Mlynarczyk, S.M., & Crane, L.F. (1985b). Predictors of acute confusional states in hospitalized elderly patients. Research in Nursing & Health, 8, 31–40.

Williams, M.A., Holloway, J.R., Winn, M.C., Wolanin, M.O., Lawler, M.L., Westwick, C.R., & Chin, M.H. (1979). Nursing activities and acute confusional states in elderly hip-fractured patients. Nursing Research, 28, 25–35.

Williams, M.A., Ward, S.E., & Campbell, E.B. (1986). Issues in studying confusion in older hospitalized patients (abstract). In S.M. Stinson, J.C. Kerr, P. Giovan, P.A. Field, & J. MacPhail (Eds.), New frontiers in nursing research (p. 390). Edmonton: University of Alberta.

Wolanin, M.O. (1981). Physiologic aspects of confusion. Journal of Gerontological Nursing, 7, 236–242.

Wolanin, M.O., & Phillips, L.R.F. (1981). Confusion: Prevention and care. St. Louis: C.V. Mosby.

Zarit, S.H., & Zarit, J.M. (1983). Cognitive impairment. In P.M. Lewinsohn & L. Teri (Eds.), Clinical geropsychiatry: New directions in assessment and treatment (pp. 38–80). New York: Pergamon.

Chapter
ELEVEN

Emergency Care in a Large University Emergency Department

Jane Benson Pond, R.N.C., M.S.N., C.R.N.P.
Susan G. Taney, R.N., M.S.N., C.R.N.P.

Levine's four conservation principles provide an effective organizing framework for professional nursing practice in the provision of emergency care. Emergency care is delivered in a variety of settings from freestanding centers to mobile intensive care units. The more common setting for the provision of emergency nursing care is the hospital-based department. Varying widely in age and socioeconomic and cultural backgrounds, patients arrive 24 hours a day, everyday, at different levels of adaptive change on the health-illness continuum. Emergency care is episodic and requires prompt assessment, planning, and intervention. Emergency nurses provide care based upon a holistic assessment of patients' perceived or actual physical and/or emotional threats to their integrity.

THE EMERGENCY DEPARTMENT SETTING

The emergency department (ED) of the Hospital of the University of Pennsylvania (HUP) is a clinical facility serving more than 150 patients daily. The department is operated by a highly trained staff of nurses and physicians. Triage is the entrance point for all patients. Triage is a responsibility shared by all ED registered nurses on a rotating basis; it requires sharp assessment skills. The triage nurse determines the acuity of the patient's presenting condition and classifies each patient according to a standard department criteria scale. The rate at which a patient receives further nursing and any medical intervention is determined by the classification assigned by the triage nurse.

In most urban settings only about 15 percent of all ED patients have the emergent needs of a life-threatening condition. Another 20 percent have urgent needs with conditions having the potential of becoming life-threatening (Jacobson, 1985). The vital question to be answered initially is how quickly does a patient presenting to an ED require intervention beyond the initial triage assessment. Therefore, triage can be viewed as the foundation of hospital-based emergency care.

The triage classification criteria scale is an effective tool in communicating to all health care providers the initial triage assessment status of patients. E-Stat describes the patient who is critically ill or injured, a patient with a life-threatening condition, or one with cardiac and/or respiratory arrest in progress upon arrival. E-½ classifies the patient who can wait no longer than a half hour until definitive care is given, patients with asthma, high fevers, or post-ictal states. Patients classified as E-1 may be processed through standard registration and may wait in the waiting room up to 1 hour if a large number of patients necessitates delays. Examples of E-1 conditions are fractures without neurovascular compromise, minor burns, and sickle-cell crisis without respiratory distress and with normal vital signs. E-2 classifies the patient as being able to wait in the waiting room up to 2 hours. This is especially useful on a day when the waiting time exceeds 2 hours. Irregular vaginal bleeding of moderate flow with normal vital signs and abdominal pain is an example of an E-2 condition. Patients capable of waiting more than 2 hours are classified as E. They have minor ailments, simple lacerations, or sprains. Other patients may be triaged directly to the adjacent walk-in clinic or other specialty clinics on a same-day basis (e.g., those with rashes, toothaches, weeping conjunctivitis). Each patient may be retriaged at any point in the process according to a change in signs or symptoms. For example, the patient with normal vital signs and a normal hemoglobin and hematocrit with the chief complaint of an upset stomach will be reclassified when hematemesis occurs.

PATTERNS OF CARE

The medical, nursing, and legal professional hierarchy of the hospital places great confidence in the ED staff nurse's ability to accurately perform the responsibilities of triage. Yet once the physician has read the nurses' notes for the record of the initial triage assessment and classification, he or she rarely, if ever, reads these notes again during the patient's visit in the ED. The primary nurse's recording of assessment and nursing plan beyond triage, and any interventions with the outcomes of those interventions, is ongoing and frequently the only recordings of patient responses to care. Yet the nurses' notes remain separate from the medical chart. This lack of communication is caused by a number of factors.

The factors that create a disjointed pattern of practice in the ED were identified and analyzed by a group consisting of one attending physician and three staff nurses. First, nurses are assigned to specific areas of the ED and provide care to any patients admitted to those areas. If a sudden change in a particular patient's condition occurs, a move to another area may be necessary to provide whatever specialized care is needed. Frequently nurses cannot follow their patients and must transfer nursing care to the nurse covering the patient's new area.

In contrast to this pattern of providing nursing care, physicians are assigned on the basis of patient presentation to the department. The most available physician assumes responsibility for the medical care of patients. This difference in assignment pattern, coupled with the separate charting practices, dissociates nurses and physicians. Physicians interact with many nurses in the department simultaneously and often do not take the time to discuss history, physical examination findings, laboratory results, or medical care plans with the patient's primary nurses. Because each nurse is trying to coordinate patient care with a wide variety of physicians and consultants, the concept of coordinated team care all too often remains merely a concept.

The current pattern of care is one that subverts the nurse's role as educator, patient advocate, and counselor. It is a pattern of care that subverts a nursing model and the nursing process. Nurses are often excluded from many important patient interactions including traditional nursing functions such as patient education, especially at the time of discharge. One of the features of the current pattern of practice is that over 50 percent of patients are discharged from the ED directly by a physician without the benefit of review of their care plan with their primary nurse.

On the initiation of the staff members who isolated and studied the aforementioned factors, a demonstration project exploring the development of a collaborative pattern of care of ED patients was established. Participating physicians and nurses schedule collaborative practice sessions where one physician would team with one nurse. As the collaborating interdisciplinary team assumes responsibility for a patient's care, the nurse obtains a more detailed history and comprehensive assessment. If immediate therapy is warranted, the physician and nurse institute intervention rapidly while gathering further information. After health care providers complete their assessment/examination, the information gathered is discussed and a plan of care is formulated. Should a sudden change in the patient's condition occur, the collaborative team re-evaluates and readjusts the plan of care accordingly.

PATIENTS IN THE EMERGENCY DEPARTMENT

The Environment

Patients in the emergency department are subject to rapidly changing internal and external environments. Levine (1973) maintains that "the integrated response of the individual arises from the internal environment" and that "the internal environment is susceptible to constant change"

(p. 9). This constant change comes from the challenges of the external environment. These challenges are always in the form of energy. The patient with stable vital signs and abdominal pain demonstrates an internal environmental change with onset of hematemesis.

Levine considers the external environment as an individual predicament of time and place. She states that the "environment is often seen as a passive backdrop against which the individual 'acts out' life experiences. But an individual cannot be understood outside the context of his or her predicament of time and place" (Levine, 1989, p. 326). Within the external environment, operational factors affecting patients in the ED include exposure to radiation during diagnostic studies of themselves and of others nearby. Patients with multiple infections may be treated in the open area of the ED, which may pose a potential hazard for the neutropenic patient.

Perceptual factors affecting the patient may change drastically with a sudden influx of ill or injured patients crowding and adding noise to an already unfamiliar setting. The sound of monitor beeps and alarms, of a hysterical patient or a grieving family, or of a resuscitation in progress cannot be ignored in the ED rooms that have curtains instead of walls.

Conceptual factors influencing the patients' environment include their language skills and ability to express their feelings. The newly arrived immigrant or the aphasic patient may not be able to articulate his or her needs. Value systems and cultural traditions often reflect beliefs about personal health and health care in general. A patient may have tried home remedies for a burn that has resulted in a necrotic area. Perhaps the patient believes that hospitals are only for the dying. The patient may know no other health care resources.

The emergency department is always open and does not require payment before treatment. Individual coping patterns must be assessed and considered in the patient's plan of care—they may otherwise hinder the outcome. The interrelatedness of the patient's internal and external environments is the basis for all interventions. In a collaborative team approach, the nurse is able to contribute this information during the care planning and revising stages.

Planning Care

Appropriate diagnostic tests, consultations, medications, and treatments are initiated and documented reflecting the findings of each discipline. If consultants are to see the patient, they are accompanied by the nurse for continuity in the patient's external environmental experience. The patient sees the nurse involved in every phase of care.

The goals of nursing care must be designed to "foster successful adaptation when possible" (Levine, 1973, p. 13). Therapeutic interventions are intended to favor adaptation. The patient with mild congestive heart failure can be cared for in the ED and discharged after several hours, subjectively and objectively improved. Families caring for a terminally ill patient at home may bring that loved one to the ED when breathing becomes more labored. Palliative measures are given to the patient and support is offered to the family.

Conservation is the tenet of Levine's model. Nursing care focuses upon the ability of the nurse to assist the patient in effectively adapting to a desirable status. These "keeping together" interventions are based upon scientific principles as well as each patient's unique responses to the specific situation. Determination of the patient's need begins with the triage process and is carried through until the patient is discharged. It is the nurses' responsibility to continually assess the patient and determine the urgency and acuity of his or her health care.

The Conservation Principles

The principle of conservation of energy states that energy expenditures must balance available energy resources (Levine, 1967). Nursing interventions for the patient with severe substernal chest pain include rapid assessment, followed by measures to decrease cardiac workload: oxygen, morphine sulfate, bed rest, and explanations as to what the patient can expect while in the ED. Likewise, the patient in acute respiratory distress from an acute asthmatic attack needs care immediately, whereas the child with a fever and sore throat may be seen in the pediatric clinic once airway patency has been determined. The patient who arrives in active labor can be assisted in breathing exercises while she awaits transportation to the labor and delivery unit.

The principle of structural integrity reflects changes in function accompanying alterations in physical structure (Levine, 1967). This principle guides care given to a patient with a major gunshot wound to the leg. Measures to ensure that circulation is maintained to the limb as well as the entire system are followed by stabilization of the extremity, tetanus prophylaxis, and antibiotics. Structural integrity must be considered when a patient presents with acute hypertension and complaints of blurred vision and a headache. If this is a chronic problem, damage to other end organs must be considered in the plan of care. Ambulatory burn patients are followed on a daily basis to assess their tissue response to a specific regimen of burn care.

The principle of personal integrity reflects the patients' rights and privileges (Levine, 1967); it is the maintenance of their self-respect and identity. The emergency department is often an open unit with the potential for lack of privacy and confidentiality. Often, curtains offer the only privacy. Unconscious patients may have their clothes cut away to inspect for trauma. Care must be taken to ensure that the patients are not compromised as they respond to illness in a strange environment.

Patients must be considered in the decision-making process unless their condition is life-threatening. The patient with a tubal pregnancy and a religious belief against the administration of blood products must have her beliefs respected. The intravenous drug-abusing patient may choose not to be admitted for intravenous antibiotic treatment of cellulitis, fearing withdrawal in an unsupportive environment. The mother whose small children have accompanied her to the hospital may need assistance to make care arrangements for them before she can be cared for herself. The patient with a fulminating breast lesion must be cared for without recrimination for her decision not to have surgery or radiation treatments.

The principle of social integrity addresses the concept that patients are individuals within society. They do not lose this individuality when they enter the hospital (Levine, 1967). The ED may be the only health care facility they know, or perhaps they were transported to the closest hospital by the rescue squad, even though they are well known at another neighborhood facility. They may be from out of town. If they present with complaints of a long-standing, nonacute nature, they cannot be summarily dismissed because the nurse does not think their complaints are "emergencies." In the event of accidental death, approaching a family to request their consideration of organ donation must be done gently without judgmental bias. The nurse must be knowledgeable about health resources and follow-up in the community. Patient and family teaching is very important; specific aftercare instructions must be given. The patient may need referral to the visiting nurse. Just as the patient does not exist independently in the community, neither does the ED exist independently within the health care system.

The applicability of Levine's conceptual model to emergency nursing lies in its concise, holistic approach to patient care. The ED is a complex, technical area. This fast-paced, complex, technical aspect can frequently foster compartmentalized patient care. The resultant fragmentation in communication between interdisciplinary team members and between the health care providers and patient can have counterproductive if not detrimental effects.

COLLABORATIVE PRACTICE PROJECT

The Collaborative Practice Project of the HUP ED was funded for 1 year (Summer 1988–1989) through the clinical collaboration grants that were established at the University of Pennsylvania School of Nursing in 1986 through the generosity of Mary C. Rockefeller. This funding propelled the ED project from a sporadic alternative approach to providing care to a permanent feature during set times on set days of the week. As the ED physicians and nurses had more exposure to the collaborative practice teams, interest in the project grew. Soon a few more of the ED staff nurses became involved. A few more of the attending physicians scheduled in "collaborative shifts." The ambulatory care rotation of the medical residents soon included a shift a week collaborating in the ED. Word spread through the hospital and a medical grand rounds was devoted to the subject of collaborative care. This medical grand rounds was presented collaboratively by a physician and nurse involved with the project. It was the first time a nurse presented at a medical grand rounds in the 224-year history of the University of Pennsylvania Medical School. The subject of nursing and medicine bringing together their particular expertise into a more coordinated, thorough approach to patient care became more a focus of attention upon completion of our grant year and the reporting of results.

First, we monitored quality of patient care by comparing charts against medical and nursing quality assurance (QA) standards. All Collab-

TABLE 11-1. COLLABORATIVE PRACTICE PROJECT: PATIENT EDUCATION
STATISTICS*

	Collaborative Practice Group (%)	Matched Control Group (%)
Could repeat discharge diagnosis	100	64
Could list discharge medications	98	52
Could repeat follow-up plan	98	48

*The routine patient-satisfaction survey of ED patients showed 96 percent of the collaborative practice patients rating their care better than on previous ED visits.

orative Practice Project charts were in compliance with QA guidelines. A statistical analysis was then done of the patient education outcomes that were monitored all year. Upon the patient's discharge from the ED the nurse would review the diagnosis, the discharge instructions, and the follow-up plan with him or her. Forty-eight to 72 hours after discharge the research assistants in the ED called each patient cared for by a collaborative practice team and a matched control patient treated in the usual manner. All patients called were asked if they could repeat their diagnosis, list discharge medications (if such had been given), and repeat the follow-up plan (Table 11-1).

One of the participating physicians stated:

It brings home the fact that the ED nurses with whom I work are experienced professionals who are very invested in both the care of their patients and in the efficient functioning of their department. Their outlook is different from that of the physicians—they are more holistic. They invite greater patient participation in the health care process and, through their participation in this project, are increasing patient compliance with treatment plans. . . . Most impressive to me is the fact that many of the patients have asked that their nurse be their primary caregiver in follow-up.

The participating nurses stated:

This approach to patient care is far more effective and efficient than our usual pattern of care. . . . In my experience the length of patient stay is actually decreased and the patients are better informed about their diagnosis and treatment.

The patients spontaneously express gratitude for being treated like a whole human being . . . and now they want to take more responsibility for their care and follow-up planning.

Nurses and physicians who have come into contact with this project show an increased understanding of each other's health care disciplines.

USE OF LEVINE'S CONSERVATION MODEL

Using a conceptual model of nursing as an approach to providing professional nursing care in an environment so closely interacting continuously with the discipline of medicine strengthens the basis for communication between the health care providers and the patient. Although the ABCs of resuscitation (airway, breathing, and circulation) are automatic in the initial patient assessment, the conservation model leads the nurse to develop an individualized care plan for the total patient.

The model is concise and easily implemented. No special assessment forms are needed. Patient care plans can be incorporated on the ED nursing record. The principles serve as goals of nursing care. They are easily communicated between caregiver from shift to shift as well as from the field to base station.

The Standards of Emergency Nursing Practice of the Emergency Nurses Association (ENA) provide measurements by which the quality of nursing practice can be evaluated. Standards relating to the practice of emergency nursing reflect specific foci with outcome criteria. "Practice is the assessment, diagnosis, and treatment of human responses to perceived, actual, or potential physical or psycho-social problems that may be episodic, primary, and/or acute" (ENA, 1983, p. 3). Standard III states: "Emergency nurses shall organize data in a systematic manner to coordinate relevant activities of themselves and other team members" (ENA, 1983, p.17). Levine's conservation principles provide such an organizing framework.

Case Presentation 11–1

A 21-year-old moderately obese woman presented ambulatory to the ED triage area complaining of intermittent lower abdominal pain over a 2-month period of time. The pain was increasing in duration and intensity for 1½ weeks. She was having nausea, vomiting, constipation, and general malaise. Her last normal menstrual period was 7 weeks prior to this visit. She was having a scant yellow vaginal discharge. She denied significant past medical-surgical history, drug use, use of birth control, previous pregnancies, alteration in urinary tract function, fevers, or chills. Her vital signs were stable. She was given a triage classification of E.

Taney was the collaborating nurse of the collaborative practice team working the day this patient sought health care. The patient was placed in an examination room at the same time the team was ready to add another patient to the team care approach. Taney and the physician entered her room, greeted her, and introduced themselves as the team that would provide her health care that day. The physician then left to perform a physical examination on another team patient. Taney initiated the interview with the new patient to obtain a more detailed history.

After confirming the initial triage record, this young woman went on to describe herself as a high school graduate employed for the past 3 years as a bank teller. She lived with her parents. Her meals were frequently of the fast-food variety. She was engaged to a young man who recently returned from overseas military service. She was sexually active and used no contraceptive method. She denied having previous gynecologic infections or inflammatory process. She denied having multiple sexual partners.

Taney applied Levine's model utilizing the conservation principles to assess the multiple acute changes in this patient's internal and external environment.

DEFICITS IN ENERGY INTEGRITY

1. Fever: rectal temperature 100.7°F
2. Orthostatic hypotension:
   Lying pulse = 92; Blood pressure = 112/70
   Standing pulse = 124; Blood pressure = 100/58
3. Nutrition: General poor eating habits; further compromise of nutritional status with current nausea and vomiting

DEFICITS IN STRUCTURAL INTEGRITY

1. Constipation: This patient's normal bowel pattern was daily bowel elimination. An acute change in bowel pattern may be directly related to dehydration.
2. Amenorrhea: Last normal menstrual period was 7 weeks ago. Patient was having sexual intercourse without contraception. She was also complaining of breast swelling and tenderness. Considering the provocative factor, it was possible that she was pregnant.
3. Vaginal discharge with suprapubic abdominal pain: Had she contracted a sexually transmitted disease (STD)? Her lover did not use condoms, putting her at risk should he be a carrier.
4. Weight: Patient is 60 pounds overweight.

DEFICITS IN PERSONAL INTEGRITY

1. Health maintenance: A few identified deficits here, as mentioned before: (a) patient had compromised nutritional status secondary to poor eating habits, (b)__ patient's unprotected sexual practices may pose a threat, and (c) patient has never had a gynecologic examination.
2. Fears about present health status: (a) Patient was afraid the abdominal pain indicated that "something was wrong with the baby." She wanted very much to be pregnant and to have a healthy baby. (b) She was afraid the constipation was now a permanent abnormality. While discussing her fear of a permanent bowel pattern change she revealed that she had tried a chewable laxative without results.
3. Family and roles: Patient said she felt (a) that her mother would be pleased if she were pregnant, (b) that her father would go along with anything as long as it made her happy, (c) that her fiancé loved her, and would be happy about the pregnancy, and (d) that he would marry her as planned, as soon as he got a job and they saved some money. These were assumptions she made without discussing any of these issues with her significant others. This may have posed obstacles to effective interpersonal communication.

DEFICITS IN SOCIAL INTEGRITY

1. Her communication style and behavior based on assumptions could set her up for any number of scenarios. Would her family indeed be pleased if she were pregnant or would she end up on the street?

2. Her frequent absenteeism from work over the past few months put her job in jeopardy. She was afraid to speak with her boss concerning her health status, as she thought he might fire her.

Based on this assessment the trophicognoses (Fawcett et al., 1987) for this patient are (a) dehydration, (b) risk for pregnancy and STD, and (c) health maintenance knowledge deficit. The goals of the nursing care plan should be structured to "foster successful adaptation when possible" (Levine, 1973, p. 13).

ENERGY INTEGRITY CONSERVATION

An intravenous infusion was initiated to rehydrate the patient, as she was not able to tolerate oral fluids. She was positioned in a recumbent posture until tachycardia and hypotension upon standing were corrected. Her knees were flexed to relieve tension on abdominal wall musculature, thus providing comfort. The physician was consulted concerning fever and oral fluid intolerance. A goal to decrease fever, nausea, and vomiting was set. Antipyretic and antiemetic agents were administered.

STRUCTURAL INTEGRITY CONSERVATION

Once a rehydrated state was re-established and nausea and vomiting ceased, the patient could move toward improvement in nutritional status and return to normal bowel patterns. She was instructed on altering her diet. The high fat and sugar content kept her overweight. She was told of the health risks of obesity. A pregnancy test was drawn and sent; its results later confirmed she was in the early stages of pregnancy. The pelvic examination performed by the physician revealed a thick yellow discharge from the cervical os and cervical motion tenderness. She had pelvic inflammatory disease (PID). Antibiotic therapy was initiated as ordered. Instruction was given as to the need for consistent, thorough follow-up for this STD. She was referred to the prenatal clinic for follow-up.

PERSONAL INTEGRITY CONSERVATION

Conversation concerning the patient's health maintenance revolved around her desire to have a healthy baby. She was interested in the information offered to guide her to improving her current health status. The importance of ongoing health maintenance, including regular gynecologic examinations with Pap smears, was stressed. The transmission of STDs was discussed. She needed to discuss this with her sexual partner because he had to be treated, to prevent possibly reinfecting her. Her mother and fiancé had accompanied her to the ED. Upon her request they were included in the evaluation and health teaching process. Open communication was facilitated between the patient and her significant others.

SOCIAL INTEGRITY CONSERVATION

With the beginning of open communication, it was established that the patient was loved by her family and fiancé. Her fiancé agreed to undergo treatment for the STD after learning about the disease. Once her abdominal pain and the vomiting subsided, the patient planned to return to work. She wanted to work through her pregnancy. She was given a note for her employer stating she had sought health care that day. She stated she would discuss her plans with her employer to ensure her job was not at risk.

The patient was discharged rehydrated, without fever, tolerating oral fluids. She left the ED with her fiancé's arm around her. Her mother spoke of the joy she felt: She was becoming a grandmother for the first time. There was conservation of the four integrities.

Case Presentation 11–2

A 34-year-old homosexual man was brought to the ED by ambulance with an acute change in mental status. He was accompanied by his lover, with whom he lived. The patient had been experiencing fever, chills, polyuria, polydipsia, nausea, vomiting, and diarrhea over the past 2 weeks. A social worker at a local hospital, he has missed work the past 10 days. He had refused to seek medical care from their private physician. When he exhibited confusion and periods of incoherent speech, his lover called a friend and coworker of the patient, a licensed practical nurse, who called the rescue squad soon after arrival at the couple's apartment. She came along to the hospital and helped to provide support to the patient's lover as he gave the history.

The patient was in a state of delirium. His rectal temperature was 105.4°F. His pulse was 142 beats per minute; he was in a sinus tachycardia when placed on cardiac monitoring. Respirations were 38 per minute and of the Kussmaul type. His breath had the fruity smell of ketosis. He was hypotensive with a blood pressure of 90/40. His skin was hot and dry with poor skin turgor. His capillary glucose level was greater than 500 mg per dl.

Taney was the nurse of the collaborative practice team that day. We had just arrived when this patient presented; he was the first patient of the day. His internal environment was in a state of imbalance so profound that he did not have the energy to raise his head from the pillow. His perceptions of the external environment were not oriented to person, place, or time. He was making incoherent sounds and speaking a few incoherent words. He could localize pain but did not have the strength to push a noxious stimulant away. When considering the integration of living processes, physiologic and behavioral responses are not separate entities but are one and the same (Levine, 1989). The nursing assessment was documented according to the four conservation principles.

DEFICITS OF ENERGY INTEGRITY

1. Dehydration: Severe as indicated by vital signs and the hyperosmolar state of hyperglycemia.

2. Acidosis: Suggested by the Kussmaul respirations and ketotic breath and confirmed by arterial blood gas measurement of a pH of 7.1.
3. Depleted strength and distorted perceptions: The unstable internal environment has caused gross energy depletion.

DEFICITS OF STRUCTURAL INTEGRITY

1. Hypotension: Potential for decreased capillary bed profusion, thus compounding hyperosmolarity and fluid shifts and causing hypoxia and a decreased ability to remove metabolic end products at the cellular level.
2. Sepsis: High fever and other vital signs indicating a systemic infectious process. White blood cell count was elevated.
3. Nausea, vomiting, and diarrhea: Severe gastrointestinal upset further compounding the dehydration effects.

DEFICITS OF PERSONAL INTEGRITY

The patient's condition at the time of hospitalization was such that he could not coherently express his fears. His lover was human immunodeficiency virus (HIV) seropositive but felt well with no symptoms of acquired immune deficiency syndrome (AIDS). The patient had tested negative twice, the last test being 6 months ago. Although they were practicing safe sex, the patient was very anxious regarding his lover's seropositive HIV status. The patient had no significant past medical or surgical history. He maintained a healthy diet and exercised regularly. He had regular medical check-ups. He never had fevers or colds, was usually very active and bright. Yet, 2 weeks before becoming ill, the patient was depressed and withdrawn and had verbalized hopelessness.

DEFICITS OF SOCIAL INTEGRITY

The patient had refused to seek medical attention. He had repeatedly ignored or rebuffed his lover's urges to seek health care. He apparently had had an argument with their private physician a few months prior to onset of his illness. Soon after that he began voicing distrust of this physician and of "insensitive, big-business health care" in general. He also was moody because a close friend had died of the complications of AIDS. He may have felt that his closest social support, his lover, was soon to become ill and follow the same course as this friend.

"Survival depends on the adaptive ability to use responses that cost the least to the individual in expense of effort and demand on his or her well-being" (Levine, 1989). With this in mind, conservation strategies were formed for this patient.

ENERGY INTEGRITY CONSERVATION

Intravenous hydration was initiated with physiologically stable saline at a rapid rate. The collaborating physician calculated the amount of insulin needed to begin to open the energy-producing pathways of glycolysis and the Kreb's cycle, and the sodium bicarbonate needed to correct the severe acidosis. Oxygen at 3 liters per minute via nasal prongs was initiated in an attempt to decrease the rate and effort of respirations. The respiratory pattern would continue until acidosis was corrected.

STRUCTURAL INTEGRITY CONSERVATION

The patient was placed in a Fowler's position—low enough to promote cerebral perfusion, yet high enough to protect the airway of a vomiting, delirious patient. An antipyretic agent and a powerful combination of intravenous antibiotics were administered. A Foley catheter was placed to monitor kidney function and urinary output. An intensive care bed was readied for this patient.

PERSONAL INTEGRITY CONSERVATION

This patient needed an environment as free of noxious stimuli as possible, a difficult goal to achieve in an intensive care unit. His nursing care required reassurance and warmth. Having his partner stay involved in planning and providing health care would help orient this patient and improve his altered mental status and keep his loved one in a vital supportive role. After marked improvement in and conservation of his other integrities, therapy with a psychologist would possibly help him sort through and come to terms with his fears and other emotionally charged issues.

SOCIAL INTEGRITY CONSERVATION

The patient had lost trust in his family physician. Since he had new-onset diabetes mellitus he would need to establish a solid relationship with a primary care provider. As soon as his delirium passed, the clinical nurse specialist in the diabetes clinic would be consulted to start diabetes teaching and fostering of an ongoing trusting relationship. The patient was always accustomed to independence. After recently expressing distrust in the health care system, dependency on that very system was a reality that may be difficult for him to accept; it was important that he and his family understand this. He should be encouraged and supported with honesty and respect, but without having the desires of others imposed upon him.

Case Presentation 11–3

A 46-year-old woman was brought to the ED by her two brothers after she exhibited violent behavior. She had thrown a chair at the television and had threatened her mother with a knife. She had a psychiatric history. Diagnosed schizophrenic at the age of 15, she had had numerous psychiatric hospitalizations. Her last hospitalization had been 8 months earlier. Since then, she had been living with her mother and visiting the mental health center once a week to get a fluphenazine decanoate injection and see her case worker. Her last visit was 4 days ago. She was feeling increasingly anxious and agitated over the past few weeks and had been experiencing brief periods of auditory hallucinations, especially at night. Her medication was being adjusted to relieve these symptoms, but her brothers did not know the dosage.

The patient was immediately brought to the padded isolation room, as she needed both physical and chemical restraint. She thrashed out an anyone who approached her. Her shouts, facial grimaces, and eye movements indicated auditory and visual hallucinations. Her brothers, two security guards, and the collaborative practice team brought her from the car to the isolation room, where she was placed in four-point leather restraints. She was reassured that as soon as the hallucinations had subsided and her behavior was controlled the restraints would be removed.

Apical pulse rate was 114 and regular. Respiratory rate was 24 with deep effort. It was impossible to get a blood pressure or temperature initially. She was very diaphoretic. She was medicated with haloperidol (Haldol) 5 mg and lorazepam (Ativan) 2 mg intramuscularly. Psychiatry was consulted immediately. The four conservation principles served as the framework for this patient's nursing assessment.

DEFICITS OF ENERGY INTEGRITY

1. Sustained sympathomimetic effect of paranoid psychosis resulted in increased heart rate, with increased cardiac output and increased respiratory rate with bronchodilation. If not checked, this will deplete energy reserves.
2. Dehydration was a potential from the profuse diaphoresis; patient's family also reported she did not eat or drink much that day.

DEFICITS OF STRUCTURAL INTEGRITY

1. Potential circulatory compromise for areas distal to leather restraints.
2. Temporal lobe seizures may have been the cause of her rapid eye movements and rage.
3. Hypotension is a potential side effect of neuroleptic drugs such as haloperidol (Haldol).

DEFICITS OF PERSONAL INTEGRITY

The effects of this patient's acute paranoid psychotic state extended into both internal and external environments. Her yelling and violent outbursts are attempts to escape from threatening sounds and visual images, both internal and external. She had lost the ability to differentiate the real from the unreal.

Her behavior placed her at risk to impulsively harm herself. Many threatening auditory hallucinations vacillate between commands to harm others and commands to harm oneself.

DEFICITS OF SOCIAL INTEGRITY

Destroying family property and threatening bodily harm to members of her family during acute psychotic episodes jeopardized her current living situation. Her family had petitioned for involuntary psychiatric commitment for hospitalization. Would they be willing to have her return home after inpatient treatment ended? She had never been able to hold a job. She would not be able to adequately support herself if her family abandoned her out of fear.

This patient's behavior was an attempt to adapt to a rapidly changing environment. Regardless of cause or effect, nursing maintains the integrity and wholeness of the person.

ENERGY INTEGRITY CONSERVATION

Administering a chemical restraining agent in the form of a rapid-acting tranquilizer brought about the depressant effect of blocking the sympathetic neurotransmitters norepinephrine and dopamine. This was done to relieve the sustained fight-or-flight response that was depleting this patient's energy reserve. The slower-acting neuroleptic drug would further alter neurotransmitters to control agitated, aggressive behavior.

Once agitation subsided, frequent intake of oral fluids was encouraged. Intravenous fluids may be necessary if the patient refuses to drink.

STRUCTURAL INTEGRITY CONSERVATION

Frequent neurovascular checks must be done of both hands and feet while four-point leather restraints are in place.

Periods of quiet punctuated by outbursts of rage and uninhibited speech with or without rapid eye movements could indicate temporal lobe seizures. Core body temperature can rise dramatically if the hypothalamus is affected by these events. A rectal temperature should be taken every few hours if temporal lobe seizures are suspected. Events such as these need further investigation with electroencephalogram and perhaps magnetic resonance imaging studies.

PERSONAL INTEGRITY CONSERVATION

Although she was not responding in a way that indicated coherent understanding of what was being said to her, constant reassurance and explanation of any interventions had to be offered quietly yet firmly. In an attempt to preserve the patient's dignity, speaking or acting in a judgmental way was avoided. It was possible that she would continue to hallucinate and respond inappropriately even if her outbursts subsided. Speaking to her in a calm, respectful way provided her with a nonthreatening environment in which to respond once she became oriented. In the meantime she stayed physically restrained to protect her from causing harm to herself or others.

SOCIAL INTEGRITY CONSERVATION

Communicating honestly with this patient's family was key to their understanding her temporary violent outbursts. Keeping them informed of responses to medication, progress in the examination, or placement in a psychiatric hospital helped to diminish the alienation siblings may have felt from their sister. We called the patient's mother at home a few times to keep her informed and involved. This provided support to the patient's traumatized significant others who may have grown afraid of their mentally ill family member.

CONCLUSION

The use of a nursing model such as Levine's strengthens communication among health care providers and improves the way nursing care is transmitted to and received by patients. In an atmosphere of collaboration each participant—health care provider and patient—is rewarded with respect and active contribution to the adaptation process. Both the internal and external environments of the patient are affected in such a way as to promote a move toward homeostasis. This is the goal called conservation or, from the medical model point of view, health maintenance. The promotion of wholeness is the goal of the human interaction called nursing (Fawcett et al., 1987).

REFERENCES

Emergency Nurses Association. (1983). Standards of Emergency Nursing Practice. St. Louis: C.V. Mosby.

Fawcett, J., Cariello, F.P., Davis, D.A., Farley, J., Zimmaro, D.M., & Watts, R.J. (1987). Conceptual models of nursing application to critical care nursing practice. Dimensions of Critical Care Nursing, 6(4), 202–214.

Jacobson, S. (1985). Decision-making in the emergency department. Comprehensive Therapy, 11(4), 16–23.

Levine, M.E. (1967). The four conservation principles of nursing. Nursing Forum, 6, 45–59.

Levine, M.E. (1973). Introduction to clinical nursing (2nd ed.). Philadelphia: F.A. Davis.

Levine, M.E. (1989). The conservation principles of nursing: Twenty years later. In J. Riehl-Sisca (Ed.), Conceptual models for nursing practice (3rd ed.). Norwalk, CT: Appleton & Lange.

Chapter
TWELVE

Ambulatory Care of
the Homeless

Jane Benson Pond, R.N.C., M.S.N., C.R.N.P.

Why use a conceptual model? After all, as a nurse practitioner I was taught to use the medical model when assessing patients. It is systematic and concise. At first, this approach seemed effective. However, I soon became frustrated with the inability to focus on nursing concerns. As a nurse I needed more than a simple assessment of body systems to plan my patients' care. I needed a sense of the person's life to be able to consider the provocative facts, evaluating each patient's adaptive changes on the health-illness continuum.

I must admit that this paradigm shift to the internalization and utilization of a model did not come easily. After a comprehensive graduate-level course in conceptual models, I was still not convinced. It was only after attempting to design a nursing assessment tool for use on an inpatient obstetric unit that I began to conceptualize my "private image of nursing" (Reilly, 1975, p. 566). I knew that my practice was more than the sum of the basic physiologic checklists. The physicians had obtained that information: maternal health history, obstetrical history, and history of present illness. As a nurse, I needed to know how this patient was going to function at home after delivery, taking care of a newborn and three other children. What were the demands on her time? What were her coping patterns? How would she deal with her responsibilities at work? The answers to these issues would be provided within the assessment based on a nursing framework; then, she and I would be able to develop a plan of care based on this information.

As my own practice developed and moved from an inpatient unit to ambulatory care settings with a more diverse patient population, I realized that Levine's conservation principles provided an effective organizing framework for my practice.

167

THE HOMELESS PROJECT

Homelessness and its related health issues have been the topics of many current publications (Bassuk, 1984; Brickner et al, 1985; Bowdler, 1989; Ferguson, 1989). It is a national dilemma and the numbers of homeless men, women, and children are rapidly increasing. As a nurse practitioner, the homeless are my patients. According to Levine (1988), "We are privileged by our license to provide an important service to the community. We are accepted in a rare relationship by utter strangers who place their well-being in our hands" (p. 7). Homeless patients come to me because they have difficulty taking care of themselves. They face multiple developmental and situational crises: (1) prevalence of acute and chronic health and social service problems, (2) lack of a stable living condition, (3) economic disadvantages, and (4) continual emotional deprivation.

According to Philadelphia Health Management Corporation (PHMC) and the 1987 Mayor's Task Force on Homelessness (1989), the estimate of homeless people in this city of 1.6 million, is between 5000 and 10,000. Approximately 3000 individuals and families are sheltered each night in a variety of public and private agencies. The remaining numbers exist in such marginal conditions that they must be considered in the population as well. All of these people have unmet health needs.

Philadelphia's Health Care for the Homeless Project was originally a demonstration project funded by the Robert Wood Johnson/Pew Memorial Trust Foundations. It provides health and social service care to the homeless through outreach teams of nurse practitioners, community health nurses, and social workers who regularly visit numerous shelters and other sites where this population congregates. This project, developed to provide a model of care to the homeless, is currently funded through the Stewart B. McKinney Homeless Assistance Act (1987). Outreach teams are located in various areas of the city and two suburban counties.

THE HOMELESS PATIENTS

Ongoing research at PHMC continues to support its report *Homelessness in Philadelphia: People, Needs, and Services* (Fox, Axelrod, & Loeb, 1985), which states that the multifactorial issues surrounding homelessness have a profound effect on the health status of these individuals. According to statistics from PHMC's homeless programs, the approximately 15,000 patients seen over the last 6 years present with serious health needs from the lack of basic health maintenance, ranging from immunizations and prenatal care to the long-term management of acute and chronic health problems: cardiopulmonary disease, substance abuse, smoking, infections, major and minor trauma, peripheral vascular disease, and gastrointestinal disorders.

Other factors such as extreme poverty, family violence, mental illness, and increased drug and alcohol use further complicate the health status of homeless patients. They are frequently undernourished; have dental disorders; are at increased risk for sexually transmitted diseases (STDs) and acquired immune deficiency syndrome (AIDS); are burdened with weather-related emergencies, skin infestations, chronic infections, developmental delays; and have a decreased sense of self-concept and self-worth.

An analysis of patients seen by the Health Care for the Homeless (HCFTH) clinical and social service outreach teams reflect specific health needs according to the defined populations. Children need immunizations, nutritional and developmental assessments, dental and vision care, lead screening, and surveillance for abuse and neglect. Women need routine health maintenance with attention to family planning information, pregnancy options, and perinatal care. The substance-abusing homeless must have ongoing monitoring for prevalent seizure disorders, gastrointestinal disease, hypertension, and nutritional status. Those who are mentally ill and/or dually diagnosed with a substance-abuse problem need health care directed at such environmental issues as hypo-hyperthermia, poisoning, and trauma.

Service delivery issues such as access to adequate health care must address the special needs to this diverse population. Our teams provide on-site primary and episodic care at the shelters and attempt to assist the patient through a complex maze of health and social service facilities. We are essentially guests in the outreach sites. The areas provided for use to see patients range from offices established specifically for us to unused laundry rooms. Often privacy is lacking, and we have only the bare essentials in equipment. We operate on a walk-in basis, although some patients may make appointments. Patients register to see us on a first-come, first-served basis. The nurse may briefly speak to the patients and encourage them to stay to be evaluated, but often they lack the patience to wait.

Some patients are referred to us by the shelter staff, and some are "recruited" by the clinical staff. When walking through the common area, the nurse may see a patient with a cast or bandage and inquire about the patient's ability to understand what the care requirements are with respect to this or another problem. Utilizing Levine's conservation model provides structure to plan for these complex patients.

USE OF THE CONSERVATION PRINCIPLES WITH THE HOMELESS

According to Levine, "the person cannot be described apart from the specific environment in which he or she is found" (1989, p. 325). An individual cannot be understood outside of his or her predicament of time and place (Levine, 1973, p. 13). The definition of "predicament" aptly describes life on the streets: "an unfortunate, unpleasant, or puzzling situation" (Guralink, 1988).

The external environment of homeless patients is indeed made up of puzzling situations. Using the formulation of perceptual, operational, and conceptual factors, one can begin to consider how the patient must adapt.

Perceptual indicators test information through the senses: selective signals that demand attention and those that may be safely ignored (Levine, 1989). Those signals are received in the context of self-concept, safety, and purpose. The sight of people walking over a huddled body; the odor of many bodies close together or from the garbage dumpsters that provide shelter; the sound of incessant noise in the shelter or inside your head; the dulled taste of overcooked food, cold coffee, or cigarettes; and the touch of the pavement or a chair over a day's time.

The operational environment consists of factors in the environment not perceived by the senses: for example, gases from the street vents and car exhaust fumes, microorganisms from the coughing person nearby or from shared needles in intravenous (IV) drug use.

The conceptual environment acknowledges that each person is sentimental, emotional, and capable of caring and coping. Who hugs a homeless person? Who speaks to a homeless person? If a homeless person enters a church sanctuary, is one's first thought that this person may be seeking spiritual solace and guidance—or a place to sleep? Attitudes about personal health and health care may be revealed. The patient may view the hospital as the place to die or the place where her last baby was taken from her without even a kiss. All of these challenges from the external environment affect the maintenance of the integration of bodily functions in the internal environment.

The internal environment is a balance of the integrated human functions (Levine, 1973). This stabilized flow is regulated by protective systems such as the fight-or-flight response, inflammatory reactions, and a perceptual awareness basic to survival. Alcohol, drugs, or an acute infection may inhibit these processes.

Inherent in the conservation principles is the concept of adaptation: the way the person and the environment become congruent, retaining integrity within the realities of that environment. It is the "best fit" (Levine, 1989, p. 329). The goal of nursing is to foster successful adaptation whenever possible. "Survival depends on the adaptive ability to use responses that *cost the least* to the individual in expense of effort and demand on his or her well-being" (Levine, 1989, p. 329). Conservation is effectively adapting to this state of well-being. Energy expenditures must balance the available energy resources. The balance of these resources against expenditures can best be assessed using the four conservation principles of energy, structural integrity, personal integrity, and social integrity.

The nurse's active participation in this environment supports the patient's adaptation. The nursing intervention that favorably influences adaptation is a therapeutic intervention. The interventions that can only support the status quo or that fail to halt a downward course are known as supportive interventions.

Energy resources available to the homeless individual consist of food and nutrition, frequently in limited amounts from the shelters, feeding programs, or begging; a balanced homeostatic state altered by selling plasma or by anemia from alcoholism; and rest, often unobtainable in the crowded shelter, subway, or street. Energy expenditures include constant emotional stress, fear of physical safety, and increased physical activity (walking long distances between appointments or looking for food or shelter). Physical stresses may also include energy expended in the form of delirium tremens or epileptic seizures. All of these conditions must be considered when the patient presents for care. The patient may not return for an appointment because it conflicts with a meal or the distance is too far after he or she is placed in a new shelter. This may reflect the patient's attempt to maintain energy integrity (i.e., eating as opposed to taking two buses and missing a meal).

Structural integrity relates to the process of healing. It reflects a change in function accompanying alteration in physical structure. Tissue insults to the body's defenses include burns from a heated vent, abscesses from IV drug use, lacerations from assaults, and damage to end organs from chronic diseases such as hypertension.

A sense of *personal integrity* relates to aspects of love and belonging, self-respect and identity, and consideration in the decision-making processes. The addict cannot be brow-beaten or cajoled into entering treatment until he or she is ready. When an infected injection site is treated, it must be done with respect for the patient's decisions. He or she may choose not to be admitted for necessary IV antibiotics, fearing withdrawal in an unsupporting environment. A mother may not bring her child to the clinic for fear that she will be lectured about delays in seeking care for reasons that may be out of her control. For example, if the police or 911 system are the main methods of transportation to the emergency room, it may be that they do not answer calls to the shelters on a high-priority basis. Space and territory are significant issues as well. Walking through the living space of a homeless person, whether the subway corridor or a shelter bunk, one can sense those personal touches that clearly demarcate the area as belonging to a certain person.

Conservation of social integrity deals with consideration of the patient's relationships with others and his or her place within several social communities: family, community, culture, religion/ethnic group, and health care system. Entering the latter may create conflict within one of these other groups. For example, it may not be perceived as "macho" to ask the nurse for condoms. Homelessness creates physical and emotional illnesses within an artificial system of street people. One must remember, however, that there may be strength and caring within these groups that once were lost.

SPECIAL PATIENTS

Case Presentation 12–1: Frank

Frank came to my outreach clinic at the day program and said he was "sick." What I saw was an elderly man covered in feces and vomitus; his face was flushed and there was alcohol on his breath. Upon speaking with him, he revealed his age as 15 years younger that I would have guessed. He had a long history of manic-depressive illness controlled by medication and therapy, and had been a recovering alcoholic for many years. With a master's degree in engineering, he had worked productively for several years, developing control systems for a major utility at its nuclear power plant. A change in the popularity of nuclear energy forced the plant to close and he could no longer cope with being unemployed, losing his marriage as well. He had returned to drinking and had been on the streets for several years. I began to assess Frank, using the conservation principles.

ENERGY DEFICITS

Frank had increased heart rate and respirations, fever, and postural hypotension indicating dehydration. His lungs had basilar rales, indicating an oxygen deficit. Infections were superimposed on excoriated areas of his groin as a result of the diarrhea and inability to use toilet facilities or get clean clothes. He was living on the street, panhandling for alcohol, and trying to keep out of the way of the police and those who would try to assault him in his debilitated state.

STRUCTURAL DEFICITS

Alcoholism had probably altered Frank's liver function, resulting in multiple petechiae and bruises, which also could have been exacerbated by falling or body insults. Poor circulation was indicated by stasis ulcers on his lower extremities, and his ataxic gait indicated a peripheral neuropathy beyond his intoxication. He was edentulous, rendering him less capable of normal nutrition. He had several minor lacerations in various stages of healing. His manic-depressive illness could be interpreted as a structural deficit.

PERSONAL INTEGRITY DEFICITS

Frank's appearance and physical condition made even those accustomed to patients in similar conditions uncomfortable. He was initially refused entry to the center, which was established to care for everyone. He was confused and his self-image was clouded by the facial and verbal expressions of those around him. He was well aware that others found him disagreeable and filthy. He appeared without hope.

SOCIAL INTEGRITY DEFICITS

Frank had no money and only limited Medicaid benefits. He had refused care by his designated physician, who had advocated imprisonment as a last recourse, even without his committing a crime! He had been in detoxification units so frequently that he was no longer allowed admission. He was isolated from his regular street companions because he was too ill to drink with them. He was fearful of any emergency room. He essentially had nowhere to go.

With this information, therapeutic interventions were planned, with the realization that they might be only supportive.

ENERGY CONSERVATION

Placement overnight was planned in a small shelter with a nurturing environment; another HCFTH nurse maintained an outreach clinic there. Frank would have limited access to alcohol and could be encouraged to take clear liquids there. An appointment was made and transportation arranged to the mental health center for evaluation and treatment of his manic-depression. He was given antibiotics, which would be started when his vomiting subsided. His superficial infections were treated with antibiotic ointment and occlusive dressings. Minimal expectations included cessation of his vomiting and diarrhea and the initiation of antibiotic therapy and psychotropic medication.

STRUCTURAL CONSERVATION

His lacerations and stasis ulcers were cleansed and dressed. Upon closer evaluation, some of his old lacerations revealed sutures that I removed to prevent incorporation into the tissue. At the mental health clinic, his tremors would be evaluated and medication might be prescribed. Minimal expectations of these interventions included prevention of further local infections at the laceration sites. Because of limited resources, it would be a while before he could get dentures. He would need a full medical evaluation, which was unavailable at the time because of the lack of physician cooperation.

PERSONAL INTEGRITY CONSERVATION

Although Frank was down-and-out, he was persistent in seeing me after being refused admission to the center. I evaluated him in my "office" with the door closed to ensure privacy, despite his overwhelming odor of which he was also aware. He was helped to shower and put on clean clothes. He was given a second set of clothes for a later change. Our encounter was not characterized by a discussion that he would die if he did not stop drinking; he knew that. We had time to discuss the next 24 hours, what might happen to him and what he could expect. I explained his medications and the reasons he needed to be evaluated at the mental health center. He was too confused to make any other decisions, and I was not sure that he would be able to negotiate the next few hours. The nurse at the shelter was given a report, and he was given written instructions tucked into his pocket. Clean clothes and respect were my nursing goals for this integrity.

SOCIAL INTEGRITY CONSERVATION

At this point, he would see only the mental health care provider. He would not be sent to the detoxification unit as he would be denied admission there because of his recidivism. He was instructed that he could see me or the other nurses at any time, even without insurance. He did not want anyone to know of his illness, so his family was not notified. He knew that unless there was a life-threatening situation, he would not be taken to the emergency room. Our goal centered on limiting his health care to the minimum until he was able to cope with an increasingly complex system.

Was I successful? Was he successful? Momentarily. That first encounter was 4 years ago, and today Frank continues in this predicament, sometimes returning to see one of our nurses at the shelter to which I originally sent him. He is constantly attempting to adapt to the changing internal and external environments that threaten his existence.

Case Presentation 12–2: Lydia

Lydia was a young woman with two small children who were currently in foster care. She came to see me about her legs, which were swollen to twice their size and had several localized infections. She had no shoes and had walked more than a mile to the clinic. She told me that her children had been placed in care because of her drug addiction. She had started using drugs after her abusing husband left the family with no support. The conservation principles provided an organizing framework for this patient.

ENERGY DEFICITS

Lydia was walking several miles daily between her outpatient detoxification program and her shelter, often arriving too late for dinner. She said she had been drug free for 2 months and was very excited about this.

STRUCTURAL DEFICITS

Skin popping had left her lower extremities swollen and marked with scars and ulcers. She had altered her circulatory system by use of her veins for intravenous drugs. Her circulation was impaired, although she had no evidence of phlebitis or systemic infection.

PERSONAL INTEGRITY DEFICITS

Lydia perceived herself as a "bad" mother, the only identity she could value. Her former mate had physically abused her, claiming she was an unfit lover. She admitted that this was the first time she had been able to articulate these feelings, because her counselor never saw her in private and she could not divulge these thoughts to her group.

SOCIAL INTEGRITY DEFICITS

Lydia had coped with stress in the past by using drugs and coped with her problems now by showing impatience with frustrating systems, often cancelling appointments. She felt isolated from her church and her sisters. The foster care system had placed her children in a suburb more than 10 miles away, and she could not see them. Her case worker then accused her of not being motivated.

Together we planned supportive actions.

ENERGY CONSERVATION

I was able to obtain bus tokens for Lydia until her welfare check came and she could budget to buy a bus pass. She would be able to travel much easier now, even to see her children.

STRUCTURAL CONSERVATION

I helped Lydia choose an appropriate pair of tie shoes and cotton socks. Together we planned how she would care for her ulcers, and I provided her with the solutions and dressings for a week. She would return to see me weekly.

PERSONAL INTEGRITY CONSERVATION

A call to Lydia's case worker revealed that the program ran several support groups for mothers whose children were in foster care. Arrangements were made to have her attend one of those. She would continue in her outpatient therapy, trying to make a private appointment on her own with her counselor.

SOCIAL INTEGRITY CONSERVATION

With her bus pass, she would be able to attend her church services. She hoped that because she had been drug free for a while, her sisters would meet her halfway.

I was disappointed, although not surprised, when she failed to show for her next visit. I did not see her for 3 months. However, when she returned, her legs were almost healed and she was off to see her children. She was still drug free and was in a work rehabilitation program. We danced around the office, hugging each other, exhilarated by these important milestones.

Case Presentation 12–3: John

John was sitting quietly in the day program waiting room. The social worker told me that he had prescriptions that he could not afford; could I help him? She added that "he must have a cold because he talked as if he has a sore throat." When he entered my office, I observed a young white man who was pale, short of breath, and covered with purplish spots on his face and arms. He presented me with prescriptions written 2 weeks earlier at the local emergency room. They were for an antifungal oral solution, an antiviral pill, and a medication for tuberculosis. It was quite obvious from those provocative facts that this patient had AIDS.

A recent major epidemic in this country, AIDS is a severe complication on the continuum of illnesses related to infection by the human immunodeficiency virus (HIV). This spectrum ranges from a subclinical seropositivity for antibodies to HIV to the life-threatening immunodeficiency diseases (Flaskerud, 1989). It is transmitted through exchange of body fluids, principally blood and semen, and from mother to fetus in utero. Whether this virus had been transmitted by intercourse with homosexual or bisexual males, through intravenous drug use and sharing needles, or by heterosexual intercourse was not important at this time; how John had become ill could be sorted out later. Utilization of the conservation principles enabled me to assess this patient's critical state.

ENERGY DEFICITS

John had an increased heart rate, dyspnea, and a temperature of 104°F, indicative of infection and an increased metabolic rate. He had a severe oral candidiasis, which had severely limited his nutritional intake. He appeared unable to walk more than five steps without stopping to rest. He had spent the last two nights not sleeping, sitting upright in the men's room at the bus station.

STRUCTURAL DEFICITS

John's immune system was functioning abnormally, unresponsive to offending antigens. The prescription for antituberculosis medication indicated a prior assessment of lung involvement and probable compromise. The purplish lesions were indicative of Kaposi's sarcoma (KS), a skin cancer of multifocal origin (Flaskerud, 1989). Bilateral pitting ankle edema reflected a change in the peripheral vascular system, which could be attributed to the KS or to the patient's day-to-day existence of walking without adequate rest.

PERSONAL INTEGRITY DEFICITS

John had lost the ability to make his own decisions. He had been "kicked out of the shelter" because he was too sick, because "they say my coughing keeps everyone awake all night." He admitted to feeling like a leper. He already felt like an outcast because of his homelessness; now he felt even more alone.

SOCIAL INTEGRITY DEFICITS

John was physically and emotionally withdrawn from all interactions. He believed he had been summarily dismissed from the emergency room because he had no insurance or income. He had come to the homeless clinic because he heard we could help him with prescriptions.

There are increasing numbers of homeless persons who are at risk for

HIV/AIDS. John was not our first patient nor will he be our last. Because of the acuity of his symptoms, the supportive nursing interventions consisted of arranging evaluation in the emergency room as a mechanism for admission to an inpatient unit. The project van took him to the hospital with the assurance that when he was discharged, we would arrange support services for him. Only an hour had passed from the time I met him until he was in the hospital. He died in the emergency room.

Case Presentation 12–4: Ramona

Ramona was a young, Hispanic woman. She said she had six children, all of whom lived with their fathers or in foster care. According to her social worker, all of them were born with fetal alcohol syndrome and the youngest was born with congenital syphilis. Ramona was addicted to crack, trading her body for her "hits." She said she thought she was pregnant again. She lived in the "cardboard-condo city" beneath the subway; that is where I met her. Her boyfriend introduced me to her, confiding to me that she had a "bad discharge" and should see a doctor. Ramona was not so sure.

ENERGY DEFICITS

Ramona undoubtedly had a poor nutritional status secondary to cocaine use and marginal food intake when she remembered to eat. If she was indeed pregnant, that would also increase her metabolic rate and deplete her nutritional stores. The possibility of a superimposed infection would increase her metabolic rate as well.

STRUCTURAL DEFICITS

Smoking crack had damaged Ramona's lung tissue, sores on her legs were an insult to skin integrity, and she undoubtedly had liver impairment as a result of her long-standing alcoholism.

PERSONAL INTEGRITY DEFICITS

Ramona's substance-abuse habits had robbed her of all sense of self and independence. Prostitution was a way of life for her, and there was no privacy in this cramped area. She seemed to have given up.

SOCIAL INTEGRITY DEFICITS

Ramona was alienated from her family and traditional support systems. She had no income, nor did she perceive she needed any.

I tried to visit her every day. At first, I hoped to win her confidence through gifts of a warm coat, socks, and sandwiches. She had a bright smile, and when I suggested we go upstairs to the clinic, she demurred;

but I kept trying. After the city relocated those individuals to shelters, I lost contact with her. Today Ramona is still in the same predicament and my assessments using the conservation principles are still valid.

CONCLUSION

Obviously, homeless patients are among the most difficult to work with. Many of our patients are easily managed and are integrated into the existing health care resources. Although it is never easy, many patients become independent in their health care and less dependent on our outreach services. We consider these many successes as reflective of the dedicated nursing interventions with these challenging situations. These patients cannot be considered outside their "broad range of environmental events" (Levine, 1989, p. 329).

As the conservation principles are used to assess each patient, a comprehensive picture develops. It is more than the sum of the medical and nursing models; it becomes the basis for a shared experience that enriches both the nurse and patient, providing rational care and hope.

REFERENCES

Bassuk, E. (1984). The homeless problem. Scientific American, 251, 40–45.
Bowdler, J. (1989). Health problems of the homeless in America. Nurse Practitioner, 7, 44–51.
Brickner, P., et al. (1985). Health Care of Homeless People. New York: Springer.
Ferguson, M.A. (1989). Psychiatric nursing in a shelter for the homeless. American Journal of Nursing, 89(8), 1060–1062.
Flaskerud, J.H. (1989). AIDS/HIV infection. A reference guide for nursing professionals. Philadelphia: W.B. Saunders.
Fox, E., Axelrod, S., & Loeb, J. (1985). Homelessness in Philadelphia: People, needs, services. Philadelphia: Philadelphia Health Management Corporation.
Guralink, D. (Ed.). (1988). Webster's new world dictionary. Cleveland: Wm. Collins and World Publishing.
Levine, M.E. (1973). Introduction to clinical nursing (2nd ed.). Philadelphia: F.A. Davis.
Levine, M.E. (1988). Address to District 18 Illinois Nurses Association. Newsletter, 6, 4–7.
Levine, M.E. (1989). The four conservation principles: Twenty years later. In J.P. Riehl-Sisca (Ed.), Conceptual Models for Nursing Practice (3rd ed.). Norwalk, CT: Appleton & Lange.
Reilly, D.E. (1975). Why a conceptual framework. Nursing Outlook, 23, 556–569.

Chapter
THIRTEEN

A Tradition of Caring
Use of Levine's Model in
Long-Term Care

Sister Ruth Alyce Cox, R.N., Ph.D.

My nursing practice has been guided by the use of Levine's conceptual framework for more than 20 years. I first met Levine in 1966 when I enrolled as an R.N. student in the baccalaureate nursing program at Loyola University of Chicago. In 1968 I began graduate study in nursing of adults at Loyola, where she was one of my major professors. The program used Levine's conceptual framework as a basis for the course work in medical-surgical nursing.

Following my graduation in 1970, I became a member of the undergraduate faculty at Loyola. As coordinator of the sophomore nursing faculty, I used Levine's book, *Introduction to Clinical Nursing* (1973), as the major textbook for the course. Although Levine's primary responsibility at Loyola University was in the graduate program, she also taught with the sophomore faculty. Thus, she became my colleague and mentor, and more importantly, my friend. This relationship endures today.

In 1977 I became nursing home administrator/geriatric nurse practitioner at the Alverno Health Care Facility, and I continued to use the conservation principles in my practice. The following is a description of the use of Levine's model at Alverno.

DESCRIPTION OF THE CURRENT PRACTICE
SETTING

Alverno is a 136-bed intermediate care facility located in Clinton, Iowa. Alverno is owned and operated by the Sisters of Saint Francis in Clinton as a nonprofit health care facility for the aged. This ministry of caring for the aged was begun by the Sisters in 1912.

179

Institutions providing long-term care may be licensed as residential (RCF), intermediate (ICF), or skilled care facilities (SCF). By definition an ICF is a health-related facility designed to provide custodial care. An ICF is not considered by the federal government to be a medical facility and therefore is not eligible for reimbursement under Title XVIII (Medicare). An SCF is a medical facility designed to provide rehabilitation on a short-term basis. Most SCFs participate in the Medicare program. States vary in the numbers of each type of facility licensed. Iowa has a predominance of ICFs. Many of the residents in Iowa ICFs would be classified as skilled care in other states. The Omnibus Budget Reconciliation Act of 1987 provides a single set of standards that designate all SCFs and ICFs as nursing facilities (NFs) beginning in 1990. State governments, through the certificate-of-need process, will still determine the number of facilities or beds that may participate in the Medicare program.

Alverno, built on a hill on 7 acres of grounds, is composed of two brick buildings. One building houses the entrance, offices, lobby, living room, chapel, dining room, and kitchen on the main floor, with activities, staff lounges, storage, maintenance, and garage at ground level. This service building is connected by a short hallway to a three-story resident care building. Resident rooms are arranged on the outside of a double-halled rectangular building with centrally located nurses' stations and service units such as utility rooms, tub rooms, laundry, linen, and housekeeping rooms, and with resident lounges located between the two halls. There are 103 private rooms, 13 double rooms, and 4 suites for married couples.

The professional staff consists of registered and licensed practical nurses, a dietitian, a physical therapist, a social worker, a recreational therapist, and a pastoral counselor. Medical services are provided by the residents' personal physician. Psychiatric, podiatry, pharmacy, occupational, and speech therapy consultants visit the facility on a regular basis to provide services. The professional staff is assisted by activity, dietary, and nursing aides.

DESCRIPTION OF THE POPULATION

The residents at Alverno are the frail elderly who have multiple chronic illnesses; new admissions increasingly exhibit more acute illness. There are 22 men and 114 women, who range in age from 58 to 99 years. The average age is 85; 80 percent of the residents are age 80 or older. With regard to marital status, 23 percent are single, 13 percent are married, and 64 percent are widowed. Thirty-four percent of the residents were living alone prior to admission; 17 percent were living with a caretaker; 35 percent were admitted from acute or skilled care; 7 percent from other ICFs; and 7 percent from RCFs. The average length of stay (LOS) is 3.5 years. Seventeen percent have resided in the facility for less than 6 months; an additional 14 percent have an LOS of less than 1 year, whereas 9 percent have an LOS greater than 10 years. Nearly all have family and friends who visit regularly.

The residents have from one to eight major medical diagnoses, with an average of three chronic illnesses for which medications are administered. The average prescription use is five.[1] Most residents need assistance with some of the activities of daily living. Ninety-six percent of the residents need assistance with bathing, 32 percent must be fed, 65 percent have serious problems with mobility, 59 percent need assistance in toileting, 48 percent are incontinent, and 58 percent are cognitively impaired. These statistics reveal that this population is greatly in need of basic nursing care.

THE CONSERVATION PRINCIPLES

Conservation of Energy

The multitude of physiologic and psychologic processes that sustain life are dependent upon the energy balance of the body. This balance is determined by measuring the energy input of essential nutrients against the output of energy-expending activities. The aging process results in physiologic alterations that leave the older person's energy reserve marginal at best. Any superimposed disease process will affect the individual's energy reserve and adaptive capacities negatively. The nurse's role in the conservation of energy is to assist the resident in maintaining the energy balance. Major nursing goals related to the conservation of energy include (1) assisting the new resident to adjust to life in a nursing home, (2) improving nutritional status, (3) balancing rest and activity, and (4) controlling anxiety and pain.

Admission to a nursing home is an energy-consuming experience. No one wants to live in a nursing home. However, declining physical or mental status forces the resident or family and physician to decide on admission. All residents grieve the loss of "what was"—health, home, independence, privacy. The resident must adapt to a new environment with its own routine for daily living and become acquainted with numerous personnel and other residents. It takes 3 to 6 months for most residents to settle in and feel "at home." The first month is extremely energy expending. To facilitate residents' adjustment to a new living situation, personnel spend extra time just being present and listening to their concerns.

The second goal related to the conservation of energy is assessment and improvement of the resident's nutritional status. On admission many residents are underweight, show obvious muscle wasting, exhibit generalized weakness, and may have peripheral edema. The dietitian is responsible for assessment of the resident's nutritional status. The diet history includes information about usual meal patterns, types and amounts of food and fluid intake, food preferences and dislikes, and allergies. Residents are observed for their ability to swallow without difficulty, to manipulate eating utensils, and to feed themselves, as well as for their endurance throughout the meal.

Body weight-to-height ratio is the most readily available indicator of nutritional status. If the resident is 10 percent or more below the desired weight for height, protein-calorie malnutrition is considered severe (Gambert, 1987). Laboratory data, when available, are used for nutritional assessment. When liver and renal functions are normal, a serum albumin level below 3.5 g per 100 ml indicates protein depletion. A hemoglobin of less than 12 g per dl or a hematocrit below 35 mg per 100 ml indicates anemia. Anemia, although common in the elderly, is not attributable simply to aging. Anemia of chronic disease accounts for 75 percent of all anemia in the elderly, and the underlying cause must be identified and treated (Gambert, 1987). Other laboratory values that are used in nutritional assessment include serum glucose, electrolytes, creatinine, and thyroid profile.

The information obtained from interview, assessment, and laboratory values is used by the dietitian to tailor the liberalized geriatric diet (Iowa Dietetic Association, 1984) (1500 calories, low sodium, low sugar, low fat) to each resident's nutritional needs. Special diets are provided when the physician determines that the liberalized geriatric diet is not restrictive enough. For example, residents with unstable diabetes or renal failure may require additional dietary modifications. Nutrient-dense foods such as meat, fish, poultry, dairy products, fruits, and vegetables are served in an effort to overcome protein-calorie malnutrition. Direct observation of the resident's appetite and eating pattern with calorie counts (dietary) or estimation of percent of diet consumed (nursing) is a routine practice for all residents. Weights are obtained monthly on all residents.

The recommended dietary allowances for specific nutrients are the same for all adults over 51 years of age except for calories (National Academy of Sciences, 1980). The number of calories needed depends on the activity level of the individual. The basic metabolic rate declines progressively with age, reflecting a decrease in lean body mass. In general, the elderly are less physically active and therefore need fewer calories. However, residents with Alzheimer's disease who actively pace may need an increase in caloric intake to maintain normal weight.

Anorexia, the loss of appetite or desire to eat, is a common complaint and a major cause of undernutrition in the elderly. Age-related changes in the gastrointestinal tract result in decreased secretion of digestive enzymes, which slows nutrient absorption, and in decreased motility, which delays gastric emptying and produces a feeling of satiety. Chronic illnesses, particularly congestive heart failure, cancer, and liver disease—as well as end-stage chronic obstructive pulmonary disease and renal failure—all cause anorexia. Medications frequently depress appetite and interfere with the various mechanisms of nutrient absorption, transformation, and utilization. Chemotherapeutic agents, antibiotics, and iron preparations are easily identified as causing anorexia, but virtually any drug can contribute to inadequate dietary intake and interfere with metabolism. In long-term care the major drugs causing anorexia and contributing to undernutrition are digitalis, diuretics, laxatives, and analgesics. Additional causes of decreased food intake include depression, pain, dysphagia, decreased acuity of taste, xerostomia, glossitis, oral lesions, and ill-fitting dentures. Each problem must be addressed as it arises in order to promote nutritional adequacy (Behnke, 1986).

Obesity also indicates poor nutrition and is often the result of a lifetime of consuming more food than was needed. Most of our residents who are overweight are not interested in changing their dietary patterns and losing weight. It is nearly impossible to prevent these residents from snacking between meals, as family and friends frequently bring in food.

Maintenance of adequate fluid balance is vital. The elderly are subject to dehydration for several reasons:

1. Total body water decreases with age.
2. The sensation of thirst lessens.
3. Limited mobility makes it difficult to reach a water glass.
4. Diuretics given to treat hypertension increase fluid output excessively in persons without fluid retention.
5. Infection, hot weather, and excessive activity increase the need for fluids.

Inadequate fluid intake is the primary cause of simple dehydration in the elderly. The recommended fluid intake is 1500 to 2000 ml daily. Residents are not always willing to consume the recommended amount, and some residents have the mistaken belief that limiting fluids will decrease urinary incontinence or eliminate the need for a diuretic. An increased blood urea nitrogen (BUN) or change in mental status may indicate dehydration.

It is often difficult to assess hydration in the elderly. Decreased salivation and anticholinergic drugs make the mouth look dry, and the loss of skin elasticity makes assessment of skin turgor imprecise. Even though the elderly lose some ability to concentrate urine and diurnal urine production may be lost, when dehydration results from water depletion, the output decreases to 300 to 500 ml daily of concentrated urine (Reichel, 1983). A pale yellow urine voided a few hours after fluid consumption is indicative of adequate hydration. At Alverno fluid intake is considered adequate for the catheterized resident if the urinary output is 1200 ml daily, and in the noncatheterized resident when urine voided at midday is clear and pale yellow. Routine intake and output is instituted whenever a resident exhibits signs of inadequate output or dehydration.

Activity tolerance is a measure of the energy an individual can expend without experiencing changes in respiration, pulse rate or character, blood pressure, pain, or fatigue. Activity intolerance is common in the frail elderly patient. Therefore, the third nursing goal related to the conservation of energy is to maintain an appropriate balance between activity and rest. Finding this balance is extremely important for two very different types of resident: (1) those newly admitted who have experienced recent hospitalization or an exacerbation of their chronic illness, and (2) those cognitively impaired residents whose anxiety or boredom causes them to pace the facility halls.

The effects of chronic illness in advanced aging results in general physical deconditioning. The effort to maintain or promote independence in the activities of daily living requires a program of gradual increase in physical activity, which is tailored to the individual resident. At Alverno the assessment of a resident's activity tolerance is made by the physical therapist in conjunction with nursing. Baseline data are obtained on pulse, respirations, blood pressure, and skin color, as well as reports of weakness, dizziness, dyspnea, or pain. In general, the pulse rate of an older person does not increase as much in response to exercise or return to the resting state as rapidly as it does in the younger adult (Williams, 1985). In addition, the possibility of respiratory muscle fatigue must be considered especially for residents with cardiac, respiratory, or neuromuscular disease and those who are undernourished. An increase in the respiratory rate is the first clinical sign of impending respiratory muscle fatigue, and breathing patterns during recovery from fatiguing periods are rapid and shallow (Ingersoll, 1989).

Parameters used to determine the need to terminate an activity because of excessive energy expenditure include:

1. An increase in pulse rate of 20 beats per minute
2. Any pulse irregularity or weakness
3. An irregular respiratory rate or increase in dyspnea
4. A drop in systolic blood pressure of more than 20 mm Hg
5. A change in skin color
6. A progressive slowing of the activity
7. Leaning on an object for support
8. Complaints of dizziness or fatigue

A heart rate that fails to return to baseline within 5 minutes after activity is also an indication that the activity was too strenuous or too prolonged (Matteson & McConnell, 1988).

Sleep pattern disturbances also affect the rest-activity balance. About one third of all elderly have significant sleep-related disturbances. Although the total amount of sleep time does not change with age, the older person usually takes longer to fall asleep. A decrease in the amount of stage IV deep sleep, compensated for by an increase in stage III sleep, produces a decrease in the transition time between sleep and wakefulness; hence, the elderly are considered "light sleepers" (Kenney, 1989, p. 127). Frequent awakening is also induced by nocturia, anxiety, pain, paroxysmal nocturnal dyspnea, sleep apnea, medications such as the beta-adrenergics and steroids, and noise levels in the institutional setting.

Sedatives, tranquilizers, or hypnotics are often used as interventions for sleeplessness; however, these drugs do not promote restful sleep and often produce daytime drowsiness. Basic nursing interventions such as warm milk, a complex carbohydrate snack at bedtime, and temperature and noise control are better strategies (Bahr & Gress, 1985). Scheduled daytime rest periods or naps are therapeutic for the frail elderly patient.

The management of anxiety and pain is an important aspect of the conservation of energy. Many memory-impaired residents exhibit a high level of anxiety that can be observed by a facial expression of worry, frequent pacing and continuous movement. Chronic pain associated with arthritis, osteoporosis, and peripheral neuropathy is common. Both anxiety and chronic pain are managed by nonpharmacologic means whenever possible. If proper positioning, massage, heat, and distraction (visitors, music, special activities) fail to relieve the discomforts residents experience, anti-anxiety or pain medication is indicated. The nurses are responsible for adjusting the medication schedule so that the smallest possible dose given routinely will allay the symptoms yet allow the resident to be alert and able to participate in the activities that make up life at Alverno.

Conservation of Structural Integrity

The aging process produces degenerative changes in all body systems. In the absence of disease, organ systems normally age at different rates; these structural changes result in varying degrees of alteration in function. Loss of vision and hearing, joint stiffness, and shrinking in stature are obvious to those affected. However, age-related decreases in function in other body systems may go unnoticed as the elderly quite normally adjust their life-styles to accommodate their functional abilities.

The aged are also subject to chronic illness, which produces structural changes in the body. Often it is difficult to differentiate the indicators of pathology and disease from normal aging indices. In spite of these physical changes, the majority of the elderly living in the community can and do maintain active, independent lives.

With advancing age there is a general increase in disability due to chronic illness, which necessitates nursing home care for those with severe limitations in functional ability. Nursing goals relating to the conservation of structural integrity include:

1. Maximizing functional capacity and maintaining or promoting mobility
2. Preventing injury through safety precautions
3. Preventing infection
4. Maintaining skin integrity

The loss of lean body mass that occurs with aging is related to changes in muscle composition and function. A gradual reduction in the number and size of muscle fibers and an increase in connective tissue causes the muscles to become less elastic. Muscle atrophy limits the amount of tension a muscle can endure. Ligaments and tendons also shorten and become sclerotic. This limits the effective range of motion in the hips, knees, elbows, wrists, neck, and vertebrae, as these joints all become somewhat flexed (Kenney, 1989). In addition, some residents have serious functional limitations following a cerebrovascular accident or because of degenerative arthritis.

Achieving maximal functional capability begins with a thorough assessment completed by the physical therapist and nurse. Assessment parameters include the following:

1. Walking independently or using a cane or walker
2. Rising from a chair
3. Transferring from bed to chair and from chair to chair or to bed
4. Position sense and balance
5. Range of motion (ROM) exercises
6. Strength and endurance

Residents who are independently mobile are encouraged to participate in scheduled daily exercise groups to help minimize the effects of functional limitations resulting from aging. An individualized physical therapy program of active and/or passive exercises is designed for residents who are not independently mobile. The program may include gait training, assisted walking, strengthening exercises, and ROM exercises. Nursing is responsible for maintaining proper body alignment and providing ROM exercises for all bed and wheelchair-confined residents.

The second nursing goal related to the conservation of structural integrity is the prevention of injury through the promotion of a safe environment. Osteoporosis predisposes bone to fracture with minimal or no trauma (Reichel, 1983). Loss of bone substance, especially trabecular bone, increases rapidly in postmenopausal women. Half of all women will have a compression fracture of the spine by 75 years of age (Hallal, 1985), and an 80-year-old woman has a 1-in-5 chance of sustaining a fracture of the neck or the femur (Kenney, 1989). Fractures of the distal radius are also common. To prevent falls it is essential that the environment be free of clutter, that spills be wiped up immediately, and that halls be nonskid and well lighted without glare. Uneven lighting casts shadows on the floor, and a resident may fall trying to step over a nonexistent object. Grab bars and raised toilet seats or shower chairs with arms are necessary environmental aids for bathrooms. Chairs should have solid seats with arms that provide leverage for rising to a standing position. Residents also need to be taught to use these aids properly.

Because many residents have visual impairments and marked limitations in mobility, falls are common. All falls are recorded on an incident report and analyzed to identify residents at risk. Risk factors for falls include advanced age, use of assistive devices (cane, walker, or wheelchair), medications that cause orthostatic hypotension, and cognitive impairment (Lund & Sheafor, 1985). Whenever possible, interventions are provided to reduce the residents' risk for falling. For example, residents with limited mobility or orthostatic hypotension are instructed to ask for assistance when they get out of bed. Soft restraints may be used on residents who have little sense of balance, but restraints will not prevent falls. Although falls seldom result in serious injury, they can lower a resident's confidence, generate insecurity or fear of walking, and create an increased dependence on staff for assistance (Hallal, 1985).

Prevention of infection is the third nursing goal related to the conservation of structural integrity. Infections are a major cause of morbidity and mortality in the elderly. The risk of infection in a long-term care facility is 5 to 10 percent per resident-month (Garibaldi, Brodine, & Matsumiya, 1981), or approximately one infection per resident per year. This population is at risk for two reasons. First, the efficacy of the immune system decreases with age. Cell-mediated immunity decreases, and fewer antibodies are produced in response to an infective agent or vaccination. Second, most residents have multiple medical conditions (congestive heart failure, chronic obstructive pulmonary disease, diabetes mellitus, dementia) that predispose them to infection (Smith, 1987).

Infection often presents atypically in the elderly. Fever and leukocytosis may or may not be present. Often the only indications of infection are anorexia, weakness, nausea, fatigue, or acute confusion. Thus, whenever there is a change in the resident's general state of health or behavior, the threat of infection must be considered (Gambert, 1987).

The most common nosocomial infections in long-term care are urinary tract and respiratory tract infections, infected decubiti, and gastroenteritis (Smith, 1987). The most prevalent type is urinary tract infection (UTI); 60 to 90 percent of UTIs follow catheterization. An indwelling catheter, while undesirable, may be necessary for the management of incontinence if a resident with a neurogenic bladder is predisposed to skin breakdown. A closed catheter system is used whenever possible. However, an ambulatory resident may need to use a leg bag in order to remain independently mobile. Catheters are irrigated and/or changed only when necessary. Routine meatal-cleansing is no longer considered necessary. The majority of catheterized residents will have significant bacteriuria, but the use of antibiotics is warranted only when clinical signs indicate active infection (Smith, 1987).

Respiratory tract infection (with influenza) is the fourth most common cause of death in the elderly and the second most prevalent nosocomial infection in long-term care. The demented resident and those who have difficulty swallowing are at risk for aspiration pneumonia. Residents with cardiorespiratory disorders are at risk for pneumococcal pneumonia. All residents are encouraged to have the pneumonia vaccine once and the flu vaccine yearly.

The major infections encountered at Alverno are UTIs, influenza, occasional conjunctivitis, and herpes zoster (shingles). Hand washing remains the single most effective nursing practice for the prevention of the infections.

Maintaining the resident's skin integrity is the fourth nursing goal for the conservation of structural integrity. Age-related changes often impair the skin's ability to serve as a protective barrier to the environment. Thinning of the epidermis leaves the skin prone to cracks and fissures. A decrease in ground substance and water content of the dermis results in dryness and loss of turgor. The blood supply to the skin lessens as the density of the dermal capillary networks is decreased, and increased capillary fragility results in easy bruising. The overall result of these structural changes is a fragile skin that may be slow to heal (Kenney, 1989). In addition many residents are incontinent of urine and feces, and/or have diabetes mellitus or congestive heart failure with edema, all of which predispose them to skin breakdown and delay healing.

Bathing must be frequent enough to keep the resident clean yet not so often as to increase dryness. In order to prevent skin breakdown in the incontinent resident, a regular schedule for toileting is used. Fluid intake is increased to 2000 ml daily (if possible) to decrease the incontinence and infection caused by concentrated urine, and residents are taken to the bathroom every 2 to 3 hours.

Very few residents develop decubiti in the facility. All residents have their position changed frequently. Residents who are undernourished or incapable of easily moving about in bed are placed on a water mattress.

Occasionally a resident may be admitted or returned from the hospital with a decubitus. The nursing goal is to heal the decubitus as quickly as possible. Increased protein intake, gentle cleansing, débridement when necessary, and the application of a hydrocolloid dressing such as Duoderm usually results in rapid healing. Pressure sores on the heels or toes of diabetic residents sometimes do not heal because of vascular problems. These may require surgical management and perhaps amputation.

Conservation of Personal Integrity

Self-identity is intrinsically bound to wholeness, and all individuals cherish their sense of self (Levine, 1973). The essence of long-term care is helping people manage the very personal daily activities that lie at the core of their sense of independence and well-being. This need for assistance threatens their sense of self-identity and self-esteem, and personnel must make a concerted effort to protect the resident's personal integrity.

The Residents' Bill of Rights supports personal integrity through federal and state legislation and regulation (Health Care Financing Administration, 1989). These rights are explained upon admission and reinforced by professional staff whenever necessary. Nursing goals related to the conservation of personal integrity include:

1. Respecting persons, their privacy, and property
2. Maintaining or enhancing self-esteem through good personal hygiene, grooming, and dress
3. Fostering independence through choice and rehabilitation
4. Promoting self-identity for those who are cognitively impaired
5. Obtaining advanced directives for treatment

Respect for the resident is shown first in the term of address. Residents are asked how they wished to be addressed. Nearly all of our residents prefer to be called by their first name. The fact that many of our residents, families, and staff have known each other for many years may account for this widespread acceptance of familiarity. Respect is also shown in the manner of approaching a resident, and nonprofessional personnel are taught not to use terms such as "honey," "dear," or "gramps." Privacy is protected when personnel knock before entering a resident's room, and modesty is honored during personal care and assistance.

Research on clothing for the disabled indicates that personal appearance influences self-identity and self-esteem (Ruston, 1982). Being dressed appropriately in one's own clothing helps to promote a sense of normalcy and well-being. All residents, unless acutely ill, are expected to be dressed for breakfast and to remain dressed until bedtime. A suggested clothing list is provided for the resident. It is also suggested that clothing should be easy to put on and take off, have sufficient fullness for easy mobility, and be laundered easily. Housecoats and dusters are not considered appropriate daytime wear. When necessary, laundry personnel will modify a resident's clothing with Velcro closures or make wrap-around skirts for ease in dressing.

Most residents go regularly to the beauty shop in the facility. Two beauticians provide this very important service to all who are able to tolerate sitting upright long enough for a shampoo and set or a permanent. For those unable to go to the beauty shop, the nurses' aides wash the residents' hair in the shower and set it with soft curlers. The appearance of the residents is important to the entire staff, and good grooming is a comfort to family and friends who visit.

Residents are encouraged to personalize their rooms with a favorite chair (preferably a recliner for comfort and rest), lamp, pictures, and family photographs. It is difficult for a resident to select from the possessions of a lifetime items that will fit in a single room. Couples occupying a suite usually bring some of their living room furniture. Facility drapes and bedspreads are chosen to coordinate with wall color and to brighten the room. In addition to their rooms, most residents have claimed a territory of their own in the halls and lounges, and this territory is usually respected by personnel and other residents. As Levine (1973) stated, "The space one claims for oneself both separates one from, and integrates one into, the social organization" (p. 462).

Many aspects of routine daily life in a nursing home are controlled by the organization necessary to facilitate institutional operation. However, allowing individual choice, and thus some control over one's own life, is essential in conserving personal integrity. Residents actually have more choice in social activities than in physical care activities. At Alverno a resident may select preferred social activities from a variety of options. Residents are always invited, but never required, to participate in the activity program. In the area of personal hygiene, the choice is between a tub bath and a shower given in the morning or evening. No bath at all (the preferred choices of some) is not an option. The resident has a choice of foods offered, but not about mealtime. In dressing, the choice is between two outfits, not between dressing or not dressing. Shortly after admission, the nurse or aide asks the resident to describe his or her former lifestyle, including type of clothing usually worn, hygiene practices, time of arising and going to bed, and usual daily activities. Whenever possible, former routines are incorporated into the plan of care, and choices often relate to lifetime habits. Although these choices may seem minor, they do serve to give the resident some measure of control over nursing home life.

For the cognitively impaired resident, conservation of personal integrity focuses on promoting self-identity through activities that focus on present reality as long as such focus does not create further agitation or anxiety. A variety of approaches (reality orientation, reminiscence, music, gardening, pets, and religious programs) may be used for individuals and groups. The use of touch and hugs helps residents feel that others truly care about them.

The issue of advanced treatment directives is an important consideration that supports the conservation of personal and social integrity. After admission a nurse consults with the resident and family about their wishes for providing or withholding treatment in the event of acute illness or sudden cardiopulmonary arrest. The statement on affirmation of life (Catholic Health Association, 1987) is available from the social worker, and residents who are capable of making their own decisions are encouraged to have a lawyer help them complete a living will if they so desire. All residents are assured that the family and physician will be notified promptly whenever there is a serious change in a resident's condition, and options for providing or withholding treatment will be discussed again.

The following material on advanced treatment directives is included in preadmission materials.

1. "Supportive care only" orders: A "supportive care only" order is a decision to provide care and treatment to preserve comfort, hygiene, and dignity, but not to prolong life. Supportive care is not considered to be part of the concept of euthanasia or as causing death, but rather should be viewed as not extending life in hopeless situations. The primary aim of a supportive care plan should be to promote the dignity of the person and to minimize pain or discomfort.
2. Cardiopulmonary resuscitation (CPR) is designed to prevent sudden unexpected death. There are certain circumstances in which it may be appropriate to withhold CPR, such as when a resident's condition has been determined to be terminal and when death is imminent or expected. "Do not resuscitate" (DNR) means that in the event of a cardiac or respiratory arrest, no cardiopulmonary resuscitation measures will be initiated.

Long-term care facilities in Iowa are mandated to use CPR in case of emergency unless there is a signed order from the physician indicating the resident's and/or family's desire not to resuscitate. In that case, a "supportive care only" order is used. Please note that the order may be changed at any time by a signed order from the physician. The family and/or legal representative should discuss these options with the physician.

Obviously, fractures and non-life-threatening illnesses must be treated appropriately. When residents are seriously ill, most families opt for the use of an antibiotic to treat infection; some request hospitalization and others request care in the facility. Resident and family wishes are supported and made known to the physician, and the proper orders are obtained. In the final analysis, nearly all of our residents are provided only care and comfort when dying.

Conservation of Social Integrity

"Individual life has meaning only in the context of social life" (Levine, 1973, p. 17). Social life is extremely important in long-term care as residents leave solitary or family living to join a community of peers who are also in need of nursing care. Nursing goals related to the conservation of social integrity include providing meaningful social activities for residents and staff, and considering the family and resident as a unit.

Many residents of Alverno have lifelong friends who are also residents. These friends help the new resident adjust to institutional living. Information about families and friends, as well as aches and pains, is shared with staff, other residents, and families.

Social and religious activities are held daily, and residents select activities that coincide with their personal preferences and interests. Some of the favorite activities are birthday parties, picnics, cards, bingo, music appreciation, reminiscence, growing plants, pets, coffee hours, crafts, drama, guessing games, entertainment provided by community and school groups, and daily Mass and other religious services. Birthday and anniversary parties are videotaped, and residents enjoy "watching themselves on TV." Young mothers in the Newcomers' Club bring their preschool children to visit monthly. Residents love to hold and hug and be hugged by the children. Cuddly puppies and kittens from the Humane Society are brought to the facility weekly, and families with pets often bring the pets to visit. Residents who are able often go "home" for a visit with their families. In warm weather activity personnel take the residents on van rides to familiar places in Clinton. In the late afternoon, many residents wheel themselves to the front desk to await the daily paper. All of these activities help the resident to maintain ties with the local community and promote social integrity.

Nursing home placement is often difficult for the family, and staff members make a concerted effort to help the family adjust and become part of the Alverno community. Many families soon realize that nursing home placement has relieved them of heavy caregiver burdens, and family relationships become easier and more enjoyable. Families interact with one another and the staff, participate in family nights, and often attend group activity programs. Residents without close family ties are "adopted" by staff members who remember birthdays and other important events.

In addition, the long-term care facility has a social structure of its own. Both resident and staff participants negotiate their roles and goals, and they invoke their rights and duties. The flow of gossip among participants is continuous. Underlying the entire social structure, however, there exists between residents and staff an abiding sense of love and concern for others that marks the Alverno Health Care Facility as a caring community.

Case Presentation 13–1: L.D.—A Resident With Alzheimer's Disease

L.D., an 82-year-old widow, was admitted in February 1989 because severe cognitive impairment made living independently in her own apartment hazardous, and her family was unable to provide the supervision she needed. Her admitting medical diagnoses were probable Alzheimer's disease, diabetes mellitus (diagnosed August 1988), and long-standing glaucoma. The physician's orders were American Dietetic Association diet of 1600 calories, no added salt; medications, 1 mg of haloperidol (Haldol) as needed, 2.5 mg of glyburide (Diabeta) daily, 500 mg of acetazolamide (Diamox) daily; timolol maleste (Timoptic) 0.5 percent and Propine eyedrops twice a day; and do not resuscitate. Her laboratory test results were all within normal limits except for her fasting plasma glucose (FPG) which ranged from 95 to 220 mg per dl. Her chest x-ray examination showed a 2-cm lesion in the right lung. Admission nursing data revealed that L.D. was 5 feet, 5 inches tall and weighed 137 pounds. She was severely confused and could not answer any questions on a Mini-Mental Status Examination. Although she was unable to speak in complete sentences, she was able to make her wants known. She appeared agitated, wandering in the hallway looking for her son. Her confusion and agitation increased in the evening. L.D. needed complete supervision of her daily activities. She had inflamed bunions on both feet, and the skin between her toes was fissured.

CONSERVATION OF ENERGY

The elements for L.D.'s nursing care that related to the conservation of energy were new admission, agitation, wandering, and impaired glucose metabolism. Transfer to an unfamiliar environment is threatening to one who is cognitively impaired, and an increase in confusion is expected until the environment becomes familiar. In addition, L.D. had lived alone for many years, and she was upset by having so many other people around her. She was agitated; her facial expression showed strain, and she constantly walked in the hall looking for her family. She exhibited "sundowning" (increased confusion in the late afternoon and evening), which is typical of the Alzheimer's resident.

Because of the nature of her medical problems, most nursing interventions were supportive rather than therapeutic in nature. Supportive nursing interventions included keeping L.D. in the area near her room until she became familiar with the environment, assessing the type of her wandering, and trying to find a balance between activity and rest. Her wandering was considered goal-directed rather than aimless, as she kept asking if anyone had seen her son. She was allowed to wander through the hall as a means of dissipating her anxiety. Rest periods were provided by having a staff member sit and talk or watch television with her. She slept well at night, and her rest-activity needs were easily managed without the use of Haldol.

L.D.'s weight was appropriate for her height, and her laboratory work was normal; thus, her nutritional status was considered adequate. She was able to feed herself. She consumed her entire diet and did not seem to miss the snacks she had consumed at home. Her glucose levels were monitored weekly. Although these levels fluctuated, they remained within an acceptable range.

CONSERVATION OF STRUCTURAL INTEGRITY

The root of L.D.'s disability lies in structural damage of the neurons, which results in organic behavior beyond her control. Nursing interventions that compensate for her disabilities are relegated to the other conservation principles. Diabetes mellitus, too, causes structural changes of the macrovascular and microvascular systems. There is some controversy about what constitutes "good" diabetic control in the elderly, and many clinicians take a flexible approach to managing the older patient with this disease. The goal is to prevent wide swings in blood glucose levels. Attempts to reduce glucose levels to those acceptable for a younger person may be dangerous because the elderly are at high risk for developing hypoglycemia (Gioiella & Bevil, 1985). The physician determined that a flexible approach to diabetic management was appropriate for L.D., and the acceptable range for FPG was from 90 to 200 ml per dl.

L.D.'s foot problems and the need for safety were the major determinants of care related to the conservation of structural integrity. She had inflamed bunions of both feet, cracks between the toes, dry skin, and a fungal infection of the toenails. Weak pedal pulses indicated impaired blood flow to the feet. Because injury to the feet can lead to gangrene and amputation in the patient with diabetes, the following therapeutic interventions were promptly instituted. Warm soapy soaks followed by careful drying were used to cleanse away the dry skin and prevent infection. The fungal infection was treated by the podiatrist. Her son bought her a pair of wider shoes, and her hose were changed after each foot soak. The cracks between her toes were healed within 1 week, and she developed no further foot problems.

Safety is always a factor for the resident who wanders. A Wanderguard bracelet (which sets off an alarm on all exit doors) was applied until it was determined that L.D. made no effort to leave the unit unless accompanied by family or staff. She was allowed to walk about as much as desired. Unfortunately she fell in her bathroom, fractured her hip, and was hospitalized for surgical repair 1 month after admission.

CONSERVATION OF PERSONAL INTEGRITY

The major factors influencing L.D.'s nursing care were her impaired cognitive status with loss of memory and self-identity, impaired communication, and her need for supervision of all her activities.

Although L.D. was confused and unfamiliar with Alverno, she needed to be treated as an adult with constant reassurance and reminders about where she was and what she should do. A simple, set routine of care was established, her questions were answered repeatedly, and she was kept on the unit in an effort to provide an environmental structure that would minimize confusion and maximize her functional abilities. In time the environment became familiar through constant repetition.

Communicating with the memory-impaired person is important in preserving personal integrity. Simple rules of communication employed include:

1. Wait until the resident is attentive.
2. Be at eye level when possible.
3. Speak quietly and directly to the resident.
4. Use short sentences with nouns.

The memory-impaired patient frequently uses pronouns rather than nouns in conversation, and this makes it difficult to understand the conversation or what the resident wants. Reality-orientation techniques were used, as this did not seem to increase L.D.'s confusion.

L.D. was accustomed to having her personal hygiene needs met by her family, whom she recognized. Being helped by strangers was frightening to her, but with a consistent, nonthreatening approach, she was able to accept staff assistance. She was pleased whenever someone told her she looked nice.

CONSERVATION OF SOCIAL INTEGRITY

L.D.'s son and daughter-in-law met with the nurses to incorporate L.D.'s usual daily routine into her plan of care. Her daughter-in-law's mother had resided at Alverno for the past 2 years, so the family was familiar with the nursing home environment and comfortable with their decision to admit L.D. to the facility. They visited her daily, and their presence was comforting to her.

To meet L.D.'s social needs, she was assigned to Friendship Circle, a small group program for residents with Alzheimer's disease, designed to provide a "pleasant present." The program is patterned on ideas gleaned from the literature on group work with residents with Alzheimer's disease. Under the leadership of the social worker and activities department, seven cognitively impaired residents met three afternoons a week for socialization and mental stimulation. A theme for the day was selected and activities related to the theme were chosen to fit each participant's physical and mental abilities. The leaders may use BiFolkal kits[2] or develop their own props, discussion questions, and activities. L.D. especially enjoyed themes that focused on food preparation and other household activities.

RESPONDING TO CHANGE

Care of L.D. After Surgical Intervention.   L.D. returned to Alverno following a 10-day hospitalization for the surgical pinning of her left hip. She was non–weight bearing. Her x-ray films showed severe osteoporosis. Her hemoglobin had dropped to 10 g and her FPG levels ranged from 250 to 400 mg per dl. The physician ordered an American Dietetic Association diet (1200 calories, no added salt), 10 mg of glyburide in the morning and 5 mg in the evening, and a daily fasting glucose. DNR instructions were also given. L.D. still recognized her son and daughter-in-law, but she was severely disoriented to time, place, and all other persons. She was quiet and withdrawn during the day, and extremely agitated during the evening and night. Although she was incontinent, her Foley catheter (in place during hospitalization) was removed the day she was readmitted to Alverno. L.D.'s care was revised based on these new data.

CONSERVATION OF ENERGY

The factors that influenced L.D.'s nursing care on readmission were her elevated blood glucose blood levels, increased confusion, and inability to perform daily activities. The destabilization of diabetes with rising glucose levels may be precipitated by any stress such as injury, infection, or hypokalemia produced by diuretics (Reichel, 1983). The stress of transfer to the hospital with its unfamiliar environment, the surgical hip-pinning, and the transfer back to the nursing home all served to elevate L.D.'s blood glucose beyond an acceptable level. Her diet was decreased to 1200 calories and her glyburide increased substantially. As L.D. was non–weight-bearing, she was unable to lower her glucose through exercise. Her glucose level continued to be excessively elevated, and she was started on regular Humulin insulin on a sliding scale.

L.D. was restless and often tried to climb out of bed at night. She needed to be restrained at night. She was given 1 mg of haloperidol (Haldol) in the early evening. However, this drug did not alleviate her nighttime restlessness, so it was discontinued.

She now needed complete nursing care, including feeding. The elderly, confused resident is in danger of aspiration. L.D. was always seated in a geri-chair to support her head in an upright position during feeding, and she was kept in the upright position for 1 to 2 hours following each meal. She continued to consume all food and fluids offered until she suffered a stroke in mid-May.

CONSERVATION OF STRUCTURAL INTEGRITY

New factors to be considered for L.D.'s care included:

1. Her surgical incision
2. A non–weight-bearing status with need for ROM exercise
3. Incontinence
4. The possibility that she would develop a UTI following the use of a catheter

Therapeutic nursing interventions focused on keeping the incision clean and dry until healed, with careful transfer from bed to geri-chair to prevent further trauma to her fragile bones. She was placed on a water mattress to relieve any pressure on bony prominences that could contribute to decubiti formation. ROM exercise was instituted four times daily, and her position was changed routinely. She continued to be incontinent, and scrupulous skin care was provided. The surgical incision healed slowly, as is common in diabetics, but she did not develop a wound infection or a UTI.

CONSERVATION OF PERSONAL INTEGRITY

The trauma sustained by L.D. resulted in her becoming severely disoriented to time, place, and person. She was unable to actively participate in any activities or watch television, and one-to-one activities were instituted. Personnel were assigned to sit with L.D. and to talk softly to her or play soothing music while holding her hand. This seemed to quiet her so that she could rest comfortably. She was always treated with dignity and dressed daily in her own clothing. In spite of her confusion, the staff tried to maintain her usual day-night routine, hoping that eventually her confusion might decrease. It never did.

CONSERVATION OF SOCIAL INTEGRITY

Although L.D. was unable to enjoy any socialization, her family continued to visit daily, and she recognized them. Her stroke in mid-May left her semiconscious. Both physicians and family came to the facility to discuss treatment options. The family did not want L.D. hospitalized, and once again they affirmed their preference for supportive care only. L.D., a Catholic, was anointed; within 48 hours she died peacefully with her son at her bedside.

UTILITY OF LEVINE'S CONSERVATION MODEL

Levine's (1973) holistic conceptual model, which focuses on the adaptation of an individual interacting with the environment, is congruent with the philosophy of Alverno and our view of nursing. At Alverno we emphasize caring over curing (although interventions that cure or alleviate illness are never neglected), functional ability over disease pathology, and "high touch" over "high tech." Levine's identification of therapeutic and supportive nursing interventions supports these emphases.

The model provides direction for nursing practice and staff development. The conservation principles provide an organizing framework, an easy-to-remember guide, for promoting wholeness within the limits imposed by the aging process and the consequences of chronic illness. The broad focus of the four conservation principles is comprehensive. The identification of common recurring nursing problems and goals in long-term care gives direction and unity to nursing practice that fosters quality care. The model allows for the contributions made by all of the members of the interdisciplinary team.

The use of a model that focuses on nursing is important in long-term care. Because federal regulations for long-term care facilities require that the plan of care be based on the physician's orders, an effort must be made to focus on nursing concepts as well as on the medical diagnosis. Levine's model focuses on nursing but does not negate the pathophysiology of chronic illness. Levine has always emphasized the need for nursing to be based on up-to-date scientific knowledge. The conservation principles allow each level of practitioner (nurse's aide, LPN, RN) to provide care based upon the knowledge appropriate for the level of practice—care that focuses on the conservation of the resident's wholeness.

I began using this model 20 years ago because I was a student and later a colleague of Levine. After years of practice in various settings and further education with exposure to other nursing models, I have continued to use the conservation principles because they are a natural fit for the long-term care setting, and the emphasis on holism supports Alverno's tradition of caring.

NOTES

1. The average prescription use refers to the number of different medications a resident takes per month. Each medication is considered one prescription; one dose of a prn drug counts the same as one drug given routinely several times a day. The national average prescription use is 6.1 (HCFA, State Operations Manual, Provider Certification, Transmittal No. 149, January, 1982).

2. BiFolkal kits are program resources designed for group work with the elderly. Each theme-related kit contains slides, props, script, and program ideas to stimulate reminiscence. (BiFolkal Productions, 809 Williamson St., Madison, WI 53703.)

REFERENCES

Bahr, R.T., & Gress, L. (1985). The 24-hour cycle: Rhythms of healthy sleep. Journal of Gerontological Nursing, 11(4), 14.

Behnke, M.C. (1986). Anorexia. In V.K. Carrierei, A.M. Lindsey, & C.M. West (Eds.), Pathophysiological phenomena in nursing—Human responses to illness (pp. 99–121). Philadelphia: W.B. Saunders.

Catholic Health Association. (1987). Christian affirmation of life. St. Louis: Catholic Health Association.

Gambert, S.R. (Ed.) (1987). Handbook of geriatrics. New York: Plenum.

Garibaldi, R.A., Brodine, S., & Matsumiya, S. (1981). Infections among patients in nursing homes: Policies, prevalence, problems. New England Journal of Medicine, 305(13), 731.

Gioiella, E.C., & Bevil, C.W. (1985). Nursing care of the aging client—Promoting healthy adaptation. Norwalk, CT: Appleton-Century-Crofts.

Hallal, J.C. (1985). Osteoporotic fractures exact a toll. Journal of Gerontological Nursing, 11(8), 13.

Health Care Financing Administration. (1989). Resident Rights Requirements. 42 CFR Part 405 et al., Section 483.10. Federal Register, 54:21.

Ingersoll, G.L. (1989). Respiratory muscle fatigue research: Implications for clinical practice. Applied Nursing Research, 2(1), 6.

Iowa Dietetic Association. (1984). Simplified diet manual (5th ed.). Ames, IA: Iowa State University Press.

Kenney, R.A. (1989). Physiology of aging: A synopsis (2nd ed.). Chicago: Year Book Medical Publishers.

Levine, M.E. (1973). Introduction to clinical nursing (2nd ed.). Philadelphia: F.A. Davis.

Lund, C., & Sheafor, M.L. (1985). Is your patient about to fall? Journal of Gerontological Nursing, 11(4), 37.

Matteson, M.A., & McConnell, E.S. (Eds.). (1988). Gerontological nursing concepts and practice. Philadelphia: W.B. Saunders.

National Academy of Sciences, Food and Nutrition Board. (1980). Recommended dietary allowances (9th ed. rev.). Washington, DC: The Academy.

Reichel, W. (Ed.). (1983). Clinical aspects of aging (2nd ed.). Baltimore: Williams & Wilkins.

Ruston, R. (1982). Dressing for disabled people (Rev.). London: Disabled Living Foundation.

Smith, P.W. (1987). Nursing home–acquired infections. Post Graduate Medicine, 81(6), 55.

Williams, T.F. (Ed.). (1985). Rehabilitation in the aging. New York: Raven Press.

Chapter
FOURTEEN

Developing an Undergraduate Program Using Levine's Model

Joan Grindley, R.N., Ed.D.
MaryBeth Paradowski, R.N., M.S.N.

In 1975, Allentown College of Saint Francis de Sales in Center Valley, Pennsylvania, accepted the first nursing students into its undergraduate program. Students studied in a curriculum based on the philosophy of Christian humanism and the conservation principles of nursing as explicated by Levine (1973). Christian humanism is the philosophy guiding the college and directing its mission. After careful deliberation, Levine's conceptual model was selected by the faculty as a model that was congruent with the college philosophy and the faculty's beliefs about nursing.

SELECTING THE MODEL

In choosing a model on which to base the nursing curriculum, it is important that those developing the program select a model that is compatible with the mission and philosophy of the college. Christian humanism embraces a holistic approach emphasizing the importance of the individual's physical, intellectual, moral, social, aesthetic, and religious development. Levine's model, which focuses on the unity and integrity of the individual, complements and reinforces the college's beliefs.

Levine's model fits also with this faculty's belief that a nursing curriculum must have a solid base in the biologic sciences as well as in the social

199

and behavioral sciences. In planning the curriculum, the faculty wanted to provide a balance among the courses that would assist students in appreciating and understanding the complex components of human nature. They had, however, a special interest in the biologic sciences, influenced by the fact that the program's first chairperson had doctoral preparation in physiology. Levine's principles, with an emphasis on physiologic responses related to conservation of energy and of structural integrity, were especially suitable.

The decision to emphasize the biologic sciences was a fortuitous one in light of future developments in health care. Drew (1988) notes that nursing programs have neglected to stress the study of the biologic sciences while favoring the psychosocial. This neglect and lack of appreciation for the significance of science in nursing practice has led to permitting less well prepared persons care for patients with very complex problems. Some nurses' knowledge base has not kept pace with the challenge brought about by rapid changes in science. Much earlier, Levine (1971) expressed her concern that technology had the potential to depersonalize our interaction with patients. She pointed out that nurses were the practitioners who must see to it that care was holistic and humanistic. Given the complex nature of patient conditions today, a firm foundation in the sciences is essential to providing professional nursing care.

PLANNING THE CURRICULUM

Although the faculty had considerable freedom in the selection of a nursing model and in making decisions about non-nursing courses and their placement, they were nevertheless required to adhere to the distribution requirements dictated by the college for all students regardless of major. These requirements reflected the college philosophy: Allentown College seeks to produce the Christian humanist for our time; the cultured person committed to a Christian understanding of existence at all levels, both natural and supernatural; the individual in whom the ideals of truth and love find intimate union and meaningful expression (Bulletin of Information, 1989).

The course distribution was (and is) consistent with the college's belief that the goal of education is to develop the total person who appreciates and contributes to the world around him or her. To achieve this goal, the college has required that all students, including nursing students, enroll in classes in philosophy, theology, the humanities, and the sciences. This supports Levine's (1984) approach that students must be involved in the whole range of courses available in the college, not because these courses prepare the student for the nursing major but because they prepare the student for the practice of holistic nursing and for lifelong learning.

Individuals are unique and can be appreciated fully only if one understands all the environmental forces that have shaped them and that continue to influence them as they move through life. The faculty at Allentown College believe that a commitment to practice holistic nursing can be made only by the nurse who can comprehend what the concept of holism encompasses. The faculty believe, along with DeBack and Mentkorowski (1986), that the effect of a broadly based education is sustained across time and in a variety of settings, producing nurses whose practice is more likely to be conceptual, independent, and geared toward supporting the individuals' ability to accept responsibility for themselves.

The typical curriculum plan for the undergraduate nursing student can be seen in Table 14–1. For the class that entered in 1990, a foreign language course became a new requirement. Selected courses from all disciplines emphasize modes of thought (MOT) that focus on critical thinking and the ability to engage in analysis of concepts. In 1984, Levine decried the shortsightedness of faculty who excluded such courses in preference to those subjects believed to be more useful to the nurse. Devising and sustaining a curriculum is never easy but faculty members must be conscious of the fact that they are educating a person for life, not for a limited goal.

TABLE 14–1. ALLENTOWN COLLEGE OF SAINT FRANCIS DE SALES TYPICAL PROGRAM: NURSING MAJOR (BSN) EFFECTIVE 1990–1991

Fall Semester	Spring Semester
First Year	
General Chemistry	Introduction to Organic and Biologic
Introductory Biology	Chemistry
Communications and Thought I	Microbiology
Foreign Language	Communications and Thought II
Introduction to Psychology . . . OR . . .	Introduction to Sociology
Physical Education	Foreign Language
	Physical Education
Second Year	
Anatomy and Physiology I	Anatomy and Physiology II
The Nursing Process I	The Nursing Process II
Education	Humanities 2
Introductory Theology . . . OR . . .	Philosophy
Humanities 1	
Physical Education	
Third Year	
The Nursing Process and the Family Unit I	The Nursing Process and the Family Unit II
Human Development	Mathematics
Intermediate Theology/Ethical Theory	Free Elective
Humanities 3 . . . OR . . .	Humanities 4
Fourth Year	
The Nursing Process in Critical and Long-Term Care	Complex Problem Solving and Management Roles
Values Seminar	Independent Study
Literature	Free Elective
Free Elective	Senior Seminar

A review of the curriculum plan shows that it has similarities to many of the existing baccalaureate program plans. The emphasis on the biologic sciences provides the basis for understanding Levine's conservation principles focusing on energy and structural integrity. Since conservation is dependent on the body's ability to adapt—to respond to factors that disrupt physiologic balance—the students must be able to understand the complex inter-relationships guiding the body's physiologic functioning. Support for the remaining principles, conservation of personal and social integrities, is found primarily in the psychology and sociology courses as well as in the humanities, philosophy, and theology.

In the early nursing courses, faculty members reinforce what has been taught in courses such as English, psychology, or philosophy. Reinforcing what is learned in English courses—the importance of accuracy in both oral and written communication—is emphasized. In almost all nursing courses, students must write papers, using the Publication Manual of the American Psychological Association (1983). In their assessments of patients and in their developing plans of care, students are asked to apply concepts learned in psychology and sociology. The faculty help students to understand and appreciate how knowledge acquired in the study of other disciplines relates to nursing.

The wisdom of selecting one model to guide the curriculum may be questioned. Certainly this approach influences how the student views his or her patients. In our setting, each step of the nursing process is guided by the conservation principles. This may be perceived as limiting the students' options; however, the choice of one model is not unusual in other disciplines. Psychologists are rarely eclectic: they are, for example, psychoanalytic, Rogerian, behavioral. Philosophers may follow Aristotle or the existentialists. Each discipline has its theorists and each theorist its disciples. This is not to say that we must necessarily be guided by the practices of other disciplines, only that there is an acceptable precedent. Nursing has a history of borrowing other disciplines' models; it is time for nursing education to be consistent in presenting its own models to students for learning (Jacobs-Kramer & Huether, 1988). Our faculty made the decision to use one nursing model realizing that other elements would have an impact on the use of the conceptual framework. As faculty members have joined the program, they have accepted that their teaching had to be adapted to the model being used. This adjustment does not mean that in their own practice they are not free to use the model of their choice.

Organizing the nursing courses around the model and including other elements that the faculty considered important was done by clearly stating curriculum strands. The strands helped to organize the curriculum and included the integrities. In all nursing courses, students are expected to use theoretical and empirical knowledge from previous courses in concert with Levine's conservation principles to maintain the integrities of human beings. The process of nursing intervention is discussed as a collaborative process whereby the dependent state of the patient is for the most part, a temporary one in which both nurse and patient collaborate to preserve, maintain, or restore wholeness.

USING THE MODEL

The student is introduced to the model in the first nursing course in the sophomore year or, in the case of the RN student, in the required transition course. Initial class meetings are directed toward a brief introduction to conceptual models in nursing. A history of the development of nursing theory is discussed as well as some of the reasons for having a theory base in nursing. To be sure that students understand that there is more than one approach to constructing nursing theories and to help them to recognize the names of several of the better-known theorists, a selection of models is discussed. This approach is consistent with the observations of Jacobs-Kramer and Huether (1988), who state that the baccalaureate students should be exposed early to the various nursing models and should have an opportunity to discuss them. The first term defined is *health*, accompanied by the rationale underlying Levine's definition (Levine, 1973). The student is helped to understand that nursing intervention is geared toward assisting the patient to achieve wholeness or health.

The importance of understanding the interrelatedness of all systems is emphasized, as is the fact that there is a definitive pattern that guides the growth and development of the organism. The concepts of homeostasis and homeorrhesis are discussed so that students can appreciate the significance of alterations in the patterns and the effects of changes occurring in both internal and external environments. The disruption of patterns can result in disease unless the body is able to cope through adaptation. Students are taught that adaptation is the organism's way of dealing with change and that nursing intervention may be required in order for the process to be successful.

For the student just beginning studies in nursing, the total curriculum can be overwhelming. Having one model to use as a guide, one that explains phenomena in an understandable and logical way, can do much to dispel anxiety and to help organize the approach to care. With greater maturity and a more comprehensive knowledge base, students will be able to accept other models and make their own choices relative to their own practice. This is not expected to occur until the student has had some experience as a graduate nurse.

Within the nursing courses, students are, however, exposed to different theories from other disciplines. These theories can be used in conjunction with Levine's model. In caring for children, students may use Erikson's (1964) psychoanalytic theory as they assess, plan, and implement care for a child. Levine's conservation principles are broad enough to be used in conjunction with other conceptual frameworks. Erikson has stated that the developmental task of the toddler is to acquire a sense of autonomy. In providing care that supports this level of development, the nurse is conserving the child's personal integrity, helping the child to counteract threats to personal autonomy. The developmental task of the adolescent, according to Erikson, is to attain identity—both a group identity and a personal identity. In accepting this as a bona fide developmental task, the students will plan care with their patients in such a way as to help them conserve both social and personal integrities. There is no conflict in combining the two, and they complement each other.

This process as outlined is different from that described by Levine (1988) in her discussion of how nursing uses concepts from related disciplines in developing nursing theory. We are using concepts from other disciplines to help students plan care based on a broad knowledge base and to confirm that there is common ground shared by those whose discipline focuses on mankind. Full integration of these concepts is predicated on careful research in which the ultimate goal is to identify how they can become unique in nursing practice.

The nursing process is another important curricular strand, and in each step the student is guided by the integrities. Assessment is done by collecting data that relate to each of the integrities. For patients confined to bed, assessment of their skin is important to determine the extent to which structural integrity may have been compromised. In addition, data related to conservation of energy, specifically diet and nutritional needs, must be assessed. As bed rest limits patients' ability to interact with other persons, assessment of the personal and social integrities is also necessary. Taking the history of patients with emphysema will include collecting information that addresses their consumption of energy, the impact of the disease on their personal and social integrities, and a review of diagnostic data so as to understand the status of their structural integrity. Assessing the child with a diagnosis of rheumatoid arthritis will focus on energy requirements as well as on the impact of the disease on structural integrity. In addition, questions will be asked about school attendance and peer interaction in an effort to determine if assistance is required in maintaining social and person integrity.

Levine (1987) has expressed some reservations about the current nursing diagnoses; however, we have found that the nursing diagnoses accepted by the North American Nursing Diagnosis Association (NANDA) can be used in conjunction with the model (Carroll-Johnson, 1989). Students are expected to use nursing diagnoses approved by NANDA as they go through the steps of the nursing process, and to draw implications for planning and intervention using Levine's conservation principles. For example, the diagnosis *potential activity intolerance* or *fatigue* would arise from initial assessment and alert the student to plan for conserving the patient's energy. The diagnosis *impaired verbal communication* will suggest the patient's personal and social integrity may be compromised. The patient's structural integrity will be a concern if the diagnosis is *potential for infection* or *impaired tissue integrity*. Each nursing diagnosis can be related to one or more of the integrities, and its use in conjunction with Levine's model serves to reinforce student understanding of how the patient's wholeness is being affected by environmental factors.

Planning and implementing care must also occur in conjunction with each of the integrities. One intent of care is to conserve by acting therapeutically. According to Levine (1973), being therapeutic is having a forward-moving positive influence on the patient's adaptation to environmental interactions. There are times, however, when nurses cannot influence the course of adaptation and their role then becomes supportive (Levine,

1973). Students are assisted in differentiating between these two approaches and in planning appropriate interventions. Evaluation of the nursing process is done by determining the extent to which the integrities and energy have been conserved. The interaction of the two—nursing process and the conservation principles—provides a reasonable, logical framework within which the student can practice nursing. This approach allows for the limited knowledge base of the young student and is easily expanded to accommodate the increased understandings and skills of the older student and the experienced practitioner.

INTEGRATING THE MODEL

The undergraduate curriculum is basically an integrated curriculum. In today's health care environment, integrated curricula provide the only reasonable approach to meeting the demands of providing care to very complicated patient populations. Maintaining the integrated curriculum is a constant challenge, however, as faculty members change and the external health care system becomes increasingly complex. Organizing the curriculum within the parameters of a strong theoretical framework is essential to maintaining its integrity.

In the undergraduate program at Allentown College, Levine's conservation principles provide the basic organizing theme. The holistic nature of the person is the focus of the first nursing courses taught in the second year. The basic concepts of health are explored relative to human interaction with the environment, both internal and external. Students learn about therapeutic communication, about patient teaching, and about the role that the nurse plays relative to the conservation principles. Some class content addresses the process of hospitalization, how to identify associated stressors, and how to work with the patient to conserve his or her energy and the integrities. Another class addresses the adaptation required by older patients as they adjust to those alterations in life-style that accompany reduced income and physiologic change. In the clinical settings that at this level are adult oriented, students assess needs and plan for care using the integrities as an integral part of the process.

In the third year, the focus is on the family as a unit as well as on the individuals within that unit. That year provides the greatest challenge to the integrated curriculum approach, since it involves learning concepts related to maternal-child nursing, adult health and illness, and psychiatric-mental health. Students assist the family as it deals with threats to the integrity of the unit or to the individuals composing that unit. Emphasis is on collaborating with family members to promote, maintain, or restore health. Specific content is taught using concepts, and these in turn are related to the conservation principles. An example of this teaching method would be a class on conserving the integrity of the patient's gastrointestinal system by examining problems related to nutrition. This topic lends itself to discussion of normal nutrition in the family unit as well as to examination of selected conditions that constitute problems such as failure to thrive, bulimia, inflammatory bowel disease, or pica during pregnancy. As each of the specialty areas of clinical practice is addressed, students can see how the stessors can affect the total family unit as well as the individual within the unit.

In the class where faculty and students discuss problems associated with mobility, the focus might be on the patient in advanced stages of pregnancy or the patient with Parkinson's disease. The child with cerebral palsy is used as an example of one whose mobility has been impaired, as is the person whose mental health has been disturbed to the point where he or she cannot interact with others. In each instance, students use the nursing process as they plan care to conserve each of the integrities and promote energy conservation. In this third year, the involvement of the family is stressed. Family members contribute to the assessment data base and participate in the planning and implementation process. The welfare of the individual as well as that of the total family unit is taken into consideration. Teaching emphasizes that holistic care encompasses not only the patients of the moment but also those who are significant to them.

In their senior year, students bring together previously acquired knowledge and skills adapting them to the needs of patients in the range of new settings—that is, critical care, community health, and rehabilitation. In the latter two instances, students continue to plan care using the conservation principles while at the same time incorporating these principles of community health and rehabilitation nursing. Incorporating these principles is not so incongruous as it may initially appear to those whose perception of Levine's model is that its use is restricted to hospital settings. The community health nurse has special concerns related to environmental factors that influence the health of the community. Levine (1989) expresses similar concerns that patients are affected by external factors in their environment even though they may be unaware of them as causing changes to which they must adapt. Levine cites radiation and microorganisms as examples of factors that can influence the internal environment and require individuals to add another element to what Levine refers to as the "multidimensional" (Levine, 1989, p. 326) adaptation process. While the body responds to maintain or restore structural integrity, community health nurses not only assist the patient in this adaptation but also institute actions that will modify or alleviate the causes. Their knowledge of epidemiology and their role as nurses to the community make it possible for them to take steps to reduce or eliminate the environmental dangers.

In the rehabilitation setting, the conservation of personal and social integrity are of special import. Students examine the effect that disabling trauma or long-term illness has on the patient's sense of self and the acceptance of that self by society. Levine (1989) notes that individuals who find themselves dependent on others for care find their personal integrity compromised. Not only must they cope with assaults on their personal "selves," but they must adapt themselves to the way those in their social milieu perceive them and to how they accept their condition. Although patients with more temporary conditions also have to adjust to changes that influence both their personal and social integrities, these changes are often only temporary and transitory. Persons in the rehabilitation situation are often dealing with a condition that significantly alters their life and their place in society. Students explore the caregiver role in supporting independence as much as possible, so that patients do not expend energy unnecessarily in fighting for their independence. Students are helped to recognize their responsibility to see that patients are able to exercise control over their personhood. The caregiver also has a responsibility to help in the adaptation required for return to his or her community group.

One of the specific clinical experiences in this year is providing care in the patient's home, where conservation principles are as applicable as they are in the hospital. Students use the hospital discharge plan, the patient's family, and community services as they plan care emphasizing conservation. As with the inpatient, students follow the steps of the nursing process using each of the integrities at each step and incorporating the hospital discharge plan or questioning its applicability relative to the actual situation in which the patient is found.

Another experience, which is essentially observational, occurs in the rehabilitation hospital, where one of the student's objectives is to assess a patient using the conservation principles. The student follows through on that assessment, focusing particularly on the transition from the rehabilitation setting to home and community. In addition, by examining those factors that made the rehabilitation process necessary, the student gains a better understanding of how the predicament could have been prevented or modified. Factors considered might be those relating to the individual or to those in which the community might have a role. This process is documented in a paper.

In senior seminar, students are again presented with nursing models. They view videotapes currently available in which the theorists discuss their frameworks and relate them to present and future practice. Having had experience with one model, students are in a better position to appreciate the value of having an organized method to use in their practice. In discussing other models, they can compare the different approaches and at the same time recognize that each model addresses the same phenomena while using somewhat different approaches and emphasizing different concepts.

SUMMARY

The undergraduate curriculum at Allentown College has persisted in its dependence on Levine's Conservation Model. How it has been used has changed over the years as the faculty changes and as new people put their own imprint on the model's application to situations. Questions are raised, content reviewed, and courses modified to meet the changes that occur in the surrounding environment. Adherence to the philosophy of Christian humanism continues, and its compatibility with Levine's model is confirmed after a long partnership.

The adaptability of the model is one of its greatest strengths. The conservation principles have easily stood the test of time and the impact of technology. Individuals continue to be unique; they cope with ever-increasing assaults on their energies. The constant barrage on their integrities by the world around them reinforces the fact that the nurse must be ever alert to the potential and actual impact of these assaults. Holistic care touches the individual, the family, and the community. Levine's principles are applicable not only to individuals but also to a larger group, the others who are significant to them.

REFERENCES

Bulletin of Information. (1989). Center Valley, PA: Allentown College of Saint Francis de Sales,

Carroll-Johnson, R.M. (Ed.). (1989). Classification of nursing diagnoses: Proceedings of the eighth conference. Philadelphia: J.B. Lippincott.

DeBack, V., & Mentkorowski, M. (1986). Does the baccalaureate make a difference? Differentiating nurse performance by education and experience. Journal of Nursing Education, 25(7), 275–285.

Drew, B.J. (1988). Devaluation of biological knowledge. Image, 20(1), 25–27.

Erikson, E.H. (1964). Insight and responsibility. New York: W.W. Norton & Co.

Jacobs-Kramer, M.K., & Huether, S.E. (1988). Curricular considerations for teaching nursing theory. Journal of Professional Nursing, 4(5), 373–380.

Levine, M.E. (1971). Holistic nursing. Nursing clinics of North America, 6(2), 253–264.

Levine, M.E. (1973). Introduction to clinical nursing (2nd ed.). Philadelphia: F.A. Davis.

Levine, M.E. (1984). A conceptual model for nursing: The four conservation principles. Quality Factors in Quality Health Care: Papers from the Dorothy Rider Pool Annual Workshop Series, 1, 29–40.

Levine, M.E. (1987). Approaches to the development of a nursing diagnosis taxonomy. In A.M. McLane (Ed.), Classification of nursing diagnosis: Proceedings of the seventh conference (pp. 45–51). St. Louis: C.V. Mosby.

Levine, M.E. (1988). Antecedents from adjunctive disciplines: Creation of nursing theory. Nursing Science Quarterly, 1(1), 16–21.

Levine, M.E. (1989). The conservation principles of nursing: Twenty years later. In J. Riehl-Sisca (Ed.), Conceptual models for nursing practice (pp. 325–338) (3rd ed.). Norwalk, CT: Appleton & Lange.

Publication manual of the American Psychological Association (3rd ed.). (1983). Washington, DC: American Psychological Association.

Chapter
FIFTEEN

Developing a Graduate Program in Nursing
Integrating Levine's Philosophy

Karen Moore Schaefer, R.N., D.N.Sc.

The graduate nursing program at Allentown College of Saint Francis de Sales is built on the undergraduate program, which, as discussed by Grindley and Paradowski in Chapter 14, is based on Levine's Conservation Model. The nursing component of the graduate program is designed, using Levine's conservation principles, to maintain the integrities of human beings. The nurse works toward the restoration and promotion of health and the prevention of disease. "The individual's integrity, his one-ness, his identity as an individual, his wholeness—is his abiding concern, and it is the nurse's responsibility to assist him to defend and to seek its realization" (Levine, 1971a, p. 258).

The graduate faculty recognized early in the developmental phase of the program that asking graduate students to accept one model as the basis of their practice would not be consistent with the beliefs that nursing was not ready for a single model. It was agreed that a single model may not be appropriate for all the research efforts of our students. However, we did agree that Levine's model would be an excellent framework for the development of the content of the graduate nursing courses. Therefore, each course is developed based on the National League for Nursing's criteria for graduate education, with at least one objective of each course incorporating Levine's Conservation Model (Table 15–1).

THE GRADUATE CURRICULUM

The graduate students of Allentown College are required to take 45 credits of course work representing nursing, the basic sciences, and elec-

TABLE 15-1. OBJECTIVES OF GRADUATE NURSING COURSES

Course	Objective*
Biology 501/502	Acquire the ability to translate knowledge and understanding of human physiologic phenomena to nursing care of patients at a level commensurate with advanced knowledge and in accord with Levine's integration concepts.†
N502 Advanced Nursing	Interpret conceptual issues according to Levine's philosophy.
N503 Nursing Theory and Models	Compare the major concepts identified by nursing theorists to those identified by Levine.
N506 Medical-Surgical Nursing	Implement a plan of care using knowledge of physiology, medical-surgical nursing, and Levine's Conservation Model.
N507 Medical-Surgical Nursing	Evaluate Levine's Conservation Model as a framework for practice.
N611 Clinical Specialist I	Develop a framework for the CNS‡ using Levine's model.
N612 Clinical Specialist II	Develop coping patterns for CNS role maintenance using Levine's model.
N614 CNS Practicum	Use Levine's model as a unifying framework for implementing the CNS role.

*The research courses do not have an objective related to Levine. The guidelines for the student's research project state that the student is encouraged to use Levine's Conservation Model as a framework for his or her study. If Levine's model is not appropriate for the research, the student may select and/or develop an appropriate framework.
†Written in the course overview.
‡CNS = Clinical nurse specialist.

tives (Table 15–2). The students have the option of selecting clinical experiences with the adult in the medical-surgical area, in critical care, or in the community. Additionally, they select a functional area from administration, education, or clinical specialization. The students take two research theory courses and select a faculty member to work with them as they complete the required research. We believe that the basic science knowledge and the research skills are essential to advanced practice and the student's ability to achieve the skills needed to develop nursing knowledge and improve nursing practice.

Consistent with the philosophy of Levine, a strong background in physiology and research is required. Levine's conservation principles direct the nurse to think about the physiology of the patient's responses (conservation of energy and structural integrity) and use the scientific process to draw conclusions and make judgments about the patient's organismic responses. Levine (1975, p. 38) has also said that "science pursues new ideas and celebrates new insight. Science can be creative." With this in mind the students are encouraged to respond to their intuitive thoughts and to take the risks needed to be creative. These skills are fostered using the following techniques: (a) free association, (b) in-class summarizing of

TABLE 15-2. MSN CURRICULUM AT ALLENTOWN COLLEGE
OF SAINT FRANCIS DE SALES

Year	Fall	Spring
One	Biology 501	Biology 502
	N 503 Theories and Models	N 603 Christian Social Principles
	N 506 Clinical I	N 507 M/S* Nursing II
	N 502 Advanced Nursing	N 501 Proseminar
Two	N 504 Research Seminar	N 605 Research Guidance
	Functional I	Functional II
	Elective	Practicum
		Elective

*M/S = Medical-Surgical Nursing, Care of the Adult in the Community, or
Care of the Adult Critical Care.

reactions to class discussions or required readings, (c) videotaping of oral presentations, (d) describing responses to abstract art for the purpose of demonstrating alternating rhythms (Mayeroff, 1971) and each nurse's own unique contribution to each health care predicament, and (e) validating the use of propositions and hypotheses derived from models in their practical experiences. Although the steps of the research process are discussed in a linear fashion, the uses of creativity and intuition in the identification of a conceptual framework are introduced early in the program. Students are encouraged to think at "random" while providing structure to the research process.

"It is a well known principle of learning that new knowledge is established only slowly in direct proportion to its perceived relevance to the person's life" (Levine, 1982, p. 29). Students in the graduate program are encouraged to identify an area of clinical specialization that is consistent with their goals of practice as an advanced practitioner and to acquire expertise in this area by developing course requirements and clinical objectives with a focus on the selected area. The following is a discussion of how the content of a core course is developed using the works of Levine. The reader is apprised that this is one instructor's approach to meeting the objectives of the course and does not necessarily represent how other instructors may choose to meet the required outcomes.

ADVANCED NURSING

Integration of Levine's Philosophy

Advanced Nursing is a course designed to introduce the graduate student to major concepts of concern to nursing that will be developed in greater depth as they move through their clinical and functional courses. An attempt is made to socialize the student to the roles of graduate student and advanced practitioner by encouraging a discussion of the two roles and using primarily the seminar approach to learning. Requirements of the course include the development of behavioral objectives, a concept analysis paper, and a debate paper of a randomly assigned topic from the affirmative or negative position. Students are expected to supplement the required reading with readings about the concepts within their specific area of clinical specialty. In-class summary writing is used as a mechanism to develop students' writing skills using a journalistic approach, to reinforce their learning relative to their practice, and to provide the instructor with immediate feedback regarding the effectiveness of teaching approaches and student learning (Meyers, 1986).

LEADERSHIP

The first concept discussed is leadership. This provides a mechanism through which the roles of graduate student and advanced practitioner can be discussed. Discussion of the concept is approached using the steps of concept analysis (Walker & Avant, 1983). In this way the students become familiar with the approach to use in the development of their papers.

> The nurse's craft speaks in a language of its own—the silent language of human exchange which is eloquent and exciting without words. It is something like this which has made the 'role model' seem so essential in nursing intervention can be transmitted by the activity of an excellent nurse. (Levine, 1975, p. 40)

Emphasis is placed on the role of leadership through excellence in practice, the quintessence of graduate education.

Collaboration in practice and research is discussed with attention to the advantages and disadvantages. "Rather than build fences that separate us from our medical colleagues, let us instead join forces to explore the clinical issues we must confront together" (Levine, 1987, p. 51). Collaboration is examined conceptually to include nurses, administration, and other health care workers (physicians, nutritionists, pharmacists). This concept is extremely important at a time when budgets are being cut and there is an increased demand for the nurse's time.

NURSING PROCESS AND DIAGNOSIS

Levine (1973) supports the use of the scientific process to collect and analyze data about patients to make a judgment about their care needs. Because of the generic nature of the word *diagnosis*, she suggests the use of the word *trophicognosis* as a term similar to *diagnosis* and *prognosis*. Trophicognosis is defined as "a nursing care judgment arrived at by the scientific methods" (Levine, 1966, p. 57). Levine (1987) believes the person is an "individual with strengths and individuality, certain of selfhood, unique, proud, and more than just a target that will respond" (p. 250). Her conservation principles are used by the nurse to determine the interventions for the patient with the goal of restoring and maintaining wholeness. Interventions are either therapeutic (promoting an improved status) or supportive (maintaining the status quo). Evaluation of the interventions are determined by the nurse observing for an organismic response (Levine, 1973).

The students study Levine's approach to the nursing process and nursing diagnosis. In class they are urged to critique her approach; whether or not they agree with her philosophy, they are to support their arguments with verified knowledge. They are challenged to respond to the notion that the nursing process may not be consistent with the concept of wholeness (Barnum, 1987). Contrasting these approaches to the contemporary literature on nursing diagnostic taxonomies creates a lively discussion often ending with more questions than answers. Levine (1980) has noted that "the nursing process demands the continuous collecting and evaluating of information, but that provides only the 'bits' of an interaction, the little pieces that can be brought together into a sense of wholeness and reality only in the fluid and creative reaches of human caring" (p. 197).

CARING

Caring may be defined as "feeling interest and concern" for another. "There is a limit to the degree to which nursing care can be converted into technological maneuvers; and that limit is irrevocably and without apology established by the intense and persistent needs of human beings in search of their humanity" (Levine, 1971b, p. 39). Caring is the essence through which nursing promotes and maintains that which is human.

A number of theorists have explored the phenomenon of caring (Carper, 1979; Leininger, 1988; Paterson & Zderad, 1976; Watson, 1988), each from a slightly different perspective. Common to all described experiences of caring is the need for a relationship that is reciprocal (Estabrooks, 1989). Caring involves interaction, and nursing is interaction (Levine, 1973). Nursing, therefore, is caring.

Students explore the definitions, antecedents, and consequences of caring, and are encouraged to explain the relationship of caring to maintaining the wholeness of the individual (Levine, 1973). Because a number of subconcepts are identified as part of caring, students begin to explore what it is that makes the caring in nursing different from the caring that is part of other human service professions. For example, using the conservation principles, the students are able to identify that the caring by social workers focuses on social integrity, whereas the caring by nurses includes all the integrities. Because nursing practice should be based on verified knowledge, research related to caring is discussed relative to its contribution to what is already known about caring (Levine, 1988a).

PERSONAL WORTH/SELF-ESTEEM

On personal worth, Levine notes:

> The defense of self is not reaching beyond, but rather a reaching into the person. Everyone seeks to defend his or her identity as a self, in both that hidden, intensely private person that dwells within and in the public faces assumed as individuals move through their relationships with others. (Levine, 1989, p. 334)

> Conservation of Personal Integrity is the "keeping together" of the self,

created of self identity, self respect, self awareness and the selfhood that is private and known only to ourselves. (Levine, 1984, p. I-38)

The knowledge of being a whole person is intensely private, and the patterns of behavior which individuals assume throughout their lives cannot be left behind when they become ill. (Levine, 1971a, p. 260)

We measure ourselves and our experiences against a social environment that helps establish the boundaries of our lives and helps establish ourselves as unique persons. (Levine, 1989, p. 336)

Considering Levine's comments on the self as being unique, whole, and intensely private, the students examine self-esteem and self-worth from the perspective of the patient, nurse, and the patient-nurse interaction. The effect that life's normal transitions and illnesses may have on the perception of self are considered in depth. From the perspective of the graduate student, the expected outcome is that the nurse will facilitate the maintenance of the individual's selfhood through illness and life's normal transitions. The depth and breadth of understanding the energy, structural, personal, and social factors that influence selfhood makes the graduate students' approach to patient care unique. Their understanding of self according to Levine provides a basis for a discussion of ethical practice. "But he (the patient) must be accepted for what he is without moralistic judgments which, in bringing censure, fail to value his sense of self worth" (Levine, 1971a, p. 260).

ETHICS

"Ethical behavior is not the display of one's moral rectitude in times of crisis. It is the day to day expression of one's commitment to other persons and the ways in which human beings relate to one another in their daily interactions" (Levine, 1977, p. 846). A discussion of ethical practice includes the nurses' behavior in relationships with others (patients and their families, nurse colleagues, other health care providers) as well as the public issues related to how the advanced practitioner can influence allocation of resources, use of technologic equipment to support life, and the options available to substance abusers. "For all the certainty people may have of that appropriate role in their independent life, the introduction of the dependency of entering the health care system creates issues and conflicts that must bring consonance between the reality that confronts them and the expectations others may have of them" (Levine, 1989, p. 336).

Some of the specific issues laden with ethical choices are integrated into the course through assigned debate papers. Two particularly difficult decisions randomly selected by the students are as follows:

1. Resolved that individuals with acquired immune deficiency disease have the right to withhold information about their diagnosis (one student discusses the affirmative and one the negative).
2. Resolved that the professional nurse has the responsibility to report colleagues engaged in substance abuse (one student discusses the affirmative and one the negative).

At the end of the semester, each student has 5 minutes to discuss his or her argument and is given the opportunity to answer questions from peers. This exercise is not graded, thus giving the student a chance to be freely expressive without the fear of failure.

Levine (1973) asserts that the individual has the right to be a participant in his or her care. Patients should be involved in the decisions about their care, and care should never be administered without the full knowledge of the patient. Ways to ensure full disclosure for the patient are studied within the framework of informed consent in research and informed consent in care. Levine's belief was reaffirmed when she stated, "She brings her faith healings to patients who have not requested it, and without 'informed consent' on the part of the child recipients or parents. Imposing this type of treatment without the full understanding of the patient is a violation of nursing's ethical code and the human rights of the child and parents" (Levine, 1979, p. 1380).

SPIRITUALITY

"We measure experience against a social environment that helps us establish the boundaries of our lives. . . . We need the homely comfort of welcome in a community, a religious group, a social circle of friends, a political system, and a nation" (Levine, 1984, p. I-38). Spirituality is discussed as a part of being whole. Spiritual existence influences the cultural patterns that are part of the conceptual environment (Levine, 1973). Spirituality therefore influences the individual's behavioral patterns. Levine (1988b) has described what could be her own experience with spirituality as faith, selflessness, sharing, a source of insight and feeling, and participation.

Students go beyond the notion of religion to learn about spirituality. Definitions and measures of spirituality are examined. Students often conclude that Levine accepts spirituality as part of and much the same as wholeness. They contrast and compare the concept of wholeness with spirituality and discuss nursing interventions to support the spirituality of themselves and the patients.

HEALTH

Some of the earlier criticisms of Levine's Conservation Model indicated that the model was useful only in the acute care setting with the focus on the ill patient, and therefore did not have universality (Fitzpatrick & Whall, 1983). On health, Levine (1987, p. 49) has stated, "It is not necessary to deny the role of the nurse in health maintenance and disease prevention to acknowledge that the nurse is vital—an absolute necessity—in the care of the sick, the injured, the disabled. A diagnostic classification that does not recognize that fact fails the large population of nurses who work with the sick and the people who desperately need their skill and expertise."

Students explore the viability of some of the health models (Pender,

1987) and consider the wisdom of Levine. Questions such as the following are addressed:

1. Is illness simply a part of health?
2. Are health and illness polar opposites necessitating that each be handled separately?
3. Are health promotion and health prevention part of illness care?

Students are reminded that the perception of self is affected by illness and that health therefore remains a relative value. Where would we place the patients with diabetes who return for periodic nursing assessments to determine how they are adapting to their predicament, only to find that they acknowledge their disorder but certainly do not see themselves as ill? The students' minds are stretched to consider a full range of responses.

STRESS/COPING

Levine does not believe that stress is the basis of all disorders (see Chap. 1). To assume such a relationship is to proclaim ignorance. Sufficient evidence exists that suggests that stress can affect how individuals respond, both positively and negatively. Thus, patient responses become the major focus of the discussion on stress. "Coping refers to the way in which the individual responds to a given social instant . . . the 'coping' processes lack precision and distinction, largely because they arise from pasts that are hidden not only to the observer but to the observed as well" (Levine, 1989, p. 335). "Coping patterns (they are not mechanisms in the wholistic sense) are judged by the social acceptance of the behavior that is manifested" (Levine, 1989, p. 335).

The students examine nursing interventions that promote adaptation (relaxation, exercise, nutrition, recreation, humor, music, imagery, and other forms of distraction) and maintain wholeness. Adaptation is the process of change, and conservation is the product of adaptation (Levine, 1989). The outcomes of care interventions will always be specific to the predicament, focusing the student again on the notion of individualizing care. "Although it is unlikely that an outcome can be specifically anticipated, knowledge of the major characteristics of the process may make the influence of adaptation potentially meaningful as a source of understanding human behavior in the context of a defined habitat" (Levine, 1989, pp. 326–327).

SUMMARY

Levine's philosophy has been used to guide the content of one of the care courses in the graduate program at Allentown College of Saint Francis de Sales. Levine's statements are used as a basis of comparison to other nurses as scholars who have addressed a specific concept. Students learn about Levine's conservation principles through an understanding of her philosophy; at the same time they learn how other nurses view a specific concept and, in some cases, how they have developed their own nursing models. This approach to developing course content has proved effective in helping the students learn Levine's philosophy of nursing and her approach to nursing care through conservation.

REFERENCES

Barnum, B.J. (1987). Holistic nursing and the nursing process. Holistic Nursing Practice, 1(3), 27–35.

Carper, B.A. (1979). The ethics of caring. Advances in Nursing Science, 1(3), 11–19.

Estabrooks, C.A. (1989). Touch: A nursing strategy in the intensive care unit. Heart & Lung, 18(4), 392–401.

Fitzpatrick, J.J., & Whall, A.L. (1983). Conceptual models of nursing: Analysis and application. Bowie, MD: Robert Brady Co.

Leininger, M.M. (1988). Leininger's theory of nursing: Cultural care diversity and universality. Nursing Science Quarterly, 1(4), 152–160.

Levine, M.E. (1966). Trophicognosis: An alternative to nursing diagnosis. In American Nurses' Association Regional Clinical Conference (Vol. 2, pp. 55–70). New York: American Nurses' Association.

Levine, M.E. (1971a). Holistic nursing. Nursing Clinics of North America, 6(2), 253–264.

Levine, M.E. (1971b) The time has come to speak of health care. American Operating Room Nursing Journal, 13, 37–43.

Levine, M.E. (1973). Introduction to clinical nursing (2nd ed.). Philadelphia: F.A. Davis.

Levine, M.E. (1975). On creativity in nursing. Image, 3(3), 15–19.

Levine, M.E. (1977). Nursing ethics and the ethical nurse. American Journal of Nursing, 77(5), 845–849.

Levine, M.E. (1980). The ethics of computer technology in health care. Nursing Forum, 19(2), 193–198.

Levine, M.E. (1982). Bioethics of cancer nursing. Rehabilitation Nursing, 9(2), 27–47.

Levine, M.E. (1984). A conceptual model for nursing: The four conservation principles. Quality Factors in Quality Health Care: Papers From the Dorothy Rider Pool Annual Workshop Series, 1, 29–40.

Levine, M.E. (1987). Approaches to the development of a nursing diagnosis taxonomy. In A.M. McLane (Ed.), Classification of nursing diagnosis: Proceedings of the seventh conference: (North American Nursing Diagnosis Association (pp. 45–51). St. Louis: C.V. Mosby.

Levine, M.E. (1988a). Antecedents from adjunctive disciplines: Creation of nursing theory. Nursing Science Quarterly, 1(1), 16–21.

Levine, M.E. (1988b). Myra Levine. In T.M. Schorr, & A. Zimmerman (Eds.), Making choices; Taking chances. St. Louis: C.V. Mosby.

Levine, M.E. (1989). The conservation principles of nursing: Twenty years later. In J. Riehl-Sisca (Ed.), Conceptual models for nursing practice (325–337). Norwalk, CT: Appleton & Lange.

Mayeroff, M. (1971). On caring. London: Harper & Row.

Meyers, C. (1986). Teaching students to think critically. London: Jossey-Bass.

Paterson, J.G., & Zderad, L.T. (1976). Humanistic nursing. New York: John Wiley and Sons.

Pender, N. (1987). Health promotion in nursing practice. Norwalk, CT: Appleton-Century-Crofts.

Walker, L.O. & Avant, K.C. (1983). Strategies for theory construction on nursing. Norwalk, CT: Appleton-Century-Crofts.

Watson, J. (1988). New dimensions of human caring theory. Nursing Science Quarterly, 1(4), 175–181.

Chapter
S I X T E E N

Creating a Legacy

Karen Moore Schaefer, R.N., D.N.Sc.

When I think about the use of models to guide nursing practice, I am reminded of a research assistant who was continually amazed about the amount of information she was able to obtain when using an assessment tool developed from a nursing model. She was forever convinced of the value of using nursing models to collect useful data for providing nursing care to her patients.

Levine (1973) unknowingly developed a model to organize nursing knowledge that has found its way back into the nursing arena and is regaining credibility as a model for nursing care. Because change is a predictable concept, the elements of the model will continually require modification, clarification, and expansion to remain a contemporary framework. The basic concepts (adaptation, wholeness) and commonplaces (person, health, nursing, environment), for the most part, will remain as identified, although their descriptions may change. To expand on the idea of Levine, there are several areas that need to be addressed.

AREAS IN QUESTION

ENVIRONMENT

Chopoorian (1986) identified the need to reconceptualize the environment. She argues that nursing's focus on the individual or group cannot be faulted, but the social, political, and cultural worlds that surround the patient and have a tremendous impact on the human condition are insufficiently considered by the majority of practicing nurses. Because most nurses practice within an organization, the nurse's care is further restricted by the rules and regulations of that particular organization. With an increasing emphasis on cost-effectiveness, nurses are in danger of becoming even more focused on individual and/or group care.

219

In describing the conservation of social integrity, Levine (1973, pp. 17–18) stated:

> Every individual shares a number of social communities—his family, his friends, his employment, his church, his ethnic group, his city, town, or village, his state, his nation, and, in a time of instant communication, even his world. The ways in which the individual relates to each of these groups influences his behavior. . . . In a broader sense, the social integrity of individuals is tied to the viability of the entire social system. Only a society which provides individuals with adequate food, gainful employment, educational opportunities, and excellent medical care is one in which health, in the sense of wholeness, can be obtained.

According to Levine (1973), each individual is viewed as having his or her own environment, both internal and external. The internal environment is the physiologic and pathophysiologic aspects of the patient. The external environment, those factors that impinge upon and change the patient, are defined according to the three levels described by Bates (cited in Levine, 1973): (1) perceptual—aspects of the world that individuals are able to intercept or interpret through the senses; (2) operational—things that physically affect individuals although they cannot directly perceive them, such as microorganisms; and (3) conceptual—cultural patterns characterized by spiritual existence and mediated by symbols of language and thought, history, and value systems.

The external environment and social integrity are not the same. However, the conservation of social integrity provides a basis for the nurse to consider environmental factors that affect the patient and may indeed be far removed from the immediate environment. It is within this framework that nurses could consider more of the social, cultural, environmental, and political factors that might affect the human condition and over which they could have some control. For example, nurses can support the passing of legislation in Congress that will have a direct effect on the availability of health care for the aged, the homeless, and those with AIDS.

Nurses do and should continue to consider the effects of environmental disasters on individuals' needs and the availability of health care to meet those needs. When a major industry lays off a large number of employees, it is reasonable for the nurses to consider threats to the employees' integrity and the possible organismic responses. For example, anxiety may produce chest pain, which in the worst-case scenario may mean that the employee has suffered a myocardial infarction. Even without structural disintegrity, the employee may experience a disruption in personal integrity (altered self-esteem secondary to inability to provide for the family), an alteration in social integrity (inability to engage in social activities because of insufficient funds and/or poor self-image), and reduced energy because of the mental anguish associated with losing a job and the energy required to find a new job or retrain for a different job. By using the conservation principles to identify potential responses to industrial disruption or environmental disasters, nurses will be able to provide care for a larger population whose integrity is threatened.

These examples suggest that Levine's Conservation Model has the components needed to expand the description of the external environment. Qualitative studies will help to clarify the environmental issues nurses can influence to help maintain wholeness.

The term *internal environment* is troublesome if only because *environment* means something that surrounds. Conceptually this seems odd in that the internal environment does not surround but lies at the center of the individual. However, the reader is reminded that Levine (1973) described the internal environment as the *internal milieu*, which means that the environment is *at the center of*. It is true that the internal environment consists of physiologic and pathophysiologic forces. Theorists and researchers should continue to explore and define the exact relationship between the internal and external environments with particular emphasis on the responses over which nursing will have some control.

NURSING ASSESSMENT DATA BASE

Taylor (1987) is the only nurse who has published a formalized attempt to identify a data base using Levine's model. As it exists it is somewhat incomplete and limited. Her data base is significant only to the patient with neurologic disorders, it fails to operationalize all the elements of trophicognosis identified by Levine (1966) as necessary for the identification and implementation of a plan of care, and it has not been tested for reliability and validity. Despite its shortcomings, it is a beginning attempt to operationalize Levine's Conservation Model through assessment and could provide a basis for the development of more focused yet comprehensive tools.

As discussed by Schaefer in Chapter 9, an assessment tool is perhaps the most important measure of wholeness. Using the elements of trophicognosis, nurse practitioners and researchers are encouraged to develop assessment measures based on Levine's Conservation Model and to test for a reliable and valid data base common to all patients presenting with a need for nursing care.

NURSING DIAGNOSES

Because of the generic nature of the word *diagnosis*, Levine (1966, 1987) has presented arguments for not using the term *nursing diagnosis*. She does not, however, object to the idea of nursing diagnoses; in fact, she believes that there is a way to use the conservation principles as an organizing framework for the identification of patient problems–nursing diagnoses if it is done right (Levine, personal communication, September 21, 1989). She supports the development of nursing diagnoses from the clustering of provocative facts that recur in practice and become the focus of nursing intervention (the process of inductive reasoning).

Taylor (1987) does suggest that the provocative facts are analyzed and extrapolated and that sets of defining characteristics are clustered and identified as appropriate nursing diagnoses. Stafford (personal communication, May 8, 1989) uses the organismic responses as a basis for identifying the defining characteristics of the nursing diagnoses, and argues that her experience with the care of patients with cardiac disease suggests that this approach works.

Consistent with Levine's (1987) belief, it is important for nurses to identify how the defining characteristics cluster repeatedly in practice in order to validate their significance to the practice of nursing and maintaining the wholeness of the patient. Both Taylor (1988) and Stafford (1989) provide reasonable approaches to the identification of nursing diagnoses using Levine's Conservation Model. Continued testing of the reliability and validity of these diagnoses will provide additional scientific support for the practice of nursing. Identification of nursing diagnoses will facilitate the keeping together of the patient with the assistance of the nurse when the patient is no longer able to adapt on his or her own.

NURSING INTERVENTIONS

The conservation principles have been identified for the nurse to organize care delivery for the individual who responds in an integrated yet singular fashion. Research described by Foreman in Chapter 10 supports that the nurse must use all the conservation principles in order for nursing interventions to be successful. Success of the interventions is measured by observing the patient's organismic response.

Using knowledge from research and experience, nurse scientists can test the effect of interventions using the conservation principles. Results of these studies will provide practicing nurses with alternative approaches to care and a scientific basis of their practice. The major goal is to identify the interventions that will maintain wholeness and support adaptation, given the unique predicament of the individual, the family, or both.

EVALUATION—QUALITY ASSURANCE

Taylor (1974) has used the conservation principles to measure outcomes of patient care. Her approach could be applied to any group of patients with common problems. Using outcomes has the advantage of serving as a measure of both cost and quality, providing patients with information about the expected outcomes of their nursing care.

In addition to using the conservation principles for outcomes of care, it is proposed that the principles can be used to develop an administrative quality-assurance model. For example, the conservation of *energy* focuses the administrator on productivity issues, which have a direct effect on cost. *Structural* issues address the equipment (technology) and supplies, as well as human resources, needed for the organization to function in a cost-effective manner. *Personal* issues focus the administrator on the need to run an organization that considers the individual needs of the employee, measures to ensure job satisfaction, and the need for a management style (decentralized versus centralized; shared governance) that supports the human element of an organization. *Social* issues help focus the administrator on how well the organization is meeting the needs of the community or the social system, while at the same time considering the effect of the community and the social system on the organization.

Ultimately the organization functions as an open system with the primary goal of maintaining the integrity of the system and the integrity of the individuals who function within the system (the employees and the patients). If the system is threatened, the administrator identifies alternative strategies to promote adaptation of the organization for social good. With careful planning the conservation model can provide the basis (philosophy and objectives) for effective administrative use of the conservation principles for developing a quality-assurance management model. Nursing leaders are challenged to expand and test the conservation model in the administration of health care.

THEORY DEVELOPMENT

Some thoughts on the development of the theory of redundancy and the theory of therapeutic intention are presented by Fawcett in Chapter 2. Levine (personal communication, September 21, 1989) would like to continue to work on the development of these theories but is unsure of the direction she will take.

The notion of therapeutic intention is very exciting. Not only will the nurse have a repertoire of tested interventions, given that a theory provides specific information about care delivery, but also the nurse should have information about the expected organismic responses. With this in mind the theory provides direction for quality-assurance activities and measures of cost-effectiveness. For example, if nurses show that specific therapeutic interventions create a therapeutic change (organismic response) in function, cost-effective care will have been provided. However, as the theory is developed, the way it differs from the conservation principles will need to be explained.

The theory of redundancy, because of its ability to explain why individuals have two of a number of organs and/or a series of adaptive responses, may provide information on alternative but effective measures of care. Levine (Chap. 1, p. 6) believes this theory helps to explain aging, but it may also explain the compensatory responses found in patients with congestive heart failure (Schaefer, Chap. 9, pp. 120–121). This theory is less clear than therapeutic intention because the thinking has not been related successfully to nursing practice. Continued work is needed before it can be considered for use.

CONCLUSION

As a model, the conservation principles are useful as a framework for a variety of patient populations. This book includes chapters describing the use of the model in a broad range of predicaments and with patients of a variety of ages. Practitioners and researchers are challenged to continue to use the model and test its significance in nursing practice.

REFERENCES

Chopoorian, T.J. (1986). Reconceptualizing the environment. In P. Moccia (Ed.), New approaches to theory development (pp. 39–54). New York: National League for Nursing.

Levine, M.E. (1966). Trophicognosis: An alternative to nursing diagnosis. In American Nurses' Association Regional Clinical Conference (Vol. 2, pp. 55–70). New York: American Nurses' Association.

Levine, M.E. (1973). Introduction to clinical nursing. Philadelphia: F.A. Davis.

Levine, M.E. (1987). Approaches to the development of a nursing diagnosis taxonomy. In A.M. McLane (Ed.), Classification of nursing diagnoses: Proceedings of the seventh conference: North American Nursing Diagnosis Association (pp. 45–51). St. Louis: C.V. Mosby.

Levine, M.E. (September 21, 1989). Personal communication.

Stafford, M. (May 8, 1989). Personal communication.

Taylor, J.W. (1974). Measuring the outcomes of nursing care. Nursing Clinics of North America, 9(2), 337–349.

Taylor, J.W. (1987). Organizing data for nursing diagnoses using conservation principles. In A.M. McLane (Ed.), Classification of nursing diagnoses: Proceedings of the seventh conference: North American Nursing Diagnosis Association (pp. 103–111). St. Louis: C.V. Mosby.

Appendix
A

Instructor's Guide to *Introduction to Clinical Nursing,* * Edition 2

Myra Estrin Levine, R.N., M.S.N., F.A.A.N.

CLINICAL NURSING—WHAT ARE THE EDUCATIONAL ISSUES?

Textbook Learning: Its Limitations

The likelihood that a real patient in a real clinical environment can provide the student with a *textbook* picture of a disease is so unusual that when, on rare occasion, it happens, the entire staff is alerted to come and see. The textbook cannot, by its very nature, be a *Clinical Baedeker* that guides a student unfailingly through the intricacies of real situations. No two patients are ever alike because no two human beings (unless they are identical twins, and there is some doubt even then) are so alike that they will respond in precise ways to the same factors of health or disease. Quite beyond the easily identified differences of age, sex, and concurrent diagnoses, the ever-present influence of the previous lifestyle, the psychological and emotional patterns of response, and the effects, however subtle, of previous illness all conspire to make every patient a new mystery to be solved. There is also a temporal factor which limits the use of a text be-

---

*Levine, M.E. (1973). Instructor's guide to introduction to clinical nursing (2nd ed.). Philadelphia: F.A. Davis. Reprinted with permission.

cause no text can possibly keep absolutely current with new knowledge, new treatments, and new therapies.

Perhaps the most important limitation of the use of any textbook in nursing, however, rests with the nature of nursing activity itself. The student is expected to take intellectual knowledge to the bedside, translate the knowledge into technical skills, communicate with the patient so that his unique needs are identified and fulfilled, and realistically evaluate the effectiveness of intervention. Book knowledge is essential to the performance of nursing activity, but it is only a part of the nursing process, and the real test of competent nursing care lies with the ways in which such knowledge is implemented in real situations by the nurse.

The Clinical Environment: Its Limitations

It has been fashionable to refer to the clinical practice area as a clinical laboratory. But this laboratory is very unlike those which are widely used in other science disciplines. Here the problem to be solved is not posed by the experimenter—the best he can hope to do is to identify its essential components. The clinical practice area has real patients and real emergencies—it cannot be structured to mark time while the learning practitioner catches up with its tempo and demands. The patient is the subject of the learner's objectives, but the patient is also a real person confronted by an immediate and intensely personal issue. He is present in the clinical area because he requires the ministrations and services of the institution, and from his viewpoint, the issue of educating young practitioners must always be the secondary consideration. He had never really bargained for second-class care. It is the urgency of this fact which characterizes much of the nursing education which prescribes the same kind of trial and error which is used in other laboratory milieus. However, the nurse cannot afford to be wrong because real patients with real needs cannot be subjected to mistaken or frankly error-ridden management.

Out of the stringent demands of reality comes still another characteristic of the clinical environment. No matter how diligently the instructor may try, it is not possible to organize the clinical environment into a formalized, planned learning experience. It has to be utilized as it really is. Clinical instructors are repeatedly frustrated because they are not able to find the kinds of patients which they identify as best suiting the current course content. Instructors are often told that they must plan learning opportunities but the uncontrolled and uncontrollable clinical environment can offer, at best, an invitation to seize teaching opportunities. The traditional method of assignment which sends the instructor to the wards looking for diagnostic entities leads to frequent frustration for the teacher and inevitable frustration for the student. It is reasonable to desire the availability of six or seven classic examples of diabetes mellitus, but such an occurrence is most unlikely in most institutions. Even where the supply of patients with appropriate clinical diagnoses is widespread and generous, the instructor often finds that the patients with diabetes have been discharged as soon as she wants to assign them, and the surfeit of individuals with gallbladder disease is encouraging except for the fact that the didactic materials on gallbladder disease are scheduled for the next semester. As desirable as it may be from an educational point of view to have experience with patients who are suffering from diseases being discussed that week in class, the likelihood is that the instructor will have to compromise a great deal, and that the students will not actually care for such patients until several weeks after the classroom materials have been completed.

The intense desire of nurse educators to bring order and continuity to the content as it develops in both classroom and clinical practice area is certainly well placed. But the practice of assigning students on the basis of diagnosis (and to some extent, even on the basis of desirable nursing procedures) creates issues for the educator and the student which simply cannot be satisfied in most clinical practice environments. The quality of clinical experience which each student engages in varies remarkably from one student to the next, and some leave the course feeling that they have been short-changed because they have never taken care of patients with specific diagnoses, or have never been given the opportunity to perform certain procedures. Such an orientation is more than a testimony to personal frustration. It is also an indication that the real value of the clinical experience has been diluted, and that many opportunities to learn and to grow in nursing have been overlooked while the attention was directed to goals of lesser importance.

Using a Textbook: Its Intent

Recognizing the temporal and spatial limitations of textbook knowledge does not mean that texts are not useful adjuncts to learning. A nursing text can provide an organized body of knowledge which helps to structure the additional knowledge that comes from participating in clinical experience and reading current literature. The text is not a substitute for a careful perusal of professional literature, especially publications which deal with current therapies in clinical contexts. But the text provides a foundation for understanding and evaluating the current clinical literature. It offers generalizations which are broadly relevant and as a result, retain their relevance over a protracted period of time. It establishes a baseline for further study, and should be used as a background against which lecture, discussion, and clinical conferences can be structured. It should never be used as the single source of information available to a student because no text, no matter how excellent, can ever achieve such eminence. It is a stimulant, a guideline, an invitation to further reading, further evaluation of clinical experience, and a means for bringing together the written knowledge and the student's own store of personal experience. It is a reference to be returned to when the need arises, and it should be a source for continuing inspiration to seek new knowledge and insight. It should create the desire to know more. It is never the end but always the means towards a lively involvement with new knowledge.

Using Introduction to Clinical Nursing: Its Design

Introduction to Clinical Nursing was based on the premise that nursing is learned in real situations with real patients, and therefore it was designed to provide a foundation which recognizes those limitations that are so frustrating to nursing educators. It has two major components. The first is an overview of beginning medical-surgical nursing as developed in the cursive chapters. The second is an organizing structure of nursing procedures as developed in the outlines of the models which follow each chapter.

The cursive material is dedicated to the proposition that the nurse must learn to deal with alterations in the physiological function of the human body in order to understand disease as well as its treatment. The chapters are organized around functional activities of the body, but the materials selected to introduce each chapter were chosen because they establish the rationale for nursing intervention in a broad spectrum of realistic clinical situations. Each chapter is completed by the conservation principles, used to describe a prototype disease entity. It must be emphasized that the disease entity described is a prototype—that the nursing implications described in reference to each are valid for many different diagnostic entities. In Chapter 2, for example, the care of the patient with a cerebral vascular accident is analyzed within the framework of the conservation principles. But the essential nursing objective that is explored in that chapter is demonstrable in many clinical situations. The message, reinforced by a description of the physiology and pathophysiology of the nervous system, is that the nurse responds for the patient when he is unable to respond for himself to the demands of his internal and external environment. Insult to the nervous system always limits the ability of the individual to mobilize freely in his environment, and to seek for himself the essentials required to sustain him such as food and water. For each patient the nurse must learn to evaluate what he can do best for himself, and what he must have provided for him. And while the hemiplegic individual can illustrate this nursing activity very definitely, there are many patients with other diagnoses who also require this precise kind of nursing intervention. Patients with neurologic diseases of many kinds also fit this nursing category, as well as neurosurgical patients, unconscious or comatose patients regardless of the cause, post-anesthetic patients during their recovery, orthopedic patients who are immobilized in traction or casts, and even patients who are very weak or in pain sufficiently intense that they are unable to move freely. Fortified with a nursing goal to seek opportunities for students to nurse patients who cannot adequately or accurately respond to their own needs, the instructor is not tied to finding six or eight or ten patients with a cerebral vascular accident. The same nursing activity can be found with many patients, and frequently a clinical conference which allows the students to compare the nursing implications in many different patients requiring similar nursing intervention can be very valuable. Such a conference helps to emphasize that the diagnostic entity is not necessarily the focus of nursing concern. It places abiding emphasis on the nursing role, an emphasis which nurses themselves are seeking and which will help to define the nursing process in realistic terms.

The models are designed to bring together the scientific rationale for the performance of many different kinds of nursing procedures. The long historic dependence on procedural rules remains as a persistent thread in nursing education, even while the emphasis has shifted from a task to an intellectual (and therefore professional) orientation. The rules provide a scientific rationale which makes the intent of the procedure unequivocal even though, as nurses quickly learn, the methods for performing procedures vary, often remarkably, from one institution to another. When most nursing education was hospital-based, learning the precise rules of the hospital was sufficient in order to learn the important how-to-do-it aspects of nursing care. But the trend now to use several clinical environments for a single group of students coupled with the great mobility of nurses in modern society has made the dependence on the procedural rules in a single institution insufficient for a real understanding of nursing activity. The emphasis in nursing procedures of all kinds has long been on the performance of a given procedure as an end in itself. It is essential that nursing procedures be placed into perspective in nursing education. It is not possible to learn nursing without learning procedures. The skills which the nurse must learn are the most vital and important means of communication she will ever have with her patients. The procedural skills are a communication system, and for the young student of nursing they represent the most essential means for establishing a viable interaction with patients. The nurse who develops such skills has found a silent language through which she can say to her patients, "I know how to take care of you." And the patient in return is aware that he is safe and in the care of a knowledgeable person. No text can teach the muscular skills that can only come with actual practice, but the models offer an organizational structure for nursing procedures which makes them meaningful and sensible in the strength of their scientific bases.

The second edition explores in somewhat detailed fashion the substantive nature of the four conservation principles of nursing. This material is intended to serve as a guide for understanding the way in which the conservation principles are used in each chapter of the book when the prototype diagnostic entities are discussed. It is expected that the instructor will be able to expand considerably, in the clinical environment, on the factors which contribute to an understanding of the conservation principles in patient care. The discussion is far from exhaustive and offers only a guideline for the kinds of information which may be included in each of the categories: energy, structural integrity, personal integrity, and social integrity.

The discussion of the scientific method is included because the exploration of patient needs can be organized in this accepted fashion and the consequent identification of priorities made clear to the student. When the Fiebelmann terminology is used, the use of scientific method is reduced to its simplest components. The real test of identifying provocative facts occurs within the clinical context itself, where students can be encouraged to respond to their own observations and evaluations of patient requirements.

This is a skill which nurses do possess, and do utilize although often they do not realize they are doing so. Nurses also engage in the development of testable hypotheses and base their decisions for intervention on such constructs. In the teaching-learning process, the young nurse will find this kind of organization a challenge not only to her observational skills but also to her knowledge and her ability to evaluate the consequences of her intervention in ways which are valid and meaningful for the patient.

The second chapter, "Nursing the Patient Who has a Failure of Nervous System Integration," is offered as a *beginning* clinical chapter in this text because, in spite of its complexity and difficulty, the important integrative functions of the nervous system are essential to the freedom to move, act, seek, and participate fully in life in all of its dimensions. Probably because of the complexity of nervous system anatomy and physiology, the usual pattern has been to place such considerations near the end of a course. That has often meant that the subject was dealt with rather quickly, and sometimes in a very superficial manner. The importance of mobilization and free choice of activity, however, is so central to all consideration of human behavior that it should be dealt with carefully and is an essential starting point for the understanding of nursing intervention. The model accompanying this chapter "Body Movement and Positioning" indicates the important scientific bases of mobilization, but coming as it does early in the development of the beginning course, it has some educational advantages as well. Young students come to nursing strongly motivated towards involvement in patient care. Their earliest clinical practice experiences are unfailingly traumatic and awkward, and they need assistance in overcoming the awe and confusion which is so characteristic of their beginning experiences. The opportunity to work in physical contact with real patients by assisting them to become mobilized satisfies at once the desire to be actively involved. The pragmatic problems of mobilizing patients is a real one in many clinical situations, and thus the service the students perform in these procedures is a genuine contribution to patient care—a contribution which they can recognize as viable and real from the outset of their participation. Assisting patients to get out of bed or back into bed and learning the proper manipulation to permit safe and protective bed postures will continue to be essential nursing activities throughout the clinical practice period. The emphasis placed on sustaining, promoting, and assisting with mobilization is a fundamental concept of nursing intervention and learning its importance from the outset permits the student to place such activities into a proper perspective. This kind of initial activity also assures the assignment of patient-centered tasks. The student is assigned to a patient, and assists the patient to get out of bed and into a wheelchair. While the patient is out of bed, the unoccupied bed can be made but it is made for a person the student is committed to help. It is not bed-making for the sake of bed-making, but providing the environment for the comfort of a person the student has come to know and help. From the outset, the most basic procedures can be used as communication systems—the student knows the bed she is making will be occupied and her activities are real, important to a known individual, and the total effect of her intervention becomes an experience in interpersonal relations from the very beginning of her clinical experience.

The third chapter, "Nursing the Patient with a Failure of Integration Resulting from Hormonal Disturbance," emphasizes still another essential integrative system in the body. The major nursing concept inherent in this chapter is that hormonal replacement therapy always means a substitution of a managed, therapeutic regime for controls ordinarily carried on by the autoregulating activities of the body. Such a therapeutic goal creates many aspects of nursing intervention: observation of patient behavior is essential to proper assessment of his response to therapy; such an individual must be taught to manage his own therapy; to recognize in himself the signals that indicate an adjustment must be made, and to learn when he can make the adjustment himself and when he must seek advice from his physician. Nursing such a patient requires that the individual's total lifestyle be involved in his therapy, and the nurse must recognize how intimately well-being is associated with every aspect of such a patient's life. He cannot be perceived as a disease entity, nor even as the subject of certain procedures. He must have the assistance to recognize that the factors which other people can ignore when their autoregulating systems are intact are all susceptible to personal interpretation and understanding by the afflicted individual. The diabetic patient is used as a prototype example of such a nursing problem, but the concept is valid in other diagnoses as well. It is equally important for patients suffering other hormonal imbalances which require therapy such as thyroid disease and adrenal insufficiency. In fact, the widespread use of adrenocortical drugs also produces clinical situations which must be dealt with in the same ways, although such patients may be receiving the drugs for many other diagnostic categories.

The biochemical regulation of metabolism which is disrupted by hormonal imbalance emphasizes as well the integrative influence of the hormones in establishing necessary conditions for healing. The diabetic patient and his difficulties with the healing process simply emphasize how important personal hygiene and management can be for all patients. The model associated with this chapter introduces personal hygiene because this emphatic nursing need is underlined by the needs of all patients for hygienic care. Using the knowledge gained in the preceding model (on mobilization), the basic procedures for bathing patients are based on the importance of assembling his own ability to help himself, and the degree of intervention selected by the nurse is thus a patient-centered approach because it requires decision-making on the strength of the individual patient's needs. Assisting with bathing may be understood from the simplest tasks of assisting the patient who can help himself through the entire spectrum of nursing participation to complete bed care. The toilet needs of patients are not made a special issue. The fact of restriction of activity is sufficient to establish the importance for providing the utensils for urination and defecation. When the request is brought to the student's attention by a patient, the least traumatic way of introducing this activity is simply to assist the student in performing this service for the patient. As a patient-centered service, it does not gain the aura of special importance which is associated with it when the student focuses on the procedure by itself.

Chapter 4, "Nursing the Patient with a Disturbance of Homeostasis: Fluid and Electrolyte Balance," recognizes that the importance of water and electrolytes to individual well-being is an integrative function of the body which the nurse can sustain through her intervention. The prototype entity used in this chapter, congestive heart failure, is chosen because the essential nursing issue in the care of such patients is the mobilization of fluids, and the nursing activities are fundamentally geared to the successful recompartmentalization of body fluids and electrolytes in such patients. But the question of proper fluid balance can be addressed with equal emphasis in many different diagnostic categories. All patients with kidney disease, for example or any disease process characterized by fluid imbalance and edema formation may be used to teach the same nursing concept. The necessity for balance is an essential aspect of preoperative and postoperative care and it is an abiding concern in the care of infants as well as any individual with fluid loss because of a disease process. Patients with diarrhea on naso-gastric suction procedures or simply older individuals who must be encouraged to take fluids in order to remain hydrated also illustrate this concept.

The accompanying model "Pressure Gradient Systems in Nursing Intervention: Fluids" emphasizes the many ways in which the movement of fluids can be therapeutically and procedurally utilized. The basic scientific information establishes the rationale for all procedures which are dependent upon the physical facts of fluid pressure gradients. In this context, blood pressure is a meaningful measure of the pressure gradients which are influencing the patient's own internal environment. It establishes the safety and therapeutic intent of intravenous fluid administration, and the issues of fluid intake and output so vital to so many therapeutic regimens. It establishes the scientific basis for enemata, irrigation of body organs, gastrointestinal decompression techniques, and provides a basis for understanding laboratory results on fluid and electrolyte balance. Both the importance of daily weights in patients who are in imbalance and the ways in which the nurse can identify the signs of dehydration in patients for whom it is an essential issue are emphasized.

The additional material in the second edition describing the electrophysiology of the heart and the instrumentation of the electrocardiograph is not intended to provide clinical competence in this very difficult area of nursing intervention. Rather, it is an effort to make meaningful to the young student of nursing the ways in which instrumentation reflects the physiologic behavior of the body. As an initial introduction to a complex nursing activity, the emphasis is on the explanation of the electrophysiologic manifestations of cardiac action and the remarkable way in which the instrumentation has been refined and improved to gather information on how to "read" the results of such intervention, but rather the emphasis is that vital information can be recorded and interpreted when the techniques are carefully observed and the limitations carefully evaluated.

Chapter 5 emphasizes the importance of nutritional balance in the care of patients. The major nursing concept focuses attention on the importance of a patent, motile, intact gastrointestinal system as a necessary condition for the proper absorption of important nutrients. The prototype disease, peptic ulcers, emphasizes the importance of therapeutic diet management as an important aspect of a medical regimen, and the important role that the nurse must play in providing adequate nutrition for patients. Any situation characterized by the therapeutic importance of diet can be used equally well to illustrate this kind of nursing activity. Gastrointestinal disease entities of any kind will fulfill this concept, but any interference with food intake, either because of disease or by prescription (as in the operative patient), will provide this kind of nursing insight as well. The model emphasizes the scientific basis of nutrition and the ways in which the nurse participates in providing adequate nutrition for patients.

Chapter 6, "Nursing the Patient with a Disturbance of Homeostasis: Systemic Oxygen Needs," emphasizes the importance of ventilatory and respiratory functions in providing sufficient oxygen for essential body activities. The nursing concept emphasizes the ways in which nursing intervention can support the respiratory effort of patients, maintaining the patent airway and postural adjustments to assist in providing an optimal vital capacity within the limits of the patient's disability. The prototype discussed is emphysema, but the same issues of respiratory exchange are present in all patients with pulmonary disease. The problem of adequate ventilation, however, is also illustrated in patients undergoing anesthesia, very weak and cachectic patients, patients with poor bed posture, patients with painful abdominal conditions, including postoperative patients. The model associated with this chapter establishes the guidelines for understanding the pressure gradient systems which are fundamental to normal respiratory exchange and the ways in which procedures must be designed to defend those gradients. Assisted respiration, chest aspiration, and chest drainage all are procedures which are designed so that the pressure gradients of respiration are sustained and protected.

Chapter 7 is devoted to an exploration of cellular oxygen needs. The structural nature of the blood is presented as a means of emphasizing the importance of delivery of oxygen and nutrients to the cells, as well as the removal of catabolic substances. The nursing concept is directed at the ways in which adequate circulation can be sustained in order to support cellular processes. The prototype disease, anemia, illustrates the holistic way in which the individual is affected when the cellular metabolism is compromised by inadequate oxygenation. But the same concept is also illustrated by insufficiency of peripheral vascular blood flow, the importance of circulatory integrity in sustaining cerebral and kidney function, and in any condition where occlusive disease of the vessels results in the threatened or actual destruction of tissue. All kinds of blood dyscrasias, including pernicious anemia, sickle cell anemia, or aplastic anemias from any cause, either disease or drug usage, may also be used as clinical evidence of this essential concept. The model is devoted to the local application of heat and cold since these procedures are effective because of their effort on the volume of blood flow to those tissues where they are employed.

Chapter 8, "Nursing the Patient with Disease Arising from Aberrant Cellular Growth," emphasizes the diffuse and disorganized kinds of problems which are a result of anarchic cell growth. The nursing concept emphasizes the erratic and threatening nature of aberrance in cell replication, and the ways in which intervention must anticipate and deal with the unpredictable anarchy of uncontrolled mitotic phenomena. The prototype example deals in general terms with the issues raised by malignant growth, and patients suffering from any form of neoplasm will illustrate the kinds of care such tissue destruction creates. The chapter includes a discussion of the dying patient—an area of nursing concern now generally recognized as an essential aspect of intervention. The model associated with this chapter, "Administration of Medications," establishes general guidelines for this activity. It emphasizes the biological effect of drugs of all kinds, and the necessity for cautious control of drug administration in order to make this a rational procedure. The use of drugs in the care of the patient with malignant disease is frequently based on decisions the nurse must make, for example, in the administration of analgesic medications, and thus the important emphasis must be on the knowledge of drug action, control systems which insure safety, and the intelligent decisions required in the patient's behalf.

Chapter 9, "Nursing the Patient with an Inflammatory Process," describes the two-fold goal of nursing such patients—to limit the inflammatory response in both space and time. The inflammatory process is described not only as a defense against noxious invaders but also as the initiation of the process of healing itself. The prototype description is generalized to establish the guidelines for the care of any individual with an acute inflammatory process, but the nursing concepts are valid regardless of the source or location of the inflammatory condition. The nature of the inflammation establishes the nursing concepts used in dealing with it, because the biological wisdom of the healing process must be sustained and protected through nursing intervention. The model "Establishing an Aseptic Environment" is concerned with the control systems for limiting the dangers posed by infection throughout the spectrum of nursing intervention. Aseptic control is viewed as a matter of degree, beginning with the basic concepts of cleanliness and moving through the variety of demands towards surgical asepsis and finally, protective isolation to prevent infection in patients whose own defenses are compromised by disease or treatment.

The final chapter offers some of the dimensions of the holistic response of individuals and includes some areas of recent research which have relevance and meaning for the nurses. The issue of periodic cycling of biological events emphasizes the intimate interactions between the individual and his larger environment. The questions of territory and space are determinants of response to the social demands not often recognized in hospitalized patients, and finally the discussion of sleep and sleep patterns focuses attention on an aspect of nursing care which has been largely ignored by nurses.

The second edition offers a discussion of body precept as a concept which has abiding implications for nursing care. The materials added deal with the use of such concepts as body image, part of the current research in perception. This has not often been included in nursing thought. Taking into consideration the importance of the individual's perception of himself in the framework of his environmental predicament is a way of emphasizing the unique response to life experiences. Such perception is clearly an aspect of the entire pattern of growth and development, and this view of the developmental process allows for the individualization of nursing intervention. The materials also emphasize the importance of sexuality in both the individual's definition of himself and his relationship to other human beings. The view has been adopted that the process of growth and the development of sexual definitions are integrating factors in every person's life and contribute, therefore, to a holistic understanding of nursing care.

This book was designed as an introduction to the basic concepts of nursing care. It is dedicated to the proposition that nursing intervention is based on a conceptualization of broad generalizations which are neither disease nor procedure oriented but focused instead on patient care. The same general organization can be used for the second course in medical-surgical nursing, using the next level of intervention as a basis for the nursing concepts. For example, the care of the surgical patients requires the basic concepts developed throughout this first text. The combination of ideas inherent in the care of the surgical patient, including respiratory management, fluid and electrolyte balance, nutritional needs, and control of the inflammatory process may be presented in relationship to the specific goals of recovery from a surgical procedure. The care of the patient with a myocardial infarct also necessitates the use of all of these concepts in relation to determination of care, and finally rehabilitation and restored well-being.

No course and no text can hope to be all-inclusive. But essential and pertinent generalizations in a beginning course provide a foundation upon which deeper insights and more intensive exploration can be based. There is one fact of clinical nursing education which must be acknowledged. The ingenuity and knowledge of the clinical instructor is the key to successful educational efforts. This text was never intended to replace that vital contribution. It is based on a deep-felt faith in the abilities, wisdom, and creativity of clinical instructors and the interest, curiosity, and refreshing sense of inquiry which young students bring to their nursing careers.

Appendix
B^*

Introduction to Patient-Centered Nursing Care

Myra Estrin Levine, R.N., M.S.N., F.A.A.N.

THEORIES OF DISEASE AS A BASIS FOR NURSING PRACTICE

Introduction

Nursing is a human interaction. It is a discipline rooted in the organic dependency of the individual human being on his relationships with other human beings. An "interaction" by its very nature presupposes a system of exchange between individuals: it can occur only if *communication* can occur. Language represents only one mode of communication, and, indeed, the ability to respond to the behavior of other individuals often requires no exchange of words at all. In every generation, meaningful interaction has taken place with utilization of the knowledge, tools, skills, and ideas unique to that time and place. The scientific knowledge of the modern world provides exciting avenues for the essential dialogue between human beings. It is not a substitute for the fundamental relationships which they must establish with each other. It is the means by which such relationships can be constituted. Nursing knowledge, thoroughly grounded in modern scientific concepts, allows for a sensitive and productive relationship between the nurse and the individual entrusted to her care. In the care of the sick, this has always been true, but never before has there been available

*Levine, M.E. (1973). Introduction to clinical nursing (2nd ed.). Philadelphia: F.A. Davis. Reprinted with permission.

to the nurse so rich and demanding a body of knowledge to use in the patient's behalf.

Nursing practice has always mirrored the prevailing theories of health and disease because such theories pervade every culture. Every society has made provision for the care of the sick based upon the ideas shared by the group about disease and its meaning to the individual and to the society. The earliest concepts of health and disease developed from man's seeming helplessness in a hostile environment. Buffeted by forces he could neither explain nor understand, he turned to supplication and endowed nature with supernatural qualities.

The care of the sick is closely related to the value that the society places on individual human life, and the economic and political structures of the group strongly influence those values. As scientific and technological change have created social and economic change, the value system has also undergone change. The sanctity of human life has always been a hallmark of Western civilization, and yet the impact of scientific and technological knowledge, which has permitted individuals to live longer lives, has resulted in overwhelming social problems related to the economic and health care of the aging population. Many societies have placed a premium of value on their young, productive members. Such social decisions, however, have both positive and negative aspects. The youth-orientation of American society, for example, creates implicit bias directed at older persons. The need for health care is not, as a consequence, always predicated on individual concerns but is markedly determined by the economic and political cost created by the dependency of disadvantaged populations.

The factors that influence the attitudes of any group towards its sick members are very complex. In any individual member, such attitudes are further complicated by the fact that they arise from the several sources that influence his life. His ethnic affiliation is one such fundamental tie, but subcultural attitudes, religious beliefs, and his unique life experiences also leave their mark on his concern for health and his response to disease.

In a real sense, nursing itself is a subculture, possessing ideas and values which are unique to nurses, even though they mirror the social template which created them. And like all other social institutions, the practice of nursing has faithfully reflected the changing currents of knowledge and belief within the human communication systems of which it is a part.

Nature as the Great Healer

The healing power of natural forces, still a part of all superstitious belief, strongly influenced the development of scientific medical thought. The concept of Nature as the Great Healer *(vis medicatrix naturae)* was enunciated clearly by Hippocrates, and persisted through centuries of evolving scientific knowledge. Man fortified himself in his hostile environment, and knowledge changed fear to awesome wonder.

A benevolent healing power in Nature was fundamental doctrine in the rise of the humanitarians and sanitarians of the nineteenth century. Florence Nightingale was their greatest spokesman. Perhaps no historical figure has been so poorly understood as has Florence Nightingale. She was called a "legend" in her own time, and the fantasies perpetuated about her have reinforced a legendary aura which belies the incisive, perceptive, and honest excellence of her thinking and her contribution to modern health theory. Her writings were primarily aimed at the establishment of a system of hospital care based on effective sanitation practices, and such practice, in turn, arose from an unceasing concern for the integrity and decency of the individual. *Notes on Nursing* was written for the "layman," and, in fact, Miss Nightingale never wrote a "textbook" of nursing. But this delightful volume is a treasury of wisdom and insight, and much of it is as relevant today as it was in 1859. Miss Nightingale wrote, "Shall we begin by taking it as a general principle—that all disease, at some period or other of its course, is more or less a reparative process . . ."

With this mandate, the direction of nursing care became remarkably clear: the nurse created an environment in which healing could occur. Nursing responsibility focused on procedures to establish an environment of cleanliness, safety, and comfort, both physical and mental. Thus protected and nurtured, the "reparative process" within the patient was enhanced. It was in this way that the "procedure-orientation" in nursing began. Its persistence to this day has accompanied the growth of technology in nursing, as indeed nursing has shared in technological expansion in every area of modern life. But the tradition of the procedure—of "how-to-do-it"—has become so deeply embedded in the nursing psyche that it is almost "holy." . . .

The Unified Theory of Health and Disease: Holism

A great theologian, Paul Tillich, summarized the problem confronting the modern nurse when he said that the "multidimensional unity of life in man calls for a multidimensional concept of health, of disease and of healing, but in such a way that it becomes obvious that in each dimension all the others are present."

The human being responds to the forces in his environment in a singular yet integrated fashion. The specific symptoms of a disease may emphasize some bodily functions more than others, but even to such a localized cluster of events, the afflicted person responds in a way peculiar to him and to him alone.

There are no magic scales which allow nurses to weigh the multiplicity of factors operating in a single individual. Ultimately, decisions for nursing intervention must be based on the unique behavior of the individual patient. It is the nurse's task to bring a body of scientific principles on which decisions depend into the precise situation that she shares with the patient. Sensitive observation and the selection of relevant data form the basis for her assessment of his nursing requirement. A theory of nursing must recognize the importance of unique detail of care for a single patient within an empiric framework which successfully describes the requirements of *all* patients.

The integrated function of the human organism has been described in the scientific literature since the nineteenth century. Claude Bernard recognized the interdependence of bodily function in his description of the *milieu interne*—the internal environment. Bernard identified the primordial seas, captured within the integument of the human body and providing the organism with a tightly regulated solution of substances essential to its continuing well-being. In the pursuit of understanding that accompanied Darwinian thought in the late nineteenth century, this significant contribution underscored the remarkable ability of the human organism to survive successfully in widely variant external environments. Man carried the essentials with him, safely packaged inside his skin. But it was apparent to Bernard, and to the army of investigators who followed him, that the internal environment was susceptible to constant change. In 1915, Walter Cannon, an outstanding American physiologist, coined the word "homeostasis" (*Homeo*, equal and *stasis*, condition) to describe the remarkable equilibrium that was maintained in the internal environment in the face of constant change.

The concept of homeostasis recognized that the balance maintained within the internal environment took place on a continuum of relationships, with an upper and a lower limit between which the balance was normally struck. In fact, the concept of "normal" presupposes that the values for the many different substances dissolved in the body fluids will fall somewhere between those upper and lower limits, and a value either above or below the limits indicates an abnormal condition. The well-being of the organism is thus dependent upon the balance, and in general, when the value exceeds the limits, it must be promptly restored or the life of the organism is threatened.

The concept of the "stable state," or homeostasis, has been extremely valuable in understanding the processes of health and illness. But as so often happens, the enlargement of understanding that came from this concept suggests that even this important idea represents an oversimplification of reality. The common experience of daily living testifies to the fact that individuals recognize alterations in their own sense of well-being throughout the 24 hour period. Such response is related to the periodic changes in physiological parameters which are not only "normal" but also essential for the effective, integrated function of the body. The straight line continuum suggests a static relationship which never really exists in health or disease. Waddington has suggested that the process be called homeorrhesis (*homeo*-stable; -*rhesis*, flow), a stabilized flow rather than a static state. Such a concept emphasizes the fluidity of change within a space-time continuum and more nearly describes the remarkable patterns of adaptation which permit the individual's body to sustain its well-being within the vast changes which encroach upon it from the environment. The concept of stabilized flow more accurately reflects the reality of daily change was well as the alterations in physiological activity that characterize the processes of growth and development.

The physiologists have identified many of the interactions that the body is called upon to make when the internal environment is threatened by alterations in the value of vital substances. By and large, such revisions depend on "negative feedback" mechanisms resulting in "autoregulation" of the internal environment. A negative feedback exercises control by rein-

serting into the system the results of its past performances. Wiener has described this effect as "patterns that perpetuate themselves." They are
control systems, designed to maintain the balance—and thereby the well-
being—of the organisms. Thus it is that the factors influencing a person's
response to illness do not exist as discrete entities which may be selected
and used at will. All of the forces within him exist in a dynamic relationship
to each other, seeking a state of equilibrium or balance that will best maintain a uniformity of function.

The exquisite internal balance responds constantly to external forces,
however. There is an intimate relationship between the internal and the external environments, much of it vividly understood in recent years by research in physiological periodicity and the circadian cycles. Some of the
earliest attention to the periodic nature of physiological function was
devoted to studies of sleep and wakefulness, and the familiar experience
of every individual emphasizes, even in this single area, how individual
well-being is dependent upon external environmental experience. The
fundamental integrative ability of the human organism illuminates all
understanding of human structure, function, and response to disease.

The total life process of the entire organism is dependent upon the
inter-relatedness of its component systems. In fact, the organism is a system of systems, and in its wholeness expresses the organization of all the
contributing parts. Organization means an orderly sequence, and so the organism represents a pattern of orderly, sequential *change*. Because it is
both ordered and sequential, the pattern is a *message*. So long as the pattern is consistent, it is also understandable. If change in the organism were
to occur in an undisciplined and unregulated way, then anarchy would result, and the pattern would be so disrupted that it could no longer successfully support life. Such anarchy, in fact, occurs in disease processes, and
unless the pattern can be restored, the organism will die.

Change is the essence of life, and it is unceasing as long as life goes
on. Such change is not a random activity. It is directed, purposeful, and
meaningful, and it is also eminently understandable. The change which
supports the well-being of the organism can be predicted, measured, and
observed, and therefore is a cogent message. It must be emphasized that
the message is not a single sentence. It is far too complex for that. It is always at least a paragraph and may indeed as often be equivalent to a book
or a library filled with books.

Change is characteristic of life, and adaptation is the method of
change. The organism retains its integrity in both the internal and external
environment through its adaptive 'capability. Adaptation is the process
of change whereby the individual retains his integrity within the realities of
his environments. Adaptation is basic to survival, and it is an expression of
the integration of the entire organism. The measure of effective adaptation
is compatibility with life. A poor adaptation may threaten life itself, but at
the same time the degree of adaptive potential available to the individual
may be sufficient to maintain life at a *different level of effectiveness*. Adaptation is not "all-or-none." It is susceptible to an infinite range within the
limits of life compatibility. Within that range, there are numerous possible
degrees of adaptation.

Thus, the dynamic processes establishing balance along the continuum are adaptations. All the processes of living are processes of adaptation. Survival itself depends upon the *quality* of the adaptation possible for the individual. Health and disease are patterns of adaptive change. Engel argues that the study of disease must be grounded in knowledge of it as a "natural phenomenon." Wolf says that "physicians now consider most diseases to be distinct from one another insofar as they represent patterned responses or adaptations to noxious forces in the environment." In any event, it has always been easier to describe the characteristics of a disease process than to define the absence of disease. The word disease itself comes from the old French words meaning "from ease." The earliest associations with the word indicated a much broader application than the descriptive details of a specific process of illness, and the word in its restricted medical meaning is fairly recent. It has proved to be far more difficult to define "health." While many definitions have been offered, they have always represented a struggle to be all-inclusive, and usually the definitions are lengthy and lack precision. But there is often a wisdom in the folk traditions which escapes the attention of the scholar, and such a tradition has persisted in the language used to describe an absence of disease. The word health comes from the Anglo-Saxon word *hal*, a word which meant *whole*. The multi-dimensional unity suggested by Tillich is a condition of wholeness, and the most accurate description of health is "whole"—a concept recognized by fundamental human experience.

Erikson has described wholeness as an open system. He writes, "Wholeness emphasizes a sound, organic, progressive mutuality between diversified functions and parts within an entirety, the boundaries of which are open and fluid." The unceasing interaction of the individual organism with its environments does represent an "open and fluid" system, and a condition of health, or wholeness, exists when the interactions, or constant adaptations to the environment, permit *ease*—the assurance of integrity (unity or one-ness)—in all the dimensions of life. Recognition of the open-ended, fluid, and constantly changing nature of interaction with the environment is the basis for holistic thought. The word holistic (rather than wholistic) is derived from the usual language of science—Greek; it comes from the word root, *hol*, which means entire.

The variety of conditions which characterize the internal environment represent the study of physiology and pathophysiology. The external environment, however, is often viewed as a kind of stage setting against which the individual plays out his life. The simplistic view of the external environment as a background fails to acknowledge that the individual is constantly interacting with his environment, and no real understanding of the internal environment is possible without careful consideration of the influences that are constantly at work to alter it.

Bates has suggested a way in which to view the external environment which allows the student to organize the relationships of the individual to the factors that are impinging upon and changing him. That portion of the environment to which the individual responds with his sense organs is called the *perceptual* environment. It includes all kinds of perceived stimuli—sight, sound, odor, taste, and touch, as well as orientation to space.

There are, in addition, a number of factors present in the environment which cannot be perceived by any of the sensory apparati. This Bates has called the *operational* environment. It includes such forces as radioactivity (including natural and man-made forms) and all microorganisms, none of which, of course, can be directly viewed without sophisticated instruments. The recent concern with environmental quality has emphasized the importance of the operational environment because of the effect of noxious substances in the air and water supplies and alteration in the constituents of the soil which can only be identified when they threaten living things.

The final external environment identified by Bates is the *conceptual* one. Human life is inextricably bound to a life of ideas, of symbolic exchange and of belief, tradition, and judgment which influence all human behavior. The exchange of language, the ability to think and to experience emotion are all part of the conceptual environment. Value systems, religious beliefs, ethnic and cultural traditions, and the individual psychological patterns that come from life experiences are all essential aspects of the conceptual environment.

The holistic approach to nursing care depends upon recognition of the integrated response of the individual arising from the internal environment, and the interaction which occurs with the external environment. Separate consideration of either the internal or external environments can provide only a partial view of the complex interaction that is taking place between them. It is, in fact, at the interface where the exchange between internal and external environments occurs that the determinants for nursing intervention are found. In this broader sense, all adaptations represent the accommodation that is possible between the internal and external environments.

The nurse participates actively in every patient's environment, and much of what she does supports his adaptations as he struggles in the predicament of illness. Nursing intervention means that the nurse interposes her skill and knowledge into the course of events that affects the patient. Thus, nursing intervention must be founded not only on scientific knowledge, but specifically on recognition of the individual's holistic response which indicates the *nature of the adaptation taking place*. The nurse must learn to read the message. Such assessments provide the only rational basis for judicious decision-making by the nurse in the patient's behalf. Furthermore, nursing intervention must be designed so that it fosters successful adaptation whenever possible.

When nursing intervention influences adaptation favorably, or toward renewed social well-being, then the nurse is acting in a *therapeutic* sense. When nursing intervention cannot alter the course of the adaptation— when her best efforts can only maintain the status quo or fail to halt a downward course—then the nurse is acting in a *supportive* sense.

The Four Conservation Principles of Nursing

The holistic nature of the human response to the environment provides the rationale for substantive principles of nursing. A principle is a fundamental concept that forms the basis for a chain of reasoning. Formulated on a broad base, it establishes the relationships between apparently otherwise unrelated facts. Nursing principles are fundamental assumptions which provide a unifying structure for understanding a wide variety of nursing activities.

Nursing principles are all "conservation" principles. Conservation means "keeping together" (L. *conservatio*) but this does not imply minimal activity. "To keep together" means to maintain a proper balance between active nursing intervention coupled with patient participation on the one hand and the safe limits of the patient's ability to participate on the other. The four conservation principles have as a postulate the unity and integrity of the individual:

I The principle of the conservation of energy
Nursing intervention is based on the conservation of the individual patient's energy.

II The principle of the conservation of structural integrity
Nursing intervention is based on the conservation of the individual patient's structural integrity.

III The principle of the conservation of personal integrity
Nursing intervention is based on the conservation of the individual patient's personal integrity.

IV The principle of the conservation of social integrity
Nursing intervention is based on the conservation of the individual patient's social integrity.

The Conservation of Energy

It is from the sun that all of the energy available to earth must come. The basic physical law of energy conservation (first law of thermodynamics) states that energy cannot be created or lost—it can only be transformed from one kind to another. The energy that comes from the sun is in the form of radiant and heat energy. It is captured by green plants and transformed into the chemical energy of foodstuffs, and, of course, all animal life is dependent upon green plants ultimately for its energy sources. The processes of life demand a constant renewal of energy. There can never be an absolute equilibrium of energy in the living system because the energy production systems in the living body are chemical systems, and a chemical equilibrium occurs only at death. Energy is the capacity to do work, and the process of life is a process of energy production which makes it possible for the multiple activities (work) of the systems of the body to move forward. Work must be performed (work equals force times distance) whenever the body moves, but it is equally required for the cellular and molecular activities which are characteristic of the life process.

The ability of the human body to perform the work of life is dependent upon its energy balance—the supply of energy-producing nutrients measured against the rate of energy-using activities. Once more, there is folk wisdom in recognizing this complex organism-environmental interaction which is often overlooked. Everyone who has experienced illness, even the common cold, knows that it is attended by feelings of fatigue which make it necessary to limit activity. The energy required by alterations in physiological function during illness represents an additional demand made on the energy production systems, and the fatigue so often experienced with illness is a very empiric measure of that additional demand for energy. An increase in body temperature (fever) always signals an increase in the rate of energy production. In fact, such an increase is measurable—a 7% increase in metabolism for every degree Fahrenheit rise in body temperature.

From the nurse's viewpoint, the balancing of energy input with energy output is a very essential aspect of all nursing intervention. Every disease process creates an increased energy demand that is characterized by the efforts made by the body to promote healing. Nursing procedures have always given tacit recognition to this basic need. The provisions for rest, for example, are all essentially aimed at energy conservation. The maintenance of adequate nutrition, even when the diet must be therapeutically managed, is another way in which the nurse promotes energy conservation. But the conservation of energy does not merely mean minimization of activity for the patient. It requires instead, a deliberate decision as to the allowable activity based upon the patient's energy resources. Such deliberate intervention depends upon accurate assessment of the patient's ability to perform necessary activities without producing excessive fatigue. In many ways, the nurse acts as the "banker" for the proper balancing of the patient's energy account. The nurse provides for an adequate deposit of energy resource and cautiously regulates the energy spending.

The Conservation of Structural Integrity

The process of healing is the process of restoration of structural integrity. In many ways, individuals are constantly threatened by factors in the environment which have a potential for inflicting injury. The body possesses a number of remarkably efficient defense systems which protect the individual from loss of body fluids (especially blood), introduction of pathogenic organisms which produce threatening infections, ability to move quickly away from dangerous threats in the environment (including a reflex which quickly withdraws a limb from a painful stimulus) as well as rapid adaptations to changes in external temperature, humidity, and oxygen supply. The intact organism is the only one that can move with freedom and without restraint in the environment.

All individuals learn very early in their lives to have confidence in their ability to heal. A cut or a scratch will heal, and afterward, if the damaged area is limited, there will be little if any evidence of the previous injury. More extensive wounds are healed with the deposition of scar tissue. But all encroachments on the continuity of the body structure must be eliminated and the continuity restored if the individual is to survive.

All surgical procedures are designed to restore structural integrity to the whole body, even when that means amputation of a diseased or injured part. Structural integrity is restored when the scar is finally organized and becomes integrated into the continuity of the part affected. Some kinds of diseases and some kinds of injuries do finally heal with resolution, which means there is no visible scarring. Most injuries or disease processes, however, are finally eliminated by the laying down of scar tissue. Once the scar has matured, there may be no further problem with the function of the part. There are some body organs, however, which depend for their function on a very unique architectural structure. The liver and the kidneys, for example, must retain their relationship of functional parts in order to do their work well. When scar tissue is produced by injuries to organs of this kind, their future function may be seriously compromised. It is therefore advantageous to the individual if the total amount of scarring can be minimized. Many nursing processes are devoted to limiting the amount of tissue involvement in infection and disease, and the logic of such activities rests with the total function left to the individual once continuity has been restored by the scarring process. The scar only restores continuity to the structure—it can never assume the functional role of the cells it has replaced. The conservation of structural integrity is the necessary defense of anatomical and physiological wholeness and is therefore the basis for a multitude of nursing interventions.

The Conservation of Personal Integrity

For every individual, his own sense of identity and self-worth is the most compelling evidence of wholeness. There is always a privacy to individual life which is shared through common experience, but the decision to share or not is always a guarded expression of one's private will. The need to assume responsibility for one's own decisions develops with the gradual process of growth and development, and even the young child learns to cherish the right to make some decisions that are his own.

Every person defines himself, and self-esteem is a necessary correlate for successful social life. The variety of factors which contribute to self-definitions are so complex that it is often difficult to sort them out for individual appraisal. Cultural, ethnic, religious, and socioeconomic influences form the baseline upon which individual life experiences make it possible for an individual to identify himself as a unique person. Such uniqueness is defended, because it represents a defense of the integrity, the oneness, of individual life, and every person must learn to value himself as a person.

Few life experiences represent a greater threat to that cherished self-definition than does an episode of illness, and particularly that kind of illness which requires hospitalization. Once having recognized the necessity to submit himself to the care of other persons, the individual must also come to terms with the loss of independence which always threatens his ability to make decisions for himself. It has long been characteristic of hospitalization, and in fact of all kinds of health care including that in the doctor's office, that the individual's right to make decisions in his own behalf is seriously curtailed.

While nurses have always zealously guarded the patient's privacy, that usually has meant his physical privacy. Too infrequently has the privacy of his self-image been accorded equal consideration. Admission to a hospital has always meant a sacrifice of personal integrity—others will make decisions, even unimportant decisions, which in the past, the individual has made for himself.

There has also been an unfortunate but persistent trend in health care which has overtones of moral considerations imposed upon patients by physicians and nurses. Censure of some individuals who require medical help because they have "brought illness upon themselves" is not uncommon. Some diagnoses are almost always greeted with moral censure; the care of the alcoholic and the drug addict, for example, is notoriously mixed with disapproval by professional health workers. Moral censure is often directed at obese persons, and the patient who fails to improve because the physician or the nurse feels he has not followed directions is scolded and sometimes rejected. The folk idea that illness is a moral punishment anyway only serves to increase the guilt which many individuals bring to the predicament they face.

Respect from the nurse is essential to the self-respect of the patient. That must include the willingness to permit the individual to make decisions for himself when it is possible, and at the very least to be a partici pant in the decisions that must be made. Moral censure has no place in nursing care. The most expert physical care cannot be expert nursing care unless the personal integrity of the patient is zealously guarded and defended by the nurse.

The Conservation of Social Integrity

Individual life has meaning only in the context of social life. Every individual shares a number of social communities—his family, his friends, his employment, his church, his ethnic group, his city, town, or village, his state, his nation, and, in a time of instant communication, even his world. The ways in which the individual relates to each of these groups influences his behavior. There is a relaxed kind of relationship that characterizes home life which is quite different from that displayed in public groups. But no individual can recognize his wholeness unless it is measured against his relationships with other human beings.

While the predicament of illness is often a very lonely experience, the ties the individual has with other persons continue, not only in the background but as an active determinant of his response to his therapy. In stressful times, the interactions with other persons become more important, not less. Not only does the individual continue to be involved in the concerns of other persons, but his illness itself often creates new problems which he feels intensely and which can be resolved only by the participation of all who are included in his social life. The strengths that come from human relationships are necessary strengths in times of illness, and very often the family is deeply affected by the changes which may result from the illness for a long time into the future. There is a long pattern of isolation from family and friends which has characterized hospitalization. Family members are removed from participation in the care of the patient, and they must follow the "rules" which restrict them just as the patient is bound by the "rules" which govern the hospital's unique social system. The most difficult aspect of a hospitalization, in fact, is the expectation that the patient (and his family) will adopt without question the social restrictions which characterize the institution. Nurses belong to the social environment of the hospital. Patients are dependent upon the good will and concern of hospital employees, and the attitude that the patient comes first has served as rationalization for excluding family members from genuine interaction with the patient. This had been a particularly difficult problem in intensive care units where the patient's needs are rightfully given a priority, but often at the expense of concerned and frightened relatives. A failure to consider the family and friends of the patient is a failure to provide excellent nursing care. Not only does this exclusion create emotional problems for the patient and his family, but the contribution the family must make in pragmatic ways to his future care is also sadly neglected. The patient must be viewed in the context of his family, and without concern for them, he is not accorded holistic nursing care.

In a broader sense, the social integrity of individuals is tied to the viability of the entire social system. Only a society which provides individuals with adequate food, gainful employment, educational opportunities, and excellent medical care is one in which health, in the sense of wholeness, can be obtained. An awareness of the individual's social integrity emphasizes that an episode of illness that requires hospitalization is often a very short interlude in the life-span of the individual. The social system of the hospital is a very artificial one, and concern for the holistic well-being of the individual demands attention to the community attitudes, resources, and commitment to health care in a number of settings other than that of the institution. Community health clinics, and free access to the health delivery system, form a crucial social problem. While preventive health practices are highly desirable and must be pursued, there are additional thousands of persons who are not able to obtain medical care for already existing conditions. The distribution of medical personnel—physicians, nurses, and paramedical workers—so that all geographic and economic areas of the country are equally served is a major issue of social integrity which all health professionals must try to solve. While excellent nursing care is often described as the unique interpersonal relationships of a nurse and her patient, it is also a community commitment to delivery of health care to all members of a society when they need it, and of a quality which assures all persons equal sharing of the rich resource available to the modern health worker. . . .

PATIENT-CENTERED NURSING INTERVENTION

The Vital Importance of Sound Observation

Patient-centered nursing care means *individualized* nursing care. It is predicated on the reality of common experience: every man is a unique individual, and as such he requires a unique constellation of skills, techniques, and ideas designed specifically for him. Such nursing intervention can take place only when the nurse has made an accurate assessment of his unique needs, and this, in turn, is possible only through the formulation of all relevant factors that contribute to the patient's predicament at a given time and place. There are numerous sources of information available in the determination of any single patient's requirements. The ability to utilize all the information about a patient comes with increasing knowledge and maturity in nursing, but even the beginning student can contribute to, and utilize important determinants in, the planning of nursing care.

The fundamental interaction between nurse and patient presupposes that the nurse brings to the relationship the objectivity and discipline of the professional practitioner. The nurse bears a responsibility for evaluation of the patient's condition at the time of actual contact, as well as the ability to anticipate the course of events in the immediate, and often the distant, future. Equipped with all the information available about the patient, the nurse functions in his behalf effectively only in direct proportion to her ability to make relevant observations of him and then to initiate activity that may be required as a result of the observations.

Miss Nightingale wrote, "In dwelling upon the vital importance of *sound* observation, it must never be lost sight of what observation is for. It is not for the sake of piling up miscellaneous information or curious facts, but for the sake of saving life and increasing health and comfort." In the century that has passed since these words were written, the importance of accuracy and relevance of observations has never been stated better. Because we are constantly in contact with our environment, all kinds of signals and stimuli reach us continuously. It is in the selection of those perceptions which bear relevance to the patient's progress that the nurse demonstrates the judgment that permits sound professional decisions.

The word "observation" is defined as "faculty or habit of taking notice." But the Latin noun from which the English word is derived, *observatio*, originally meant "guarding against" or "watching over." Those observations which form the structures of professional assessment are distinguished by the importance that active involvement places upon them. The skills of observation are subservient to the guardian responsibilities of the nurse who makes them. From the outset, the student of nursing should be constantly aware of the signals, both obvious and hidden, which come from her interaction with the patient. Abdellah has called these "overt" and "covert" needs, because the apparent intent of a patient's behavior may often substitute for a real intent of far greater importance and relevance to his well-being.

The professional skill of "observations" requires that the test of "relevance" always be intrinsic to the act. All observations of patient behavior take place within an environment which influences his behavior, and thus the relevance may well reflect the environment as well. A patient may not have displayed any behavior that suggested anxiety until another patient within his milieu became noisy or desperately ill, or, perhaps, died. On the other hand, a patient may become increasingly fearful as the time for an operative procedure draws near. A patient may be rested and relaxed on a morning after a good night's sleep, but irritable and tired on another morning when his sleep has been interrupted because of some distraction during the night. Nurses frequently can see measurable relaxation in patients following their morning care. There are countless situations in the environmental exchange which influence the patient's response, and they must be identified when they occur.

Another important dimension in observation is the passage of time. The expectation of change characterizes all medical and nursing goals, and therapy is decidedly based on deliberate anticipation of change. The entire semantics of medical care is formulated on concepts of change. The patient is described by relating his "progress." He may be "improving" or he may be "going downhill." He "reacts" or "responds" to a therapeutic intervention, such as a medication or a treatment. His disease is a "process" which includes the idea of an onset, a course, and a termination. Thus an observation which is relevant at one time may no longer be accurate at another. Some responses are almost instantaneous, and some are gradual and subtle. Observations of his reactions at the onset of his disease should be quite different from those when he is nearing convalescence. And observations before a treatment or a nursing process is accomplished will not be the same as those evaluating the effects of such activity after it is completed. Observations are continuous, repetitive, and changing, because they must, to retain their validity and usefulness, reflect the constant and changing nature of the individual's response to his illness. Many therapeutic designs, in fact, include a time factor as an aspect of their success. If one treatment does not bring the desired results in a specific time, then another may be tried in its stead. Only cautious observation can provide the data for making decisions of such importance.

Observations become relevant when they fit into a pattern of orderly relationships. If the patient's condition has been altered by the administration of a drug, the importance of the drug to the change is a basic part of the observation. This is true of any active intervention in the patient's progress, but it may be equally essential in assessment of the disease process. Knowledge of the expected course of a disease influences the relevance of observations because an unexpected development may presage great danger if it goes unobserved. Recognition of priorities of importance in the changing pattern of the patient's response depends on thorough knowledge of disease processes and their pathophysiological implications. Of equal importance is knowledge of the expectations of the therapeutic purpose in the medical and nursing plan for the patient. Here, too, an unexpected or untoward response may demand intervention not previously indicated.

If observation is practiced as a "guardian" activity, it is successful only when it is, in fact, used to initiate activity on the part of the nurse. Some observations are important because they contribute information that the doctor must have in planning the medical care. Others are important because they contribute information which *both the nurse and the doctor* may use in planning care. Still other observations are important because they contribute information which *the nurse* must have in planning care. Whatever their ultimate contribution to the patient's care, the measure of usefulness is dependent upon the institution of the necessary action they indicate. Observation is not an end in itself, but a tool that is used to guide patient care. As a guide to action, it constitutes an important part of the nurse-patient interaction. There is a mutuality of response which assures the paient that he is in safe hands and a continuing assessment by the nurse of the effects of her ministrations.

In addition, the sharing of knowledge gained by observation assures the necessary continuity of care from one group of nurses to the next, and from the nursing personnel to the medical personnel responsible for the patient's care. As information is accumulated, it serves as a continuing evaluation of the patient's progress. And because, for all its genius, modern health care is constantly learning and appraising, the consistent recording of observations contributes to the furtherance of knowledge. The precision of description of the patient's response to his disease and its treatment illuminates and enlarges the knowledge available concerning that disease. Thus, observations correctly made, sensibly utilized, and diligently recorded extend the "guardian" role of the observer beyond the individual who benefits directly to many who may benefit in the future.

Nursing and the Scientific Method

The volume of information presented by careful evaluation of each patient is often extensive and always complex. The problems of organizing such information into a workable formula which assures every individual of adequate nursing care, while it simultaneously produces a work load which is realistic for nursing personnel, is one of the most crucial issues that face nurses in practice. Nursing literature is replete with formulations for the development of nursing care plans. There has even been a hearty discussion whether such plans are worth producing at all. The fundamental question is one of selecting out of the multiplicity of needs for each individual those concerns which deserve priority of attention from the nurse. The long tradition of nurses being "all things to all patients" continues to obscure the readiness with which priorities can be assigned.

Much of the nursing literature has concerned itself with the concept of a "nursing diagnosis"—an idea that recurs without adequate examination of what a diagnosis really is. According to Engel, a medical diagnosis is "predictive and statistical," *and it is nothing more*. The diagnosis provides the physician with a direction; it is a broad generalization which must be uniquely and individually assessed for every patient. It is never an end in itself. The diagnosis tells the physician—as it should, indeed, tell the nurse—the kinds of examinations and therapies which he can select for the treatment of a patient, but it does not give him the explicit details for care, which come only from the most careful evaluation of the patient's symptoms, behavior, past history, and contributing factors such as age, sex, social and psychological determinants, nutritional state, and the individual's response to the treatment already administered.

There are obvious advantages to the use of a diagnostic designation since the expectations and the therapy are guided by the predictability of the diagnosis itself. In addition, there is a *language of diagnosis*. It is universally understood and can accomplish the transmission of a great deal of information in very few words. But the language of medical diagnosis, for all of its importance to nurses, is the particular province of the physician. In the past, only the physician was legally permitted to make a diagnosis. Nurses have always contributed to the process, and in many ways have made diagnostic decisions themselves, but the nurse has never been entirely free to use the language of diagnosis in reporting her findings. There are many traditions of diagnostic language usage which nurses quickly learn when they are in a clinical environment. Some of these traditions seem strange and even ludicrous, but they have nevertheless been charged with intense feeling and concern by both physicians and nurses. The nurse, for example, observing the presence of blood coming from a wound was taught to record: "Bright red drainage." To have called the drainage "bloody" was an infraction of the unspoken rule against using diagnostic language.

There is some, but only some, relaxation of that restriction in modern practice, and it derives entirely from the presence of skilled nurses in intensive care units. In such units it has become increasingly necessary for the nurse to make diagnoses, but they are frankly *medical* diagnoses, and even though the necessity exists, there is still some aura of legal restraint in this kind of nursing activity.

While the physician has immediately available a language of diagnosis, which nurses must understand and use in limited ways, there is no precise language of nursing diagnosis. This lack of precision makes it very difficult indeed for nurses to establish a method for "predictive" purposes which will meet the criteria of a diagnostic generalization.

The word *diagnosis* is freely used by many people who, in doing so, pinpoint a process in the language of cause and effect. The garage mechanic, for example, may "diagnose" a difficulty in an automobile motor. But the free use of the term by an automobile mechanic does not have the same legal restraint that the term has in health care. Only the physician may diagnose—that is his obligation and his privilege. Whatever participation nurses have is delegated by a specific physician in a specific instance.

What the nurse really needs is a method of gathering and evaluating the information about a patient which makes it possible to plan intelligently for his care. Such a method is, in fact, the essence of the physician's diagnostic responsibility. The careful gathering of information, the formulation of plans, and the carrying out of decisions based on those plans are a simple statement of the scientific method. Nurses may and should use a scientific method in the assessment of patient care.

As emphasized above, the importance of observation in this process is fundamental to its success. The guardian activity demands a cautious gathering of data—not only from what the nurse can observe for herself, but also from the information that can be gained from the patient's medical and nursing history, his laboratory and x-ray findings, his progress as recorded by the physician and by the nurse in frequent notations on the chart, and from that which is available about him from family, friends, and even his roommate in the hospital. Every source of information should be explored. The nurse must come to know everything that can be known about the patient. Quite obviously this will present a body of data which must be organized and evaluated so that priorities can be established and a sensible evaluation of progress can be made. Some of the data which are available may have grave importance for the patient's well-being, but some of it will prove to be unimportant and irrelevant. The entire problem of planning for a patient's care rests with the test of relevancy and priority.

The scientific method offers the nurse a basis for selecting essential and prior data which will structure the nature of nursing intervention. According to Feiblemann the first step in the scientific method is the awareness of "provocative facts." A fact which provokes attention is one which, falling on fertile (i.e., knowledgeable) ground, must be heeded. This represents a selection process at the outset. It means that the nurse must have a store of knowledge which serves to alert her to the implications inherent in any available data. The discovery of penicillin was stimulated by a provocative fact. In Fleming's laboratory, an agar plate on which a pathogenic organism was growing was contaminated by bread mold *(Penicillium notatum)* by accident. The researcher, noticing the contaminant, was provoked by the fact that a clear area of agar surrounded the bread mold growth. That meant that something in the bread mold had killed the pathogenic organisms in its immediate vicinity. Only a knowledgeable and alert investigator would have responded to this provocative fact in ways other than dismay that the agar plate had been spoiled by the contaminant.

In establishing his diagnosis, the physician responds to provocative facts. The patient's presenting symptoms immediately alert him to the possibilities of their cause. His attention is directed toward the explanation of those symptoms which can be either proved or disproved by various testing procedures. There are, for example, many kinds of disease processes which are manifested by a cough, fever, and a feeling of weakness and loss of appetite. Alerted by these facts, the physician will order the diagnostic tests which will finally help him decide whether the individual has pneumonia or severe bronchitis or flu or simply a very bad cold. The initial information has meaning to the physician because he has knowledge that makes it meaningful. His skill in finally determining what the patient's illness really is depends upon how he explores the condition. According to Feiblemann, the next step in the scientific method is the establishment of a "testable hypothesis." A hypothesis is a hunch; it is often a statement that says, *"if* this is true, *then* this must be true." The if-then statement must be testable because if it is not, there is no way to determine whether the initial evaluation was correct or false. On the basis of his knowledge, the results of his investigation, and the breadth of his experience, the physician makes a testable hypothesis. He decides that his patient has pneumonia and institutes therapy for it. In short, he "tests" his diagnostic decision. If the patient responds to his treatment, then he has made a hypothesis that was correct—it has been tested and the success of therapy establishes the fact that it was a valid hypothesis. However, if the treatment is not successful, then he must respond first to the provocative facts which tell him it is unsuccessful, and then reformulate a testable hypothesis which allows him to alter his treatment accordingly. By testing, he has learned that his original hypothesis was not correct, and by continuation of the scientific method, he reaches another hypothesis based, in part, on the failure of the first.

The scientific method can be used as readily by the nurse in establishing the guidelines for patient care as it is by the physician. Even lacking the precision of diagnostic language, the establishment of provocative facts and a testable hypothesis which arises from the nurse's knowledge and ability to use those facts is a method of establishing necessary care that can be easily employed in nursing.

The nurse provides care for that patient. She knows his diagnosis (it is now definitively established as pneumonia), and she has fortified herself with all the information she can learn about him. She knows, for example, that he is an elderly man, that his food and fluid intake has been meager because of a lack of appetite related to his disease, that he is weak and moves about with great effort even in bed. She knows that when he coughs, he should have a productive cough, removing the excess phlegm which has been stimulated to form in his lungs by his disease. She knows that coughing is itself a very active process which will add to the fatigue which the patient already has. She becomes "provoked" by the fact that the patient is not coughing productively. She observes that he coughs frequently, but it is a high, dry hack which does not bring the excess secretions up and that even this coughing is very fatiguing to him. The physician is apprised that the cough is nonproductive, and so to assist the patient he orders intermittent positive pressure treatments which will force the patient to bring up some of the phlegm. The nurse realizes at once that even with the assistance of the machine, the patient will be exhausted after his treatments. She hypothesizes that he will need time to rest and recuperate following his treatment. She therefore schedules other activities, such as his bath, his meals, and his medications administration in relation to his IPPB treatments so that he is certain of a rest period following each IPPB treatment. She might state the scientific method she used as follows:

Provocative facts:

1. The elderly man is diagnosed as having pneumonia.
2. He is weak and fatigued and needs the assistance of IPPB to make his otherwise exhausting cough productive.
3. Unless the secretions are raised, he will be a candidate for serious lung complications which will render the therapy ineffective.
4. To conserve his energy so that he will have energy available for the healing process, his expense of energy must be carefully regulated.

Testable hypothesis:

If the necessary removal of secretions is to be effective without completely exhausting the patient, then all nursing activities should be planned to allow for periods of rest following each IPPB treatment.

The hypothesis is then tested by establishing a protocol of care which will be understood by all persons caring for the patient. For example, if the first IPPB treatment is scheduled at 9 a.m., then the patient should be given his breakfast well before that time and the bath schedule adapted so that he will be permitted a full hour of rest following the IPPB treatment. Evaluation of the success of this plan then comes from continuing observation of the individual, including any evidence in his behavior that he is not becoming overly tired following procedures which he must have during the course of a twenty-four hour period. Through observation, the nurse will soon learn whether this hypothesis is a valid one. If it does not achieve its goal, then the indications of failure contribute to the new provocative facts, and a new testable hypothesis must then be formulated. Since our expectation is that the patient will improve with medical and nursing care, the hypothesis will also be changed when the patient's condition has improved so that this kind of conservation of energy is no longer necessary. As he gains in strength with healing, those facts will also be observed, and since he is an elderly man, he will be mobilized to his point of tolerance in order to prevent the complications which inactivity can also produce.

The success of the scientific method rests with the knowledge and skills the nurse brings to her task. The more the nurse knows, the more likely that she will find essential facts provocative and the more likely that she will be able to formulate a testable hypothesis which will provide a valid form of nursing intervention.

Modes of Communication

Nursing skills of all kinds represent a "language" which speaks more eloquently to the sick than words can possibly do. The certainty and sureness of what the nurse does for the patient tells him he is safe. The knowledge the nurse brings to bear on his problems tells him he is secure. Attentiveness and prompt fulfillment of his needs tell him that he is respected and cherished as a person.

Verbal communication between patient and nurse may range from the most casual social exchange to a complex teacher-learner relationship, and skilled verbal communication is often therapeutic as well. Frequently the beginning student finds verbal communication awkward and difficult. But, as knowledge grows, and the ability to assess patient needs increases, the uses of verbal communication become more comfortable and productive for both the patient and the nurse. The nurse becomes a teacher when her confidence in her own knowledge allows her to recognize the patient's need to learn. This, too, becomes easier with experience and increasing maturity.

Communication between other members of the health team concerned with the patient's welfare is vital to the provision of a consistent plan for care. A basic exchange must always exist between the nurse and the doctor. The nurse acts as the doctor's agent in his absence and is directly responsible for the actual performance of the therapeutic measures he prescribes. Each contributes the special knowledge and skill which defines the respective roles of the physician and the nurse, and, of course, the patient is central to their mutual concern. The nurse is obligated to fulfill the doctor's orders in an accurate and precise way, including meeting the specifications as to time and place that may contribute to the treatment.

Medicine and nursing share their historical growth in modern hospitals. Both disciplines have become increasingly complex, and both demand an exacting educational preparation. The demands of new knowledge, coupled with the technological progress of the past fifty years, have resulted in shifting to the nurse many responsibilities that once were performed only by doctors. There is good evidence that such shifting roles continue and, in fact, seem accelerated in the age of electronics. But the focus of both doctors and nurses remains on the patient and his predicament of illness. With this central concern in both professions, a fruitful dialogue, grounded in continuing communication, is possible and essential.

Many other professional workers function in the patient's interests too. These include the dietitian, the social worker, the physical and occupational therapists and, in some hospitals, the professional hospital administrator, both in the ward setting and in the hospital as a whole. Here, too, continuing communication is essential in the patient's interest, and frequently the nurse becomes the focus of communication because of her intimate involvement with the patient. The hospital chaplain, or private religious advisor, is another individual who may contribute to the dialogue that assures quality patient care.

Nonprofessional hospital workers who are concerned with many aspects of nursing care can make significant contributions to the information about a patient. Regular seeking of such communication is part of many hospital routines. The licensed practical nurse, ward aide, or attendant, and sometimes the volunteer worker are participants in regular conferences that promote the exchange of information and observation which may aid in the care of the patient. A new technician, the so-called physician's assistant, has recently appeared on the hospital scene. It must be emphasized that, even with the uncertainty of the physician-assistant role, such individuals do not perform nursing tasks and are not, in any sense, nurse workers. Any person entrusted with responsibility for patient care, including those delegated by the physician for portions of his tasks, must enter the mainstream of communication in the patient's interest.

The patient's family are concerned witnesses to his welfare, and they often can provide the staff with information that cannot be obtained in any other way. Even their expressions of disaffection or dissatisfaction may bring important knowledge to the staff, because they may communicate distressing fears and anxieties which they share with the patient. They are, in any event, so essential to his well-being that the nurse must have free channels of communication with them as part of the routine seeking of information which will benefit the patient.

In addition to the variety of ways in which information is disseminated by verbal means, the use of written records and charts represents another important method of communication. Every hospital ward has a variety of record-keeping duties that are designed to promote the free exchange of essential information about the patient between those who must participate in his care. In the past few years, the recording of nurses' observations has been severely criticized because it lacks substance and relevance. The oft-repeated accusation that nurses spend too much time on "paperwork" frequently fails to recognize that the recording of information is absolutely essential to the patient's continuing welfare. Nurse records should be succinct, but they should also be meaningful; efforts to provide shortcuts by reducing the amount of recording must be planned so that essential knowledge is still transmitted. The written record bears the additional burden of becoming a legal record, and this simply adds to the importance of relevant but accurate selection of observations recorded by the nurse. A well-kept patient history is a gold mine for every student in the care of the patient. Each individual nurse bears a responsbility to add to the record so that the clarity and incisiveness make it the valid communication system it should be.

The two-dimensional concept of a body image is an imperfect and incomplete concept of the experience all human beings share. The loss of a limb, for example, represents far more than a structural change or even a disfigurement. An amputated limb not only disrupts the acceptable landmarks of the body structure, but also threatens the individual's self-percept as a mobile, active participant in his environment. Such participation must be changed by amputation and that means a change in the body percept. The individual is not only structurally altered, the most serious loss is a functional one, and with it the individual's habitual identification of himself as a person. . . .

THE INDIVIDUAL'S TERRITORIAL CLAIM
DEFINES HIM IN THE SOCIAL GROUP

"Individuals," wrote Thoreau, "like nations, must have suitable and broad boundaries, even a considerable neutral ground between them." Not every person can retreat, as Thoreau did to Walden Pond, to establish a "considerable neutral ground" and to surround himself, thereby, with inviolate space. Yet every individual requires space, and both the establishment of his personal boundaries and their defense are essential components of his behavior.

There are many boundaries that are marked only by the intense feeling which erected them in the first place. Certainly this is true of nations; even when there is no threat to the boundary line that separates two nations, the intensity of affect is apparent when the line is crossed. The borders that create the United States are quiet borders, but nevertheless constructed of patriotic fervor. Nations with threatened borders live in an atmosphere of political uncertainty. The peace that reigns inside the American boundary lines ill equips a citizen of this country to understand the anguish that is a daily experience for an Israeli who lives in a kibbutz on the Syrian border. In every political arena where border dispute is a persistent fact, the dislocation of the group is reflected in the individuals who compose it. There are boundaries, too, of cultural allegiance that influence the political and social goals of the entire populace. Until very recently, the immigration laws of the United States reflected cultural boundaries that excluded Central Europeans and Orientals from joining the "melting pot" of American life. And social boundaries may be the most subtle, but the most powerful, of all. The civil rights movement is directed at social boundaries, and these walls which cannot be seen have proven to be the most difficult to tumble. Social boundaries are woven of the cloth of shared value systems, and irrational and ignorant as such restrictive devices may be, such borders are defended with a ferocity which even exceeds that of the patriot. The old saying that "a man's home is his castle" is incorporated into the American Constitution, in which the right to search and seizure without due process of law is expressly forbidden. . . .

The consideration of space needs of the individual as a determinant of nursing intervention is an expression of the influence of other living beings in the environment as part of the perceptual information received by the individual. There is little doubt that space requirements are influential in human behavior and that such interpretations are culturally induced and socially prescribed. When an individual comes into the hospital, he discovers that an entirely new set of space definitions are an established fact of the cultural determinants in the hospital itself. His personal territorial claim is immediately restricted to the boundaries of his "unit." If he must remain in bed, his territory has shrunk to the limits of the bed itself. "His" bedside table and chair and perhaps "his" half of the closet or dresser space establish the limits that are now his boundaries. He must learn rather promptly that encroachment on the space in the hospital is especially dangerous because the aseptic ritual establishes safe and unsafe zones, and the walls that separate them are invisible. The concern for asepsis is real, but the frequency with which he may be enjoined to respect the territorial limits of aseptic safety may be threatening in itself. If, for example, he has been "taught" not to touch a sterile dressing on his own body, the inroad on his territorial prerogative may be considerable. The unusual intensity with which many patients defend the artifacts in their immediate environment may well be related to their need to establish a bubble of "self" that supports their sense of integrity, both personal and social. Nurses are often impatient with individuals who refuse to allow a wheelchair out of their sight, even when they have no plan to use it for a length of time. But when the bedridden patient is finally given permission to expand his territory and the success of such a move depends on the ready access of a wheelchair, his defense is more than a selfish focus on his own needs. The competition for the upholstered chair in a two-bed hospital room is another example of the territorial demands made by patients.

It is hardly possible to provide nursing care without entering the personal zone of the individual. And there is never an assurance that the interpretation of such an infringement will mean the same things to all patients. They will bring their own cultural values to the hospital with them, and even though they must adopt those of the hospital during their stay, the emotional impact of this demand may be a telling one. The use of space is, of course, equally a factor in the nurse's behavior, and thus the interaction between patient and nurse may involve their mutual concerns about spacing. From Hall's analysis of the zones of interaction, the nurse can use territory as a positive contribution to the patient's comfort and well-being. One obvious source of control is the voice level. Some of the subjects of conversation between nurse and patient require the emotional level of the personal or even the far phase of the intimate zone. Raising the voice level in the personal or intimate zone has the effect of widening the distance, whereas the same behavior in the social zone decreases the distance. The essential communication involving the personal factors in the patient's care may be projected into a personal zone by the use of the voice, even if the distance maintained is a social one and thereby more comfortable for the patient. The direction of the gaze is another means of controlling the distance; during those aspects of care that require encroachment on the personal zone of the patient, the nurse can reduce the anxiety by directing her eyes away from the patient's face. In fact, this is precisely the outlet used by many patients during the bathing procedure. They rarely engage the gaze of the nurse, and by looking at a far point, reduce the distance to a tolerable level.

The culturally determined territorial rules of the hospital are temporary as far as the patient is concerned, even though the nursing personnel subscribes to them without analysis or understanding. There are instances when nurses recognize the behavior that tells them the patient is uncomfortable, but this is rarely attributed to territorial demand. Some conversations with patients, involving doctors or nurses, would produce very different results if the distance zones were understood. For example, inquiries about personal problems and needs of the patient directed from the foot of the bed may be responded to in one way, whereas the same conversation at the patient's head level will be quite different. This, too, must vary with the cultural antecedents which influence the patient's behavior. The defense of territory is an essential aspect of personal and social integrity. When the bubble of territory is challenged and disrupted as often it must be during hospitalization, the individual must mount his defense in another way or sacrifice a portion of his feelings about himself. If, in addition, his defense is not understood or tolerated, then the effect on the therapeutic process may become measurable. The patient who demands that his chair be left in sight is defending his integrity. The nurse who stubbornly ignores his request may well be defending hers.

Appendix
C

Glossary*

adaptation The process of change whereby the individual retains his or her integrity, or wholeness, within the realities of the person's environment. It is the expression of the integration of the entire organism. It is possible to have degrees of adaptation. It is not an all-or-none phenomenon.

antecedents Those things that come before.

change The essence of life. It is directed, purposeful, and meaningful, and eminently understandable.

commonplaces Usual words necessary for the description of nursing; include nurse, person, health, and environment.

communication Verbal and nonverbal meaningful exchange between individuals.

compensatory An adjective that means "counterbalancing."

concept Created when a relationship between commonplaces is described (e.g., adaptation, wholeness).

conceptual environment That part of the environment which refers to a life of ideas, of symbolic exchange, and of belief, tradition and judgment.

conservation Keeping together. The product of adaptation. The maintaining of a safe balance of nursing intervention and patient participation.

coping Patterns of behavior. Processes that arise from the past.

creativity The marriage of the art and the science of nursing.

disease Patterns of adaptive change.

energy conservation Nursing interventions based on the conservation of the patient's energy.

environment The internal and external environment.

external environment The perceptual, operational, and conceptual environments.

haptic system The perceptual system that responds to touch.

health Wholeness. Patterns of adaptive change.

holistic Entire.

homeorrhesis Stabilized flow; emphasizes the fluidity of change.

homeostasis Stable state; energy sparing state; state of conservation.

hypothesis "If this is true, than that must be true"; a hunch.

integrity Unity; oneness.

internal environment The physical and the physiologic functioning of the individual.

---

*These definitions are paraphrased from the works of Myra Levine.

261

model   A framework for the design of nursing care.

nosology   The classification of disease; represents the advantage of observation and a precision of terms to describe.

nursing   Nursing is a subculture, possessing ideas and values that are unique to nurses. Nursing is human interaction.

operational environment   The unseen and unheard parts of the individual's environment that are not perceived by way of the sensory organs.

organismic response   The capacity of the organism to become adequate to its environmental conditions.

pattern   A message of orderly and sequential change.

patienthood   Temporary condition of dependency, which through the combined efforts of nurse and patient, will terminate as soon as independence can be restored to the individual.

perceptual environment   That part of the environment to which the individual responds with his sensory organs.

person   Whole, feeling, believing, thinking, dreaming, somewhat imperfect, and unpredictable being. Unique and proud. Individual integrity and unity are axiomatic.

personal integrity   One's sense of identity and self-definition.

provocative facts   Presenting symptoms alerting one to a cause.

redundancy   Series of adaptive responses available when stability of the organism is challenged. Interplay of back-up systems.

social integrity   Life gains meaning through relationships. Nursing interventions designed to maintain these relationships.

structural integrity   Process of healing is the restoration of structural integrity. Nursing interventions that promote healing and maintain structural integrity.

supportive interventions   Activities designed to maintain the status quo or the downward course.

survival   Responses that cost the least. Survival itself depends on the quality of the adaptation possible for the individual.

territory   The space that individuals claim for themselves and the boundaries that are marked by the intense feelings that erected them in the first place.

theory of nursing   A body of knowledge must be usable in nursing practice. It must successfully describe the requirements of all the patients.

therapeutic interventions   Interventions that influence adaptation in a favorable way. Enhance the adaptive responses available to the patient.

trophicognosis   Nursing care judgment arrived at by the scientific method.

well-being   Consequence of experience in relationship to the environment. When the organism is in tune with the environment and surroundings; is whole.

whole   Oneness, integrity, of the individual; parts within a boundary that is open and fluid.

Appendix

D

Annotated Bibliography*

Brunner, M. (1985). A conceptual approach to critical care nursing using Levine's model. Focus on Critical Care, 12(2), 39–44. This article presents an example of Levine's conceptual model for the care of a cardiac patient. One modification of the conceptual model is the use of nursing diagnoses, rather than trophicognoses. A nursing care plan is given.

Crawford-Gamble, P.E. (1986). An application of Levine's conceptual model. Perioperative Nursing Quarterly, 2(1), 64–70. Levine's conservation model is used as a framework to guide care of a patient undergoing reimplantation of digits of her right hand. The four conservation principles are used as a basis for nursing care throughout the surgical experience.

Esposito, C.H., & Leonard, M.K. (1980). Myra Estrin Levine. In Nursing Theories Conference Group, Nursing theories. The base for professional nursing practice (pp. 150–163). Englewood Cliffs, NJ: Prentice-Hall. An overview of Levine's model is presented. Nursing is defined and a description of the four conservation principles is included. The nursing process is described in detail and an application of the model to a clinical situation is offered. Limitations of the model are identified. This review suggests that the authors misinterpreted much of Levine's work.

Fawcett, J., Cariello, F.P., Davis, D.A., Farley, J., Zimmaro, D.M., & Watts, R.J. (1987). Conceptual models of nursing: Application to critical care nursing practice. Dimensions of Critical Care Nursing, 6, 202–213. This article includes a brief analysis of Levine's conceptual model and identification of trophicognoses for a 57-year-old man who was dying from cardiac disease.

Foli, K.J., Johnson, T., Marriner, A., Poat, M.C., Poppa, L., & Zoretich, S.T. (1986). Myra Estrin Levine. Four conservation principles. In A. Marriner (Ed.), Nursing theorists and their work (pp. 3353–3344). St. Louis: CV Mosby. This chapter presents an overview of Levine's conservation model.

Foli, K.J., Johnson, T., Marriner-Tomey, A., Poat, M.C., Poppa, L., Woeste, R., & Zoretich, S.T. (1989). Myra Estrin Levine: Four conservation principles. In A. Marriner-Tomey (Ed.), Nursing theorists and their work (2nd ed., pp. 391–401). St. Louis: C.V. Mosby. The authors provide a biographical essay of Levine, and a focused analysis and critique of the conservation principles as a model. An extensive reference list of all Levine's publications is included, as well as references to citings of her work.

---

*Fawcett, J. (1989). Analysis and evaluation of conceptual models in nursing (2nd ed., pp. 165–167). Philadelphia: F.A. Davis. Updated and reprinted with permission.

Foreman, M. (1989). Confusion in the hospitalized elderly: Incidence, onset, and associated factors. Research in Nursing & Health, 12, 21–29. Using Levine's Conservation Model, Foreman studied variables related to the onset of confusion in elderly patients admitted to the hospital. Ten variables related to the four conservation principles were found to be associated significantly with the onset of confusion. The findings suggest that for nursing interventions to be successful, they must be guided by all four conservation principles.

Herbst, S. (1981). Impairments as a result of cancer. In N. Martin, N. Holt, & D. Hicks (Eds.), Comprehensive rehabilitation nursing (pp. 553–578). New York: McGraw-Hill. This book chapter presents an overview of Levine's conservation principles. The conservation principles are then applied to the problems the cancer patient experiences.

Hirschfeld, M.J. (1976). The cognitively impaired older adult. American Journal of Nursing, 76, 1981–1984. Care of the cognitively impaired older adult is discussed in the context of Levine's conservation principles. Theories of aging and cognitive impairment are incorporated into the discussion.

Jacob-Kramer, M.K., Levine, M.E., & Menke, E.M. (1988). Parse, R.R. (1987). Nursing science: Major paradigms, theories and critiques (book review). Nursing Science Quarterly, 1(4), 183–186. Levine uses this critique to explain how nursing spends too much time on rhetoric, and not enough time on substance. She evaluates the critiques of the models presented in the book focusing on the need for nurses to offer critical judgment of their peers in order to advance nursing. She is honest and substantive in her recommendations.

Leonard, M.K. (1985). Myra Estrin Levine. In Nursing Theories Conference Group, Nursing theories. The base for professional nursing practice (2nd ed., pp. 180–194). Englewood Cliffs, NJ: Prentice-Hall. This book chapter presents a review of Levine's conservation model. The review does not present an accurate account of the model inasmuch as several aspects of Levine's work were misinterpreted.

Levine, M.E. (1963). Florence Nightingale: The legend that lives. Nursing Forum, 11(4), 25–35. Levine describes how Nightingale's work and beliefs about nursing remain fundamental to the profession of nursing. Careful reading of the article provides the student of Levine with information about the source of Levine's philosophy of nursing. Some major points include the notion that nursing is a separate discipline from physician practice, the nurse exercises judgment in the interest of the patient, the nurse communicates "her" knowledge, and the nurse considers the effect of the environment on the delivery of nursing care.

Levine, E.B., & Levine, M.E. (1965). Hippocrates, father of nursing, too? American Journal of Nursing, 65(12), 86–88. Myra and her husband explore the philosophy of caring of the father of medicine. They do not state that Hippocrates is the father of nursing but do suggest a relationship of his approach to patient centered care that has become the focus of nursing. This article provides information of the Levines' philosophy of nursing care which is fundamental to the development of a model for the delivery of nursing care.

Levine, M.E. (1966). Adaptation and assessment: A rationale for nursing intervention. American Journal of Nursing, 66, 2450–2453. Historical developments that influenced nursing are reviewed. The role of the nurse in promoting adaptation to disease is addressed. Emphasis is placed on scientific knowledge as well as awareness of individual responses as the basis for assessment.

Levine, M.E. (1966). Trophicognosis: An alternative to nursing diagnosis. In American Nurses' Association Regional Clinical Conference (Vol. 2, pp. 55–70). New York: American Nurses Association. Trophicognosis is offered as a more accurate term to describe nursing judgments than diagnosis. The term is defined and described in detail and is contrasted with nursing diagnosis. A comprehensive clinical example is included.

Levine, M.E. (1967). The four conservation principles of nursing. Nursing Forum, 6, 45–59. The conservation principles central to Levine's conceptual model are presented in detail. General clinical examples are included to augment understanding of the principles.

Levine, M.E. (1969). The pursuit of wholeness. American Journal of Nursing, 69, 93–98. The concepts of wholeness and interaction of person and environment are discussed. Four levels of organismic response are described and examples of each are offered. Five perceptual systems are discussed and possible dysfunctions are considered. The holistic approach to nursing is presented.

Levine, M.E. (1969). Introduction to clinical nursing. Philadelphia: F.A. Davis. This book contains the first comprehensive presentation of Levine's Conservation Model. The first and last chapters present the major concepts of the model. Designed as a beginning level medical-surgical nursing text, the book includes several other chapters considering nursing care of patients with failure of nervous system integration; failure of integration resulting from hormonal disturbance; disturbances of homeostasis in terms of fluid and electrolyte imbalance, nutritional needs, systemic oxygen needs, and cellular oxygen needs; aberrant cellular growth; and an inflammatory process. Each of these chapters includes a list of objectives, essential science concepts, and the relevant nursing process.

Levine, M.E. (1971). Holistic nursing. Nursing Clinics of North America, 6, 253–264. The concept of holism is discussed and contrasted with dualistic, mechanistic approaches. The four conservation principles are delineated. The importance of organismic generalizations in nursing is presented.

Levine, M.E. (1971). Renewal for nursing. Philadelphia: F.A. Davis. This book was written for the nurse returning to nursing practice. Levine maintains that the returning nurse has retained her identity as a nurse, has matured, and has considerably more knowledge and skill than she may credit herself. In the first chapter, Levine describes the patient in terms of current concepts, such as "the patient is a person." She uses her conceptual model definition of health as wholeness throughout the book. The content follows the format of Levine's text, Introduction to clinical nursing. Each chapter identifies relevant pragmatics, including related diagnostic entities, related nursing procedures, and appropriate drug therapy. The concluding chapter focuses on the implications of recent research for improved nursing care.

Levine, M.E. (1973). Introduction to clinical nursing (2nd ed.). Philadelphia: F.A. Davis. The second edition of Levine's textbook. Format is similar to the first edition. Content is updated and greater emphasis is placed on the changing role of the nurse.

Levine, M. (1988). Myra Levine. In T.M. Schorr & A. Zimmerman (Eds.) Making choices: Taking chances. St. Louis: C.V. Mosby. In this chapter Myra writes about her life, her joys, her sorrows, her triumphs, her failures. This information cannot be annotated; it must be read. She offers the reader a chance to "get under her skin" and see the universe as she does.

Levine, M.E. (1988). Antecedents from adjunctive disciplines: Creation of nursing theory. Nursing Science Quarterly, 1(1), 16–21. Levine explains that new knowledge (insights, intuitions) is always built on accumulated knowledge. She clarifies the difference between concepts and commonplaces of a discipline, while indicating that scientific knowledge becomes adjunctive to all other disciplines comprising the health related disciplines. She traces the antecedents of nurse theorists, focusing on the "West Coast Parsonians" and the "East Coast Quantumists." She argues for a simple language of theory, and the need for pragmatism. Ultimately she suggests that theory must be understandable and useful for the practicing nurse.

Levine, M.E. (1989). The four conservation principles: Twenty years later. In J.P. Riehl-Sisca (Ed.), Conceptual models for nursing practice (3rd ed., pp. 329–337). Norwalk, CT: Appleton-Lange. This book chapter presents a revision and expansion of several concepts and propositions of Levine's conceptual model. Emphasis is placed on the concepts of conservation and adaptation and the four conservation principles.

Levine, M.E. (1989). The ethics of nursing rhetoric. Image, 21(1), 4–6. Levine explains how nurses have been "caught up" in using language they do not understand and that may in fact not be what they mean, hence is not ethical (patient vs. client; care vs. cure). Attempts to express clinical phenomena (slept well) have been rhetorical, becoming simply slogans without meaning. This has not only confused nurses' relationships with patients but also with physicians, moving nurses and physicians away from rather than closer to collaboration. She ends simply, "We must say what we mean and always mean what we say."

Levine, M.E. (1989). Ration or rescue: The elderly patient in critical care. Critical Care Quarterly, 12(1), 82–89. While the author does not discuss the explicit use of her Conservation Model or principles, she does expand on her beliefs about personhood, the sanctity of life and the alleviation of suffering. Applying ethical principles to care of the elderly in critical care, the importance of personal integrity is exemplified.

Littrell, K., & Schumann, L.L. (1989). Promoting sleep for the patient with a myocardial infarction. Critical Care Nurse, 9(3), 44–49. The authors propose that Levine's conservation principles can provide a basis for meeting the rest/sleep needs of the patient who has had a myocardial infarction. A review of the non-REM and REM sleep cycles is provided. Nursing interventions directed towards conserving energy by providing restful sleep are discussed.

Newport, M.A. (1984). Conserving thermal energy and social integrity in the newborn. Western Journal of Nursing Research, 6, 176–197. Levine's principles of conservation of energy and social integrity provided the conceptual base for the study reported in this article. The investigator compared temperature of infants placed in a warmer immediately after birth with those of infants placed on their mothers' chests immediately after birth. No temperature differences were found between the two groups of infants.

Pieper, B.A. (1983). Levine's nursing model. In J.J. Fitzpatrick & A.L. Whall (Eds.), Conceptual models of nursing: Analysis and application (pp. 101–115). Bowie, MD: Robert Brady. This book chapter presents an overview of Levine's conservation model.

Savage, T.A., & Culbert, C. (1989). Early intervention: The unique role of nursing. Journal of Professional Nursing, 4(5), 339–345. The authors provide the readers with a brief explanation for early intervention, its goals and expected outcomes. Levine's conservation principles are used to develop a plan of care for a family experiencing a developmentally disabling disorder.

Taylor, J.W. (1974). Measuring the outcomes of nursing care. Nursing Clinics of North America, 9, 337–348. A pilot project to develop criterion measures of patient outcomes of nursing care is described in a step-by-step manner. Levine's four conservation principles are used as the frame of reference for defining common nursing problems in the care of neurological patients.

Winslow, E.H., Lane, L.D., & Gaffney, F.A. (1984). Oxygen consumption and cardiovascular response in patients and normal adults during in-bed and out-of-bed toileting. Journal of Cardiac Rehabilitation, 4, 348–354.

Winslow, E.H., Lane, L.D., & Gaffney, F.A. (1985). Oxygen consumption and cardiovascular response in control adults and acute myocardial infarction patients during bathing. Nursing Research, 34, 164–169. These two reports focus on the results of studies based on Levine's principle of the conservation of energy.

Yeates, D.A., & Roberts, J.E. (1984). A comparison of two bearing-down techniques during the second stage of labor. Journal of Nurse-Midwifery, 29, 3–11. This article presents the report of a pilot study designed to determine the differences in progression of second stage labor for women who followed their involuntary urge to bear down and women who used sustained breath-holding techniques. The study, which was derived from Levine's conceptual model, revealed no differences between the two groups of women in terms of second stage labor progression.

I n d e x

A "t" following a page number indicates a table.